Medical Tox

Medical Toxicology

Edited by
Brian Patrick Murray and Joseph Carpenter

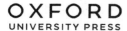

OXFORD
UNIVERSITY PRESS

Oxford University Press is a department of the University of Oxford. It furthers
the University's objective of excellence in research, scholarship, and education
by publishing worldwide. Oxford is a registered trade mark of Oxford University
Press in the UK and certain other countries.

Published in the United States of America by Oxford University Press
198 Madison Avenue, New York, NY 10016, United States of America.

© Oxford University Press 2024

Library of Congress Cataloging-in-Publication Data
Names: Murray, Brian Patrick, editor. | Carpenter, Joseph (Joseph Edward), editor.
Title: Medical toxicology / [edited by] Brian Patrick Murray and Joseph Carpenter.
Other titles: Medical toxicology (Murray)
Description: New York, NY : Oxford University Press, [2024] |
Includes bibliographical references and index.
Identifiers: LCCN 2023032651 (print) | LCCN 2023032652 (ebook) |
ISBN 9780197635513 (paperback) | ISBN 9780197635537 (epub) |
ISBN 9780197635544
Subjects: MESH: Poisoning | Emergencies | Emergency Treatment—methods |
Toxicology—methods
Classification: LCC RA1211 (print) | LCC RA1211 (ebook) | NLM QV 600 |
DDC 615.9—dc23/eng/20230801
LC record available at https://lccn.loc.gov/2023032651
LC ebook record available at https://lccn.loc.gov/2023032652

DOI: 10.1093/med/9780197635513.001.0001

Printed by Marquis Book Printing, Canada

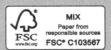

Contents

List of Figures   ix

List of Tables   xi

List of Boxes   xiii

List of Contributors   xv

1   **Beyond NAC: Acidemia After Acetaminophen Overdose**   1
Benjamin Tartter and Michael Ballester

2   **Severe Complications of Salicylate Overdose**   17
Jay Bhula and Richard Kleiman

3   **Mind the Gap: Toxic Alcohol Management**   27
Patrick Filkins

4   **Unrelenting Insulin Release: Sulfonylurea/Meglitinide Overdose**   41
Matthew Sheneman, Brian P. Murray, and Joseph E. Carpenter

5   **Some Like It Hot: Management of Toxic Hyperthermia**   49
Nicholas Titelbaum and Brent Morgan

6   **Neuroleptic Malignant Syndrome Versus Serotonin Syndrome**   65
Jasmine Gentry and Katie Lippert

7   **To Chelate or Not to Chelate: When Too Much Iron Is Too Much**   77
T. Christy Hallett

8   **How Low Can You Go? Beta-Blocker and Calcium Channel Blocker Overdoses**   85
Michael Frein and Jessica Zhen

9   **Vitamins That Kill: Vitamin A and D Overdoses**   101
Stephanie Hon

10   **Rats Hate This Stuff: Potent Long-Acting Vitamin K Antagonists**   113
Reena Underiner and Jonathan de Olano

11   **Stuffing Is for Turkeys: Management of Illicit Drug Stuffers**   127
Zachary Illg

12 **When Antidiarrheals Stop More Than Loose Bowels: Loperamide-Induced Cardiac Dysfunction**   135
Rita Farah and Brent Morgan

13 **Save a Life, Initiate Buprenorphine: Emergency Department Buprenorphine Administration**   149
Maxwell Kruse and Joshua da Silva

14 **Tricyclic Antidepressant Toxicity: Management of the Crashing Patient**   159
Matthew Oram and Joshua da Silva

15 **Don't Lose Your Ear Over Cardiac Glycosides: Cardiac Glycoside Toxicity Management**   171
Marshall Howell, Girgis Fahmy, and Emily Kiernan

16 **The (Lack of) Benefit of a Screening Urine Drug Screen**   183
Rebecca Ervin and Pradeep Padmanabhan

17 **Diphenhydramine: The Cardiac Poison**   193
Chidiebere Victor Ugwu and T. Christy Hallett

18 **A Long Way from Woodstock: Synthetic Cannabinoids**   201
Daniel Nogee

19 **Beyond Benzos: Alcohol and Sedative-Hypnotic Withdrawal**   211
Kyle Suen

20 **All Amped Up and Nowhere to Go: Caffeine and Methylxanthine Overdose**   223
Nicholas Nuveen and Melissa H. Gittinger

21 **Not So Essential Oils: Essential Oil Ingestions**   235
Ashima Goyal Gurkha and Dhritiman Gurkha

22 **ME THink You Should Not Use: Methamphetamines Intoxication**   247
Suad Al-Sulaimani

23 **The Rummy Rum Rums: Alcohol Intoxication**   259
Destiny Horton and Mohan Punja

24 **The Mu-Agonist Blues: Opioid Overdose and Withdrawal**   269
Tori Ehrhardt and Alaina Steck

25 GABA-B, the Forgotten Receptor Overlooked No More: Baclofen Overdose and Withdrawal 283
Nicholas Hoffmann and Jay Bernstein

26 Is That Chest Pain a Heart Attack, or a Line of Cocaine? Managing Cocaine-Induced Chest Pain 297
Amir Jamal Mansour, Pradeep Padmanabhan, and Besher Assi

27 Don't Poke the Snake: The Do's and Don'ts of Snake Bite Management 309
Katie Lippert and Joshua da Silva

28 You Are Barking Up the Wrong Scorpion: Bark Scorpion Envenomations 321
Karl Holt and Jonathan de Olano

29 The Shy Widow: Black Widow Envenomations 331
Matthew Eisenstat

30 Don't Get Washed Away in the Red Tide: Shellfish and Seafood-Related Toxins 339
Alyka Glor P. Fernandez and Melissa H. Gittinger

31 Acetylcholine Overload: Organophosphate and Carbamate Exposures 351
Luis Espinoza and Joshua da Silva

32 Redox Cycling Out of Control: Herbicide Ingestions 363
Nicholas Titelbaum

33 I Am All Choked Up Over Chlorine: Chlorine and Other Pulmonary Irritants 377
Emily Kiernan

34 You Are Getting Chernobyl Close to Home: Acute Radiation Syndrome and Cutaneous Radiation Syndrome 387
Girgis Fahmy and Ziad Kazzi

Index 399

Figures

1.1 Metabolism of acetaminophen to metabolites. 3

2.1 Mechanisms of acid–base disturbances in salicylate (SA) toxicity. 20

3.1 Reciprocal change in anion gap and osmol gap over time with toxic alcohol ingestions. 31

5.1 Angel's trumpet (*Brugmansia*), a plant containing belladonna alkaloids that can cause anticholinergic toxicity. 55

10.1 Chemical structures of warfarin, bromadiolone, and brodifacoum. 116

10.2 Vitamin K cycle. 117

12.1 (A) Initial ECG showing sinus rhythm with QRS widening: heart rate of 61 bpm, QRS duration of 126 ms, QTc of 337 ms.136 (B) ECG showing sustained ventricular tachycardia; HR 105 bpm, QRS duration of 201 ms, QTc of 426 ms. 136

12.2 (A) Meperidine structure. (B) Loperamide structure. (C) Haloperidol structure. 139

14.1 ECG of patient with tricyclic antidepressant toxicity. 160

15.1 Triage ECG. 172

19.1 Approach to alcohol withdrawal syndrome in the emergency department. 215

24.1 One possible dosing scheme for naloxone administration in acute opioid toxicity. 276

29.1 Typical appearance of a *Latrodectus* species in the United States. 332

34.1 Andrew lymphocyte nomogram. 391

Tables

1.1 Four stages of acetaminophen (APAP) toxicity from time of ingestion 6
1.2 Oral N-acetylcysteine dosing 9
1.3 Intravenous N-acetylcysteine dosing 10
5.1 Hyperthermia-inducing agents 52
7.1 Common oral iron formulations and their elemental iron content 78
9.1 Vitamin content of foods 109
12.1 Drugs that can potentially interact with loperamide 141
12.2 Summary of the management plan of loperamide overdose 142
17.1 Diphenhydramine toxidrome, its effects and treatment 195
18.1 Synthetic cannabinoid "street names" and packaging labels 202
20.1 Clinical findings in methylxanthine toxicity and suggested therapies 230
21.1 Toxic essential oils with significant toxicity 243
24.1 Routes and suggested starting doses for naloxone administration in suspected opioid overdose 274
24.2 Example medications for symptom management in acute opioid withdrawal 278
25.1 Toxic effects of baclofen organized by system and effects 286
25.2 Key diagnostic and differentiating factors between intrathecal baclofen withdrawal and similar presenting syndromes 290
30.1 Overview of shellfish and seafood-related toxins 342
30.2 Toxicology of marine organisms and treatment protocols 348
33.1 Irritant gases by water-solubility 380
34.1 Acute radiation syndrome dose-symptom relationship 395

Boxes

1.1   Studies and scoring system commonly utilized in
      acetaminophen overdose   7
1.2   King's College Criteria   8
3.1   EXTRIP guidelines for methanol toxicity   35
15.1 Common dysrhythmias in cardiac glycoside toxicity   174
15.2 Indications for DSFab administration   177
15.3 Dosing instructions for DSFab   178
19.1 DSM-5 diagnostic criteria for alcohol withdrawal syndrome
      (AWS)   213
26.1 Symptoms of cocaine use   301
30.1 Fish associated with ciguatera poisoning   344
30.2 Fish associated with tetrodotoxin poisoning   345
30.3 Fish associated with scombroid poisoning   346
30.4 Marine life associated with palytoxin poisoning   347

Contributors

Suad Al-Sulaimani
International Toxicology Fellow
Emory University School of
Medicine
Georgia Poison Center

Besher Assi
Medical Student
Northeast Ohio Medical University

Michael Ballester
Program Director
Assistant Professor of Emergency
Medicine
Wright State University Boonshoft
School of Medicine

Jay Bernstein
Assistant Professor of Emergency
Medicine
Wright State University Boonshoft
School of Medicine

Jay Bhula
Emergency Medicine Resident
Kennestone Regional
Medical Center

Joseph E. Carpenter
Assistant Professor of Emergency
Medicine
Emory University School of
Medicine
Georgia Poison Center

Joshua da Silva
Medical Director
Wright Patterson Medical Center

Jonathan de Olano
Assistant Professor of Emergency
Medicine
Emory University School of
Medicine
Georgia Poison Center

Tori Ehrhardt
Emergency Medicine Resident
Emory University School of
Medicine

Matthew Eisenstat
Assistant Professor of Emergency
Medicine
University of Louisville

Rebecca Ervin
Emergency Medicine Resident
Wright State University Boonshoft
School of Medicine

Luis Espinoza
Emergency Medicine Resident
Wright State University Boonshoft
School of Medicine

Girgis Fahmy
Emergency Medicine Resident
Emory University School of
Medicine

Rita Farah
Epidemiologist
University of Virginia School of
Medicine

Alyka Glor P. Fernandez
Emergency Medicine Resident
Emory University School of
Medicine

Michael Frein
Emergency Medicine Resident
Wright State University Boonshoft
School of Medicine

Jasmine Gentry
Emergency Medicine Resident
Emory University School of
Medicine

Melissa H. Gittinger
Associate Professor of Emergency
Medicine
Emory University School of
Medicine
Georgia Poison Center

Ashima Goyal Gurkha
Pediatric Emergency
Medicine Fellow
Beaumont Children's Hospital

Dhritiman Gurkha
Assistant Professor of Pediatrics
Wright State University Boonshoft
School of Medicine
Dayton Children's Hospital

T. Christy Hallett
Assistant Professor of Pediatrics and
Emergency Medicine
Emory University School of
Medicine
Georgia Poison Center

Nicholas Hoffmann
Emergency Medicine Resident
Wright State University Boonshoft
School of Medicine

Karl Holt
Emergency Medicine Resident
Emory University School of
Medicine

Stephanie Hon
Director
Georgia Poison Center

Destiny Horton
Emergency Medicine Resident
Kennestone Regional
Medical Center

Marshall Howell
Emergency Medicine Resident
Emory University School of
Medicine

Zachary Illg
Medical Toxicology Fellow
Emory University School of
Medicine
Georgia Poison Center

Ziad Kazzi
Professor of Emergency Medicine
Emory University School of Medicine
Georgia Poison Center

Emily Kiernan
Assistant Professor of Emergency
Medicine
Emory University School of Medicine
Georgia Poison Center

Richard Kleiman
Emergency Medicine; Medical
Toxicology
Kennestone Regional
Medical Center
Assistant Professor, Emergency
Medicine, Augusta University

Maxwell Kruse
Emergency Medicine Resident
Wright State University Boonshoft
School of Medicine

Katie Lippert
Emergency Medicine Physician
Wright Patterson Medical Center

Amir Jamal Mansour
Emergency Medicine Resident
Wright State University Boonshoft
School of Medicine

Brent Morgan
Professor of Emergency Medicine
Emory University School of Medicine
Georgia Poison Center

Brian P. Murray
Assistant Professor of Emergency
Medicine
Wright State Boonshoft School of
Medicine

Daniel Nogee
Medical Toxicology Fellow
Emory University School of
Medicine
Georgia Poison Center

Nicholas Nuveen
Emergency Medicine Resident
Emory University School of
Medicine

Matthew Oram
Emergency Medicine Resident
Wright State University Boonshoft
School of Medicine

Pradeep Padmanabhan
Assistant Program Director
Associate Professor of Pediatrics
Wright State University Boonshoft
School of Medicine
Dayton Children's Hospital

Patrick Filkins
Clinical Toxicologist, Emergency
Medicine Clinical Pharmacist
Georgia Poison Center
Grady Health System

Mohan Punja
Emergency Medicine; Medical
Toxicology
Kennestone Regional
Medical Center
Assistant Professor, Emergency
Medicine, Augusta University

Matthew Sheneman
Emergency Medicine Resident
Wright State University Boonshoft
School of Medicine

Alaina Steck
Associate Professor of Emergency
Medicine
Emory University School of
Medicine
Georgia Poison Center

Kyle Suen
Assistant Professor of Emergency
Medicine
Baylor College of Medicine

Benjamin Tartter
Emergency Medicine Resident
Wright State University Boonshoft
School of Medicine

Nicholas Titelbaum
Medical Toxicology Fellow
Emory University School of Medicine
Georgia Poison Center

Chidiebere Victor Ugwu
Pediatric Emergency
Medicine Fellow
Emory University School of
Medicine

Reena Underiner
Emergency Medicine Resident
Emory University School of Medicine

Jessica Zhen
Assistant Professor of Emergency
Medicine
Wright State Boonshoft School of
Medicine

1 Beyond NAC: Acidemia After Acetaminophen Overdose

Benjamin Tartter and Michael Ballester

Case Presentation

You are working at a community ED when a nurse tells you that there is an 18-year-old somnolent female with concern for acetaminophen (APAP) overdose. Vitals in triage show blood pressure 90/60 mmHg, heart rate 130 beats/min, respiratory rate 23 breaths/min, and an SpO_2 of 97% on room air. The patient is accompanied by her mother, who tells you her symptoms began within the last hour. She appears unwell, seems confused, and has vomited multiple times. The mother states that her daughter has been depressed recently. She went in to check on her in her room approximately 1 hour ago and found her minimally responsive on her bed with a large 1,000-tablet bottle of 500 mg APAP lying on the floor next to her. The patient did have some vomit on her shirt that contained pill fragments. After obtaining an appropriate initial workup, the patient's labs show an elevated acetaminophen level, an anion gap metabolic acidosis, an elevated lactic acid, and normal AST/ALT levels.

What Do You Do Now?

DISCUSSION

Background

The Consumer Healthcare Products Association estimates that 23% of adults in the United States use APAP each week. This medication has a good safety profile when taken within recommended therapeutic guidelines. Unfortunately, overdoses are common, and APAP exposures are a leading cause of calls to US Poison Centers. Whether due to intentional or inadvertent overdose, acetaminophen toxicity results in approximately 500 deaths, 56,000 emergency department visits, and 26,000 hospitalizations a year in the United States.[1] APAP-associated liver failure is a major indication for liver transplantation in both the United States and worldwide.[2] Overdose is most commonly seen in the pediatric population. Due to impaired metabolism and glutathione stores, older adults are at risk for hepatotoxicity through repeat "supratherapeutic" doses, even though acute overdose is less common.[3] Among pregnant individuals, APAP is the most common medication implicated in overdose.[4]

Toxicology and Pathophysiology

APAP is available in both oral and IV formulations. After oral ingestion APAP is rapidly absorbed in the duodenum since it is a weak acid and non-ionized in the acidic environment of stomach. Once in the blood compartment, APAP is metabolized primarily in the liver and has an elimination half-life of 2–3 hours, longer in patients with chronic liver disease and impaired metabolism. In therapeutic doses, APAP achieves peak concentration within 1.5 hours for immediate-release formulations.[5] In the setting of a single oral APAP overdose, peak serum concentrations may not be seen until 4 hours post ingestion, longer in the setting of a co-ingestant which slows gastric motility or if the APAP is in an extended-release formulation.[3]

APAP is metabolized through three main pathways (Figure 1.1). Approximately 90–95% of APAP is metabolized by the hepatic phase II metabolic pathways, where its conjugation is catalyzed by UDP-glucuronosyl transferases (UGT) or sulfotransferases. This converts APAP into glucuronidated or sulfated metabolites, both nontoxic products that are renally eliminated. From 5% to 10% of APAP is processed by the phase

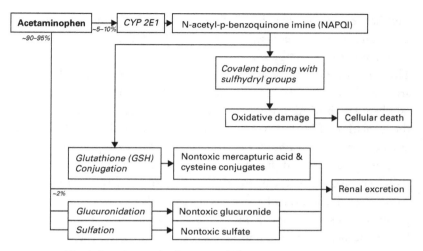

FIGURE 1.1 Metabolism of acetaminophen to metabolites.

I oxidation hepatic cytochrome CYP 2E1, which forms the highly reactive metabolite N-acetyl-p-benzoquinone imine (NAPQI). This is the metabolite responsible for end-organ damage. Approximately 2% is eliminated unchanged in the urine.

NAPQI is formed even after ingestion of therapeutic doses; however, it is rapidly metabolized via conjugation to glutathione (GSH) to form nontoxic mercapturic acid and cysteine products that are eliminated renally. In the setting of overdose, glucuronidation and sulfation pathways are overwhelmed and saturated, respectively, shunting more APAP to CYP 2E1 phase I oxidation. Additionally, the liver's stores of GSH may become depleted, particularly in patients with poor nutrition.

NAPQI exerts its toxicity through the formation of covalent bonds with sulfhydryl groups on cysteine and lysine containing molecules.[5] These protein-adducts result in chain reactions of oxidative damage disrupting mitochondrial function, which can lead to fulminant liver and multiorgan failure. Liver damage primarily occurs in the centrilobular zone-3 of hepatocytes where the highest concentration of CYP 2E1 enzymes is found. Interestingly, even though the damage is caused by oxidative stress, the centrilobular region has the least amount of oxygen because it is the furthest from the arteriole blood supply. Conversion to NAPQI can also occur anywhere else in the body that CYP 2E1 is found. This contributes to renal injury after massive overdose, owing to renal CYP 2E1.[6,7]

Ethanol has a complex relationship with the metabolism of APAP. There are two primary ways in which ethanol consumption is thought to affect APAP metabolism. In someone ethanol-naïve, the simultaneous use of ethanol with APAP is thought to be potentially protective and decrease the formation of NAPQI via competitive inhibition of CYP 2E1 because ethanol is also a substrate for this enzyme. In the setting of chronic ethanol use, it is theorized that there is an upregulation of CYP 2E1, potentially increasing the risk of toxicity these patients may experience after APAP use.[8] Regardless of the clinical effect of CYP 2E1 upregulation, patients who suffer from alcohol use disorder may be malnourished and have rapid depletion of glutathione stores as well as liver failure and impaired ability to metabolize APAP, placing them at increased risk for APAP toxicity.[6,9]

Acidemia After APAP Ingestion

An uncommonly seen but interesting phenomenon is the indolent development of an elevated anion-gap acidosis in patients with chronic APAP use. This is thought to be secondary to the build-up of 5-oxoproline (pyroglutamic acid). Most noted cases of this presentation are female patients with chronic APAP use who present with low to therapeutic levels of APAP in the serum. The mechanism for how this occurs is thought to be related to an inborn defect in the gamma-glutamyl cycle related to the breakdown of 5-oxoproline.[10] Certain conditions will predispose patients to acquiring this pathology, such as chronic renal impairment, chronic liver dysfunction, vegetarian diet, pregnancy, sepsis, and malnourishment. It is theorized that APAP ingestion can result in a more marked increase in 5-oxoproline levels in these situations because these patients are more prone to decreased 5-oxoproline metabolism. This acidosis typically responds to volume expansion with fluids and dextrose.[11–13]

Acutely, patients can develop a significant lactic acidosis shortly after massive APAP ingestions. While lactic acidosis is common in late-presenting APAP overdose as a sequelae of liver failure, in rare situations patients have been reported to present with life-threatening acidosis early after ingestion without elevation of liver enzymes. Animal studies have demonstrated APAP has a direct inhibitory effect on mitochondrial complex I and cytochrome b of complex III within 2 hours of exposure. In these settings, N-acetylcysteine (NAC) may not be sufficient as a solo therapy, and emergent hemodialysis should be strongly considered.[14]

The dysfunction of the oxidative process in the mitochondria is also thought to play a role in APAP's cytopathic effect on renal podocytes because they have decreased capacity for regeneration. This is also theorized to be why some patients develop renal failure outside of the setting of liver failure as the kidneys are heavily dependent on mitochondria to function.[15]

Workup and Diagnosis

As with any patient presenting with a toxic ingestion, it is important to determine the time of first ingestion as well as the duration of time the patient was ingesting the xenobiotic, the amount ingested, and any co-ingestants. Vital signs and a focused examination can provide important clues for possible xenobiotic exposures. There is no specific toxidrome associated with APAP toxicity, and vital sign changes are more associated with the level of end-organ toxicity and shock than with the APAP itself. Therefore, it is imperative to consider APAP ingestion/toxicity in anyone with a possible suicidal ingestion, with new-onset transaminase elevation, or in anyone presenting with abdominal pain, nausea, vomiting, and metabolic acidosis. While rare to discover an occult severe APAP ingestion, it could be lifesaving if treatment were rapidly initiated.

The clinical course for patients with APAP toxicity typically follows four stages from time of ingestion, as described in Table 1.1.[16,17]

In the acute setting, the provider should obtain a serum APAP level, liver function test, and coagulation profile. In the setting of a single acute ingestion, or multiple ingestions within an 8-hour window, the Rumack-Matthew Nomogram can be utilized. This nomogram is only applicable when the serum APAP is obtained between 4 and 24 hours from the time of the first ingestion. Optimally a serum APAP level should be obtained at the 4-hour mark. The nomogram should not be used for multiple ingestions over a greater than 8-hour period. If the

TABLE 1.1 Four stages of acetaminophen (APAP) toxicity from time of ingestion

Stage	Theme	Timeframe	Presentation
1st	Gastrointestinal phase	30 minutes– 24 hours	• Usually asymptomatic or vomiting, may have abdominal tenderness, diaphoresis, and/or dehydration • *In severe overdose*: May have hypotension, metabolic acidosis, altered mental status in the setting of normal liver function test values
2nd	Hepatic injury	18–72 hours	• May include vomiting, hypotension, and/or right upper quadrant pain
3rd	Hepatic necrosis & multiorgan failure	72–96 hours	• Significant liver dysfunction with renal damage, metabolic acidosis, coagulopathies, and encephalopathy. 　○ Right upper quadrant abdominal tenderness 　○ Jaundice and scleral icterus 　○ Purpura and other signs of bleeding diathesis 　○ Ascites 　○ Tachycardia 　○ Hypotension 　○ Altered mental status 　　■ Lethargy or coma 　　■ Grade 3 or 4 hepatic encephalopathy *The patient is most likely to die in this stage*
4th	Recovery	4 days–3 weeks	If patient survives the 3rd stage, they will begin the path to recovery during the 4th stage

nomogram indicates the APAP level is above the treatment line, NAC should be initiated.

If there is uncertainty regarding the initial time of ingestion, the number of ingestions, or chronicity of ingestions, clinicians should err on the side of caution and initiate treatment because NAC both safe and effective.

If patients do not meet criteria for treatment with NAC initially, but there is concern for delayed gastric emptying due to medical reasons or co-ingestions, or extended-release APAP was taken, there should be a low threshold to repeat serum APAP levels at the 8-hour mark and even the 12-hour mark. If the patient has taken multiple doses over a period greater than 24 hours, treatment should be guided by the amount ingested, serum transaminase levels, residual serum APAP, and risk factors for toxicity such as alcohol use disorder, malnutrition, and use of CYP2E1 inducers such as isoniazid. Consultation with a medical toxicologist and/or regional poison center is recommended. In these situations, the threshold for initiating NAC should remain low (see Box 1.1).

BOX 1.1 **Studies and scoring system commonly utilized in acetaminophen overdose**

STUDIES THAT SHOULD BE OBTAINED

- Serum APAP levels (not before 4 hours timed from ingestion)
- Prothrombin time (PT) test
- Hepatic function panel

SUGGESTED STUDIES

- Lactate
- Other suspected toxic ingestion serum levels (e.g., salicylate)
- Basic metabolic panel
- Ammonia
- 12-lead electrocardiogram
- Venous blood gas/arterial blood gas
- Lipase
- Complete blood count
- Phosphate

SCORING SYSTEM

- King's College criteria (KCH criteria)

Treatment

In patients presenting within 1–3 hours of ingestion, or with ingestion of an extended-release formulation, 1 gm/kg of activated charcoal should be administered. Caution should be taken in patients with vomiting and/or an altered mental status out of concern for aspiration leading to charcoal pneumonitis.

Acetylcysteine is the primary antidotal treatment used in APAP overdoses. It is highly effective if given within 8–10 hours of ingestion. While its effectiveness diminishes if given more than the 8 hours from ingestion, it is still recommended and is associated with improved outcomes.[18] NAC should be administered to anyone with an acute ingestion that has an APAP level above the treatment line on the Matthew-Rumack nomogram or in chronic ingestions of multiple supratherapeutic doses with elevated serum transaminase levels or an elevated INR without alternate explanation.

NAC can be administered intravenously or orally. The oral formulation smells strongly of sulfur, or rotten eggs, and becomes more tolerable when it is mixed with a soda and/or is placed in a container with a cover and ingested through a straw, thus negating the odor. Theoretically, both formulations are equally efficacious though there are significant logistical differences. The oral formulation is initially given as a loading dose of 140 mg/kg followed by 17 more doses of 70 mg/kg administered every 4 hours for a total duration of treatment of 68 hours (Box 1.2).[19] The standard dose for the IV formulation is 150 mg/kg over 1 hour, followed by

---

BOX 1.2 **King's College Criteria**

KCH criteria[4,21] is commonly utilized, and it should be noted that, if even one criterion is met, consider transferring the patient to a liver transplant center.

- Arterial pH <7.3
- Lactate >3.5 mmol/L after fluid resuscitation (<4 hours) or lactate >3 mmol/L after adequate fluid resuscitation (12 hours)
- Grade III or IV hepatic encephalopathy w/PT >100 seconds
- INR >6.5 with creatinine > 3.4 mg/dL

Note: Serum phosphate >3.75 mg/dL (1.2 mmol/L) at 48–96 hours is a predictor of poor prognosis without transplant. (2)

---

50 mg/kg over 4 hours, followed by 100 mg/kg over 16 hours, for a dedicated 21-hour protocol. Although other IV NAC protocols have been proposed, this currently is considered the standard of care.

Once NAC is initiated, the oral formulation must be given for a minimum of 24 hours, and the IV protocol should not be stopped early for any reason. Both protocols can and should be continued for ongoing signs of toxicity, as defined by an APAP serum concentration greater than 10 mcg/mL, an ALT level which is trending up or >100 mg/dL, and an INR greater than 1.4 (see Tables 1.2 and 1.3). An important consideration is that NAC itself may increase the INR slightly from baseline. Repeat laboratory values should be obtained shortly before the completion of the IV protocol to assess the need to continue treatment but should not be checked in the middle of the protocol because this will not help to guide management. Consider consultation with a medical toxicologist and/or poison center whenever ambiguity exists regarding the decision to cease NAC therapy.

In select situations, standard NAC therapy will be inadequate, and patients may benefit from advanced therapy such as hemodialysis, extracorporeal liver support, and liver transplantation. Transfer agreements must be in place to facilitate prompt transfer to a facility or unit capable of providing these treatments. There are several scoring systems used to help determine the need for a liver transplant, most notably the King's College criteria (KCH criteria).[20] Clinicians should not wait until all criteria of the KCH score are fulfilled and should consult a liver transplant center early.[4,21]

When a massive APAP overdose presents with evidence of mitochondrial dysfunction (elevated lactic acidosis) early hemodialysis should be considered in addition to NAC. According to the Extracorporeal Treatments in Poisoning (EXTRIP) workgroup, extracorporeal treatment (ECTR) is recommended if NAC is not given and the serum APAP is greater than

TABLE 1.2 **Oral N-acetylcysteine dosing**

Loading dose	Continued dosing	Notes
140 mg/kg	70 mg/kg q4h for total of 18 doses	Repeat any dose vomited within 1 hour of ingestion

TABLE 1.3 **Intravenous N-acetylcysteine dosing**

Weight	Loading dose— Given over 1 hour	2nd dose— Given over 4 hours	3rd dose— Given over 16 hours
40–100 kg (for weight >100 kg, use 100 kg dosing)	150 mg/kg in 200 mL diluent	50 mg/kg in 500 mL diluent	100 mg/kg in 1,000 mL diluent
20–40 kg	150 mg/kg in 100 mL diluent	50 mg/kg in 250 mL diluent	100 mg/kg in 500 mL diluent
<20 kg	150 mg/kg in 3 mL/ kg diluent	50 mg/kg into 7 mL/kg diluent	100 mg/kg in 14 mL/kg diluent

1000 mcg/mL; if NAC is not given and the serum APAP is greater than 700 mcg/mL with signs of mitochondrial dysfunction; or if NAC is given and the serum APAP is greater than 900 mcg/mL with signs of mitochondrial dysfunction.[14] NAC is also removed from the body during dialysis and should be continued at an increased rate.

Additional therapies have not yet been validated for standard of care use but have promising potential, the forerunner of these being fomepizole. Fomepizole is typically utilized as an alcohol dehydrogenase inhibitor in cases of toxic alcohol ingestion; however, it is also an inhibitor of CYP 2E1 and may help prevent hepatotoxicity through its interaction with the c-jun N-terminal Kinase (JNK). In cases where the patient is at considerable risk of acute liver failure due to a large overdose of APAP, fomepizole can be used as an adjunct to NAC. A recent in vitro study demonstrated that in primary human hepatocytes exposed to APAP, the addition of fomepizole appeared to prevent the cell death that would otherwise occur. Another small human study using volunteers who acted as their own controls showed that with therapeutic APAP dosing, subjects receiving fomepizole exhibit decreased formation of oxidative metabolites. The currently proposed dose of fomepizole in APAP toxicity is a single dose of 15 mg/kg IV. One proposed criterion is an [APAP] × [ALT] product of greater than 10,000.[22,23]

Long-Term Concerns

There is evidence that acute liver failure not requiring transplant in APAP overdose does not directly increase long-term mortality. This is noted in one study which interestingly excludes patients who expired within a year after discharge, as they only begin to follow patients after the first year from initial overdose event.[24] This is challenged by a cohort study from Taiwan which indicates that toxic ingestions of APAP do appear to be associated with increased all-cause mortality in the long term, especially in the younger population and within the first 12 months after discharge.[25] It is postulated that the stress which the oxidative damage caused by APAP overdose places on multiple organs throughout the body increases the patient's overall susceptibility to terminal pathology and that this risk is higher in the shorter term. There is concern that those who intentionally overdose are also at an increased probability to be diagnosed with a primary psychiatric disease and commit suicide. While patients do not necessarily require hepatology follow-up there should be strong consideration for psychiatric evaluation and care.[24,25]

Patients who have undergone a liver transplant are at increased risk from immunosuppression including metabolic and infectious complications. There is also the chance they will develop renal failure requiring hemodialysis and that they may require this for the long term. Overall, patients undergoing liver transplantation for APAP-induced liver failure can have qualities of life comparable to the general population for many years.[26,27]

CASE CONCLUSION

The patient is provided IV fluids, antiemetics, and started on IV NAC. The initial APAP level results above the upper limit of detection. After discussion with the lab to further dilute the sample, they report a level of 1100 mcg/mL. Nephrology is consulted and hemodialysis is initiated. The patient's mental status and hemodynamics rapidly improve, and NAC is discontinued after 40 hours of treatment. The patient is transferred to an inpatient psychiatry unit on hospital day #4.

- Acetaminophen (APAP) is a significant cause of acute liver failure in the United States, either through acute overingestion or chronic excess use.
- Gathering the timing of the overdose is important regarding proper utilization of the Rumack-Matthew nomogram.
- N-acetylcysteine (NAC) the first-line antidote to APAP toxicity and is known to be effective. If there is suspicion, start it sooner rather than later.
- Emergent hemodialysis is crucial to consider in patients presenting with acute kidney failure and/or lactic acidosis secondary to APAP overdose.
- If there is clinical suspicion for acute liver failure in the setting of APAP overdose, evaluate for need of liver transplant.
- When there is significant risk for liver failure secondary to massive APAP ingestion, with limited or delayed access to a liver transplant facility, fomepizole could be considered as an additive therapy to NAC. The suggested dosing of fomepizole in the setting of APAP overdose is 15 mg/kg IV once.

Further Reading

Bacak SJ, Thornburg LL. Liver failure in pregnancy. *Crit Care Clin.* 2016;32(1):61–72. doi:10.1016/j.ccc.2015.08.005

Elsayed S, Gohar A, Omar M. A review article on 5-oxoproline induced high anion gap metabolic acidosis. *S D Med.* 2021 Oct 1;74(10):468–470.

Gosselin S, Juurlink DN, Kielstein JT, et al. Extracorporeal treatment for acetaminophen poisoning: recommendations from the EXTRIP workgroup. *Clin Toxicol (Phila).* 2014;52(8):856–867. doi:10.3109/15563650.2014.946994

Hendrickson RG, McKeown NJ. Acetaminophen. In: Nelson LS, Howland M, Lewin NA, Smith SW, Goldfrank LR, Hoffman RS, eds. *Goldfrank's Toxicologic Emergencies.* 11th ed. McGraw Hill; 2019. https://accesspharmacy.mhmedical.com/content.aspx?bookid=2569&sectionid=210270383

King JD, Kern MH, Jaar BG. Extracorporeal removal of poisons and toxins. *Clin J Am Soc Nephrol.* 2019;14(9):1408–1415. doi:10.2215/CJN.02560319

Ohba H, Kanazawa M, Kakiuchi T, Tsukada H. Effects of acetaminophen on mitochondrial complex I activity in the rat liver and kidney: a PET study with ^{18}F-BCPP-BF. *EJNMMI Res.* 2016;6(1):82. doi:10.1186/s13550-016-0241-4

Shah KR, Beuhler MC. Fomepizole as an adjunctive treatment in severe acetaminophen toxicity. *Am J Emerg Med*. 2020;38(2):410.e5–410.e6. doi:10.1016/j.ajem.2019.09.005

References

1. Nourjah P, Ahmad SR, Karwoski C, Willy M. Estimates of acetaminophen (Paracetomal)-associated overdoses in the United States. *Pharmacoepidemiol Drug Saf*. 2006;15(6):398–405. doi:10.1002/pds.1191

2. Mendizabal M, Silva MO. Liver transplantation in acute liver failure: a challenging scenario. *World J Gastroenterol*. 2016;22(4):1523–1531. doi:10.3748/wjg.v22.i4.1523

3. Agrawal S, Khazaeni B. Acetaminophen toxicity. In: *StatPearls*. StatPearls Publishing; February 12, 2023.

4. Hodgman MJ, Garrard AR. A review of acetaminophen poisoning. *Crit Care Clin*. 2012;28(4):499–516. doi:10.1016/j.ccc.2012.07.006

5. McGill MR, Jaeschke H. Metabolism and disposition of acetaminophen: recent advances in relation to hepatotoxicity and diagnosis. *Pharm Res*. 2013;30(9):2174–2187. doi:10.1007/s11095-013-1007-6

6. Zimmerman HJ, Maddrey WC. Acetaminophen (paracetamol) hepatotoxicity with regular intake of alcohol: analysis of instances of therapeutic misadventure [published correction appears in Hepatology 1995 Dec;22(6):1898]. *Hepatology*. 1995;22(3):767–773.

7. Mazer M, Perrone J. Acetaminophen-induced nephrotoxicity: pathophysiology, clinical manifestations, and management. *J Med Toxicol*. 2008;4(1):2–6. doi:10.1007/BF03160941

8. Schmidt LE, Dalhoff K, Poulsen HE. Acute versus chronic alcohol consumption in acetaminophen-induced hepatotoxicity. *Hepatology*. 2002 Apr 1;35(4):876–882.

9. Bunchorntavakul C, Reddy KR. Acetaminophen-related hepatotoxicity. *Clin Liver Dis*. 2013;17(4):587–viii. doi:10.1016/j.cld.2013.07.005

10. Elsayed S, Gohar A, Omar M. A review article on 5-oxoproline induced high anion gap metabolic acidosis. *S D Med*. 2021 Oct 1;74(10):468–470.

11. Duewall JL, Fenves AZ, Richey DS, Tran LD, Emmett M. 5-Oxoproline (pyroglutamic) acidosis associated with chronic acetaminophen use. *Proc (Bayl Univ Med Cent)*. 2010;23(1):19–20. doi:10.1080/08998280.2010.11928574

12. Pitt JJ, Brown GK, Clift V, Christodoulou J. Atypical pyroglutamic aciduria: possible role of paracetamol. *J Inherit Metab Dis*. 1990;13(5):755–756. doi:10.1007/BF01799581

13. Fenves AZ, Kirkpatrick HM 3rd, Patel VV, Sweetman L, Emmett M. Increased anion gap metabolic acidosis as a result of 5-oxoproline (pyroglutamic acid): a

role for acetaminophen. *Clin J Am Soc Nephrol*. 2006;1(3):441–447. doi:10.2215/CJN.01411005

14. Gosselin S, Juurlink DN, Kielstein JT, et al. Extracorporeal treatment for acetaminophen poisoning: recommendations from the EXTRIP workgroup. *Clin Toxicol (Phila)*. 2014;52(8):856–867. doi:10.3109/15563650.2014.946994

15. Ohba H, Kanazawa M, Kakiuchi T, Tsukada H. Effects of acetaminophen on mitochondrial complex I activity in the rat liver and kidney: a PET study with ^{18}F-BCPP-BF. *EJNMMI Res*. 2016;6(1):82. doi:10.1186/s13550-016-0241-4

16. Levine M, Stellpflug SJ, Pizon AF, et al. Hypoglycemia and lactic acidosis outperform King's College criteria for predicting death or transplant in acetaminophen toxic patients. *Clin Toxicol (Phila)*. 2018;56(7):622–625. doi:10.1080/15563650.2017.1420193

17. Olson KR. Acetaminophen. In: Olson KR, Anderson IB, Benowitz NL, Blanc PD, Clark RF, Kearney TE, Kim-Katz SY, Wu AB, eds. *Poisoning and Drug Overdose*. 7th ed, pp. 73–76. McGraw Hill; 2018.

18. Shah AD, Wood DM, Dargan PI. Understanding lactic acidosis in paracetamol (acetaminophen) poisoning. *Br J Pharmacol*. 2011 Jan;71(1):20–28.

19. Smilkstein MJ, Knapp GL, Kulig KW, Rumack BH. Efficacy of oral N-acetylcysteine in the treatment of acetaminophen overdose: analysis of the national multicenter study (1976 to 1985). *N Engl J Med*. 1988;319(24):1557–1562. doi:10.1056/NEJM198812153192401

20. Cholongitas E, Theocharidou E, Vasianopoulou P, et al. Comparison of the sequential organ failure assessment score with the King's College Hospital criteria and the model for end-stage liver disease score for the prognosis of acetaminophen-induced acute liver failure. *Liver Transpl*. 2012;18(4):405–412. doi:10.1002/lt.23370

21. Yoon E, Babar A, Choudhary M, Kutner M, Pyrsopoulos N. Acetaminophen-induced hepatotoxicity: a comprehensive update. *J Clin Transl Hepatol*. 2016;4(2):131–142. doi:10.14218/JCTH.2015.00052

22. Kang AM, Padilla-Jones A, Fisher ES, et al. The effect of 4-methylpyrazole on oxidative metabolism of acetaminophen in human volunteers. *J Med Toxicol*. 2020;16(2):169–176. doi:10.1007/s13181-019-00740-z

23. Akakpo JY, Ramachandran A, Kandel SE, et al. 4-Methylpyrazole protects against acetaminophen hepatotoxicity in mice and in primary human hepatocytes. *Hum Exp Toxicol*. 2018;37(12):1310–1322. doi:10.1177/0960327118774902

24. Jepsen P, Schmidt LE, Larsen FS, Vilstrup H. Long-term prognosis for transplant-free survivors of paracetamol-induced acute liver failure. *Aliment Pharmacol Ther*. 2010;32(7):894–900. doi:10.1111/j.1365-2036.2010.04419.x

25. Huang HS, Ho CH, Weng SF, et al. Long-term mortality of acetaminophen poisoning: a nationwide population-based cohort study with 10-year follow-up in Taiwan. *Scand J Trauma Resusc Emerg Med*. 2018;26(1):5. Published Jan 8, 2018. doi:10.1186/s13049-017-0468-8

26. Muñoz LE, Nañez H, Rositas F, et al. Long-term complications and survival of patients after orthotopic liver transplantation. *Transplant Proc.* 2010;42(6):2381–2382. doi:10.1016/j.transproceed.2010.05.007
27. Åberg F, Isoniemi H, Höckerstedt K. Long-term results of liver transplantation. *Scand J Surg.* 2011;100(1):14–21. doi:10.1177/145749691110000104

2 Severe Complications of Salicylate Overdose

Jay Bhula and Richard Kleiman

Case Presentation

A 21-year-old woman is brought into the ED by ambulance after her roommate witnessed her having convulsions and becoming unresponsive next to an empty pill bottle. She has no known seizure disorder. Her medical history is significant for dysmenorrhea, anxiety, and depression. Her roommate is unsure of what medications the patient takes; however, she recalls her roommate telling her that she has been out of her antidepressant medicine for over 1 month and that she had been feeling overwhelmed and stressed lately. After speaking with the patient's mother via telephone, it is found that she has had a previous suicide attempt. Upon arrival to the ED, she remains unresponsive. Initial vital signs are blood pressure 136/74 mm Hg, heart rate 117 beats/min, respiratory rate 28 breaths/min, SpO_2 96% on room air, and a temperature of 101.8°F/38.8°C.

What Do You Do Now?

DISCUSSION

Background

This patient has unfortunately ingested a large quantity of aspirin and has developed significant salicylate toxicity. New-onset seizure, especially in the presence of abnormal vital signs, merits the consideration of a broad range of diagnoses such as electrolyte imbalance, metabolic disorders, infectious processes, neurologic or intracranial trauma, ischemia, and toxicologic exposures, among others. The patient in this scenario presents with seizures and coma, two of the most serious complications of salicylate toxicity.

The use of salicylates dates back more than 3,500 years, when its analgesic and antipyretic properties were initially discovered from the bark of the willow tree. Salicylic acid was subsequently derived from willow by the Italian chemist Raffaele Pirìa in 1838. Acetylsalicylic acid was then chemically synthesized in 1853, by the French chemist Charles Frédéric Gerhardt. Acetylsalicylic acid was subsequently registered and manufactured as the household name Aspirin by Friedrich Bayer and Company in 1899.

Salicylates have since then become universally available in several different formulations and preparations and are accessible either via prescription or over the counter. Acetylsalicylate, or Aspirin, is available over the counter in varying dosages, either as a tablet or as a dissolving powder, and frequently is combined with other over-the-counter medications. Methyl salicylate (also known as oil of wintergreen) is the most concentrated preparation of salicylate. It is found in liniment form for joint and muscle pains. Another common over-the-counter formulation of salicylates is bismuth subsalicylate, also known by its brand name Pepto-Bismol, a commonly used remedy for GI symptoms.[1]

Toxicology and Pathophysiology

Salicylates are rapidly absorbed in the stomach and then are mostly protein bound. They are metabolized predominantly by the liver via conjugation with glycine and glucuronides and then subsequently excreted by the kidneys. Under typical conditions, with standard dosing, they have a half-life of approximately 2–4 hours.[2] Salicylate toxicity occurs when the protein binding and hepatic metabolism becomes saturated. In this setting, elimination transitions from first-order kinetics to zero-order kinetics, and the half-life can then increase to as much as 30 hours. Peak plasma concentration can also take 6 hours or longer to reach.[3]

Salicylates act on the respiratory center in the medulla to cause increased respiratory rate and hyperventilation. This results in a centrally mediated respiratory alkalosis. Salicylates also cause a metabolic acidosis through the uncoupling of oxidative phosphorylation and inhibition of citric acid cycle dehydrogenases. This results in the shift in metabolism to glycolysis for energy production, resulting in increased oxygen consumption and increased heat production (Figure 2.1).[1] A compensatory increase in body catabolism and substrate breakdown is required to supply the energy needed for the increasingly inefficient production of adenosine triphosphate (ATP) from adenosine diphosphate (ADP) through glycolysis. This response is manifested by increased oxygen consumption and increased heat production (leading to hyperthermia, diaphoresis, and dehydration). It is important to note that patients may have hyperthermia from other causes as well and that hyperthermia in a salicylate toxic patient is usually an ominous sign of a possibly preterminal event.

In most cases, signs of acute toxicity are manifest when serum salicylate levels exceed 40–50 mg/dL. Fatal ingestions have been known to occur at doses of 10–30 g in adults.[4] The toxidrome associated with salicylates covers a broad range and severity of symptoms. The earliest symptoms include tinnitus, dyspnea, vertigo, nausea, vomiting, and diarrhea. The mechanism of ototoxicity is likely due to a combination of factors including alterations in calcium flux and N-methyl-D-aspartic acid (NMDA) signaling in cochlear neurons. Symptoms of severe toxicity include altered mental status, hyperthermia, noncardiogenic pulmonary edema, and coma. The CNS symptoms and complications of salicylate toxicity are due to an accumulation of uncharged/protonated salicylate molecules which readily cross the blood–brain barrier. This occurs via three separate pathways: (1) direct salicylate toxicity in the CNS, (2) neuroglycopenia, and (3) cerebral edema.[5] *Neuroglycopenia* refers to decreased glucose being available to neural cells. This is interesting because there may be a relatively normal systemic glucose level while a significantly lower level of glucose in the cerebrospinal fluid (CSF). It appears that the uncoupling of oxidative phosphorylation along with other changes in metabolism leads to increased glycolysis and then decreased glucose within the neural cells.

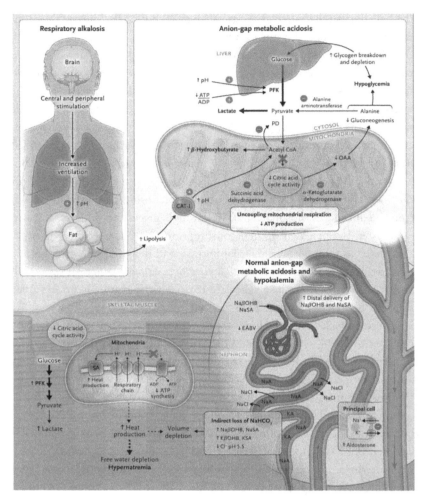

FIGURE 2.1 Mechanisms of acid–base disturbances in salicylate (SA) toxicity.

Reprinted with permission from Massachusetts Medical Society.[5]

Chronic salicylate toxicity typically occurs in the elderly population. It is thought to occur due to unintentional overdosing for the treatment of chronic conditions such as rheumatoid arthritis and osteoarthritis. Chronic salicylate toxicity overlaps with acute salicylate toxicity in presenting signs and symptoms, however the onset is slower and less severe, and serum salicylate levels are typically lower than in acute ingestions, although, due to prolonged penetration into multiple compartments, the whole-body stores are much greater than in acute toxicity. Mortality can be higher in chronic salicylate toxicity, however, due to delays in diagnosis and misdiagnosis.[2]

Workup and Diagnosis

The patient's clinical signs and symptoms should be of greatest priority in evaluating and managing salicylate ingestions. As a part of a general toxicology screen, serum salicylate concentrations as well as concentrations of other possible co-ingestants, such as acetaminophen, should be obtained. It is important to interpret the initial salicylate level in regard to the symptoms and history. It is often equally important to determine if the level is increasing. In a significant ingestion, it is common to repeat the next level 1–2 hours after the initial level, and this may continue until you have shown the level to be trending downward. Once levels are trending down, repeat levels will still be needed, but can be spaced out accordingly (every 4–6 hours and then every 12 hours) until levels are in a therapeutic range. Salicylate levels should be used and interpreted in conjunction with blood pH. and the frequency of these repeat labs often depends on the clinical status of the patient. Recommendations by your local poison center can help determine the frequency needed.[2]

As mentioned above, arterial blood gas measurements are important in assessing the severity of salicylate toxicity as they provide the blood pH and acid-base status. Depending on the time of ingestion and the stage of toxicity, blood gas analysis may show a respiratory alkalosis, metabolic acidosis, or a mixed primary respiratory alkalosis-primary acidosis. A serum chemistry may often reveal an elevated anion gap due to the accumulation of organic acids such as lactic acid and ketoacids. This causes a mixed respiratory alkalosis/metabolic acidosis. It is important to note that a normal anion gap does not rule out salicylate toxicity. This can be due to renal tubular acidosis causing metabolic acidosis and, in some cases, a falsely elevated chloride level.

Other associated lab abnormalities that should be evaluated include elevated serum creatinine, hypoglycemia, hypokalemia, and elevated prothrombin time (PT) and INR.[1] The patient may also have a normal serum glucose level with significant toxicity. They may still be neuroglycopenia, as discussed above, and undergoing significant anaerobic metabolism. The potassium is also very important and will need to be monitored closely, usually with serial levels. This will become very important when treating significant toxicity, as will the renal function.

Treatment

Treatment of salicylate ingestion ranges from mild supportive care measures to more invasive measures such as intubation and hemodialysis. Early consultation with a toxicologist is recommended. The initial focus should be on assessing, maintaining, and protecting the airway. In the case of salicylate toxicity, however, intubation and mechanical ventilation can come with profound consequences. As stated earlier, salicylic acid acts on the respiratory center in the medulla to increase respiratory rate and minute ventilation, leading to a respiratory alkalosis. This initially may help ameliorate further toxicity as it decreases the amount of protonated salicylate, and only the protonated salicylate crosses the blood–brain barrier. It is also important to recognize that a normal pH is not always reassuring. If a patient with significant salicylate toxicity has a normal pH but a low bicarbonate and CO_2, then this patient is in distress and likely expending significant energy trying to maintain homeostasis.

It is difficult to replicate the patient's hyperventilation on the ventilator, and intubation can result in hypoventilation and death. Therefore, intubation should only be considered after careful risk-benefit analysis and reserved for only the most severely poisoned patients.[5] If a patient does require intubation for salicylate toxicity, it is important to try to match their pre-intubation minute ventilation, which was likely compensating for severe acidosis. Patients who require intubation should also undergo hemodialysis as there is increased mortality in intubated patients who do not undergo dialysis.[6]

Activated charcoal is effective at absorbing aspirin and should be considered in patients presenting within 2 hours of salicylate ingestion. The initial dose is 1g/kg up to 50 g PO. Activated charcoal should not be given in patients with altered mental status or somnolence without a secured airway—in such cases, after airway securement, activated charcoal may be given through a nasogastric or orogastric tube. Great caution should be had for patients with nausea and vomiting due to the risk of charcoal aspiration. If rising salicylate levels are noted, multidose activated charcoal may be considered, with additional doses of 25 g every 2–3 hours or 50 g every 4 hours for two doses after the initial dose is given. Whole-bowel irrigation can also be considered for massive ingestions; however, no studies have demonstrated a clinical benefit.[2]

Serum and urine alkalinization with sodium bicarbonate is a mainstay in the management of salicylate toxicity. Salicylates exist in the body as either uncharged molecules that can cross membranes such as the blood–brain barrier or as charged ions that cannot cross these membranes into tissues and are more easily excreted. Alkalinization results in more of the ionized salicylic acid being trapped in the nephrons and then excreted in the urine by the kidneys. The initial dose of sodium bicarbonate is 1–2 mEq/kg IV bolus. This is followed by an infusion of 100–150 mEq in 1 L D5W, the rate of which is titrated to a urine pH of 7.5–8. At the same time, it is important to monitor the serum pH to make sure it does not exceed 7.55. It is important to correct hypokalemia to ensure efficacy of alkalinization because hypokalemia will cause hydrogen ion dumping into the collecting duct, acidifying the urine and leading to reabsorption of salicylate. Therefore, serum potassium levels should be normalized to greater than 4.0 mmol/L and checked hourly. Urinary alkalinization can be discontinued once the following endpoints have been reached: serum salicylate level is less than 40 mg/dL and down-trending over two consecutive levels, serum pH has normalized, metabolic acidosis has resolved, and the patient is asymptomatic with normal respiratory rate and effort. Blood gases and serum salicylate levels should initially be checked every 1–2 hours, and urine pH levels should be checked every 2–4 hours to ensure resolution of toxicity. Alkalinization should be restarted if serum and urine pH increase, serum salicylate levels increase, metabolic acidosis recurs, or if the patient becomes symptomatic.[1-3]

Patients may also present with hypoglycemia or even euglycemia with altered mental status due to neuroglycopenia, which is caused by a shortage of glucose available to neurons and results in altered neuronal function and thus altered mental status. Clinically, these patients should be treated with dextrose-containing fluids either as a bolus or infusion. If the patient is clinically altered, the clinician may need to try to increase serum glucose to between 150 and 200 mg/dL to try to alleviate any neuroglycopenia. Hypotension can be due to sensible and insensible fluid losses as well as systemic vasodilation. Volume resuscitation with fluid boluses should be attempted first. Hypotension refractory to fluid resuscitation can be treated with vasopressors such as phenylephrine or norepinephrine.[3]

Acetazolamide does enhance salicylate excretion, but it is contraindicated as the bicarbonate loss from plasma lowers the arterial pH, which can in turn worsen salicylate neurotoxicity.[2]

Hemodialysis can enhance salicylate removal due to the low molecular mass, water solubility, and low volume of distribution of salicylates.[1] Therefore, nephrology should be consulted early for salicylate intoxication if there is any indication the patient may require hemodialysis.

The general indications for hemodialysis in salicylate toxicity include:

- Altered mental status
- Pulmonary edema with respiratory distress and/or requiring supplemental oxygen
- Cerebral edema
- Acute or chronic kidney injury
- Intubation
- Fluid overload (preventing ability to administer sodium bicarbonate)
- Salicylate concentration of greater than 90 mg/dL in normal renal function, greater than 80 mg/dL in impaired renal function
- Severe acidosis (pH ≤7.20)
- Clinical deterioration despite aggressive supportive care

Salicylate toxicity is not as common as other ingestions, such as acetaminophen, but salicylate toxicity can be immediately life-threatening. The provider must be able to recognize certain signs of serious toxicity including hyperthermia and increased respiratory rate. The provider must also be comfortable with both acute and chronic toxicity as well as management strategies for both presentations.

CASE CONCLUSION

The patient described above represents a significant salicylate ingestion at the severe end of the spectrum. She has already had a seizure and is even hyperthermic, which can be an ominous sign. The presentation can range from subtle to this extreme, but providers need to be able to recognize and treat the entire range of presentations.

- Intubating a patient with salicylate overdose can lead to a worsening toxidrome if the patient is hypoventilating relative to pre-intubation minute ventilation; intubation should be accompanied by hemodialysis.
- Alkalinization is the most effective initial treatment of salicylate toxicity but requires close monitoring of serum potassium; dialysis is the most definitive treatment.
- Patient should be closely observed, and labs should continue to be trended during and after treatment.
- Salicylate toxicity can be acute or chronic, but the presenting symptoms can be similar.

Further Reading

Palmer BF, Clegg DJ. Salicylate toxicity. *N Engl J Med*. 2020 Jun 25;382(26):2544–2555.

Shively RM, Hoffman RS, Manini AF. Acute salicylate poisoning: risk factors for severe outcome. *Clin Toxicol*. 2017 Mar 16;55(3):175–180.

Vale A. Salicylates. *Medicine*. 2016 Mar 1;44(3):199–200.

References

1. Clegg DJ, Palmer BF. Salicylate toxicity. Ingelfinger JR, ed. *N Engl J Med*. 2020;383(13):1288–1289. doi:10.1056/nejmc2025928
2. Flomenbaum N, Hoffman RS, Goldfrank LR, et al. *Goldfrank's toxicologic emergencies*. McGraw-Hill Education; 2019.
3. Thongprayoon C, Petnak T, Kaewput W, et al. Hospitalizations for acute salicylate intoxication in the United States. *J Clin Med*. 2020;9(8):2638. doi:10.3390/jcm9082638.
4. Hill JB. Salicylate intoxication. *N Engl J Med*. 1973;288(21):1110–1113. doi:10.1056/NEJM197305242882107
5. Thisted B, Krantz T, Strøom J, Sørensen MB. Acute salicylate self-poisoning in 177 consecutive patients treated in ICU. *Acta Anaesthesiol Scand*. 1987;31(4):312–316. doi:10.1111/j.1399-6576.1987.tb02574.x
6. McCabe DJ, Lu JJ. The association of hemodialysis and survival in intubated salicylate-poisoned patients. *Am J Emerg Med*. 2017 Jun 1;35(6):899–903. doi:10.1016/j.ajem.2017.04.017

3 Mind the Gap: Toxic Alcohol Management

Patrick Filkins

Case Presentation

A 48-year-old man presents to the ED after he is found minimally responsive at the auto body shop where he is currently employed. Coworkers who called EMS reported seeing him last well at 7 pm the previous evening. According to EMS, he has a past medical history of depression and alcohol abuse disorder. They recovered an empty bottle of vodka and open bottle of radiator anti-freeze at the scene. Vitals upon arrival to the hospital are heart rate 101 beats/min, blood pressure 101/63, respiratory rate 22 breaths/min, temperature 97.3°F/36.3°C (rectal), and 99% SpO_2 on 4 L nasal cannula. On exam he appears grossly inebriated with a Glasgow Coma Scale (GCS) of 11: eyes open to verbal command with inappropriate responses and purposeful movement to painful stimuli. Exam reveals pupils that are equal, round, and sluggishly reactive to light. There are no obvious signs of trauma. Point of care glucose reveals a level of 52 mg/dL. IV access is obtained, and 25 g of IV dextrose 50% and 100 mg of IV thiamine were administered. Review of the electronic medical record reveals multiple prior admissions for ethanol intoxication and ethanol withdrawal. Additionally, he is currently prescribed sertraline, thiamine, and folic acid.

What Do You Do Now?

DISCUSSION

Background

Based on the history and clinical presentation described in the clinical vignette, the emergency medicine provider should be highly concerned for a toxic alcohol ingestion. The term "toxic alcohol" generally refers to a group of alcohols not meant for consumption. This term is a misnomer as the parent compounds are not toxic. It is the acidic metabolites produced that cause the clinical effects. Though there are many which fall into this category, methanol, ethylene glycol, isopropanol, diethylene glycol, and propylene glycol are the most encountered substances.[1] More than 18,000 toxic alcohol exposures were reported to the National Poison Data System (NPDS) in 2020. Miscellaneous alcohols were the fourth leading category in terms of number of fatalities reported to NPDS.[2]

Methanol is the simplest of the toxic alcohols, consisting of an alcohol group attached to a single carbon methyl group. It is produced through the fermentation of wood. It is commonly encountered in products such as windshield washer fluid, solid cooking fuel, colognes and perfumes, illicitly made spirits (such as moonshine fermented from wood products), and gas line antifreeze (dry gas). The most common source of methanol exposures comes from ingesting windshield washer fluid.[3] Methanol toxicity is also possible via inhalational and dermal routes.[3,4] Ethylene glycol is primarily used as an engine coolant, however it can also be found in hydraulic brake fluid, deicing agents, and other coolant solutions. The primary route of exposure is typically oral.[1,3] Isopropanol is the only secondary alcohol in this group of toxins and is primarily available as rubbing alcohol. Typical household preparations are 70% weight per volume (w/v). Other sources include hand sanitizers, cosmetics, and topical pharmaceutical preparations. Exposures are typically via the oral route.[1,3] Isopropanol remains the most common toxic alcohol exposure reported on a yearly basis.[2,3]

Toxicology and Pathophysiology

The key to understanding the pathophysiology of toxic alcohol ingestions is to understand their metabolism. The end-organ toxicity stems from the accumulation of the acid metabolites. All toxic alcohols are absorbed rapidly and follow a similar metabolic pathway to ethanol. The alcohol species is initially metabolized by alcohol dehydrogenase (ADH) to an aldehyde, and then is further metabolized by aldehyde dehydrogenase (ALDH) to a carboxylic acid. Metabolism of toxic alcohols is zero-order, like that of ethanol, and is unchanged in chronic alcohol users.[3-5]

Methanol is initially metabolized by ADH to form formaldehyde, which is rapidly metabolized by ALDH to form formic acid. This formic acid metabolite is then bound to tetrahydrofolate and is metabolized by 10-formyltetrahydrofolate dehydrogenase to carbon dioxide and water. Formic acid accumulation is responsible for the clinical effects seen in methanol toxicity, including metabolic acidosis and potentially irreversible retinal and neurologic toxicity.[3,4,6]

Ethylene glycol is initially metabolized by ADH to form glycoaldehyde and then by ALDH to glycolic acid, the primary contributor to the metabolic acidosis seen in ethylene glycol toxicity. Glycolic acid is then metabolized by lactate dehydrogenase or glycolic acid oxidase to form glyoxylic acid, which is then rapidly metabolized to oxalic acid, another toxic metabolite. Oxalic acid precipitates with calcium to form calcium oxalate crystals, which precipitate in renal tubules and lead to acute kidney injury (AKI), characteristic of ethylene glycol toxicity. Other minor pathways include pyridoxine-dependent and thiamine-dependent enzymes to form nontoxic metabolites.[3,5]

Isopropanol differs from other alcohols in that it is only metabolized by ADH to form acetone. It is a ketone not an aldehyde, thus is not metabolized by ALDH. Acetone is subsequently eliminated in urine and expelled in air. Isopropanol is known to cause hemorrhagic gastritis.[1,3]

Workup and Diagnosis

All alcohols are inebriating. Animal evidence suggests that the higher the molecular weight of the alcohol, the more inebriating. Thus, isopropanol is potentially the most inebriating toxic alcohol and methanol the least.[7] These CNS manifestations are thought to be mediated through agonism of gamma-aminobutyric acid (GABA) $GABA_A$ receptors and inhibition of the N-methyl-D-aspartic acid (NMDA) glutamate receptors in a similar fashion to ethanol.[3-5,8] Lack of inebriation cannot rule out a potential toxic alcohol exposure. Toxic effects can be seen with methanol concentrations of greater than 20 mg/dL.[9] Thus, patients may present with a potentially toxic ingestion with the absence of CNS manifestations. Additionally, chronic consumers of alcohol are more likely to be tolerant to the inebriating effects of other alcohols.

In an undifferentiated patient presenting with altered mental status, the differential can remain exceedingly broad. The presence of an anion gap metabolic acidosis is the hallmark of toxic alcohol ingestions. As methanol and ethylene glycol are metabolized, the acid metabolites begin to accumulate and increase the number of unmeasured anions on the chemistry.[3,10] The elevation of an anion gap without ketosis or lactic acidosis can indicate a methanol or ethylene glycol ingestion even in the absence of a reported history of ingestion.

The absence of an elevated anion gap metabolic acidosis cannot exclude a toxic alcohol ingestion because there may be a several-hour delay from the time of ingestion to the development of an anion gap metabolic acidosis; potentially up to 23 hours in the case of methanol.[3,11] Additionally, if patients have co-ingested ethanol, this will compete with the metabolism of methanol and ethylene glycol because ADH has a 67 times higher affinity for ethanol than ethylene glycol and a 15.5 times higher affinity than methanol.[3] A potentially early diagnostic marker for a toxic alcohol ingestion is an elevated osmol gap. The measured serum osmolality represents the sum of the activity of all osmotically active particles in the blood. Toxic alcohols are osmotically active as well, thus the presence of an osmol gap elevation can potentially indicate that an unmeasured solute, such as a toxic alcohol, is present. The osmol gap is calculated as follows[11]:

$$Osmolar\ Gap = Measured\ Osmolality - \left(2[Na] + \left(\frac{[BUN]}{2.6} + \frac{[Glucose]}{18} + \frac{[Ethanol]}{3.7}\right)\right)$$

where [Na] is mmol/L and [Glucose], [BUN], and [Ethanol] are mg/dL, and BUN is blood urea nitrogen.

There are some important caveats to consider when assessing an osmol gap. First, the osmol gap is neither sensitive nor specific for toxic alcohols. The "normal" osmol gap is defined as –14 to +10 mOsm/L. This cannot exclude a toxic alcohol because typically a patient's baseline osmol gap is unknown. Therefore, a patient with a baseline osmol gap of –12 could present with a calculated osmol gap of +8. While this is within the typical normal reference range, in this patient, it represents a 20 mOsm/L increase from baseline which may indicate the presence of a toxic alcohol.[11,12] Second, there are additional xenobiotics and conditions that may cause an osmol gap elevation including mannitol, propylene glycol, glycerol, contrast dye, lactic acidosis, ketoacidosis, and critical illness. Third, the laboratory results for the measured osmols and the sodium, BUN, glucose, and ethanol should be on the same blood draw and collected at the same time to accurately calculate the osmol gap, thus a basic metabolic panel, serum ethanol, and serum osmolality should be sent simultaneously.

The anion gap and osmol gap should be interpreted simultaneously. As shown in Figure 3.1, a reciprocal change will occur in the osmol gap and anion gap in methanol and ethylene glycol toxicity. Shortly after ingestion, there will be a significant rise in the osmol gap due to the circulating parent compounds. As time passes and the parent compounds are metabolized into their acid metabolites, the osmol gap will begin to normalize as the anion gap begins to elevate. In the case of isopropanol, the initial osmol gap elevation will be observed; however, there will be no increase in anion gap because the major metabolite is acetone. This is the basis of the

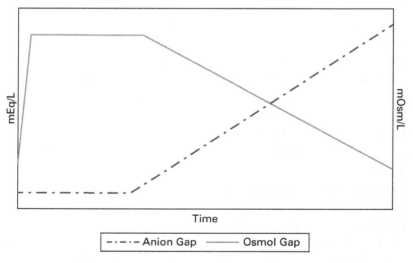

FIGURE 3.1 Reciprocal change in anion gap and osmol gap over time with toxic alcohol ingestions. It is important to note that with isopropanol, the anion gap should remain normal as the osmol gap narrows.

common phrase "ketosis without acidosis" that is associated with isopropanol ingestions.

The optimal diagnostic modality for toxic alcohol exposures is the measurement of serum ethylene glycol and volatile alcohol (e.g., methanol, isopropanol) levels. Unfortunately, these tests are usually send-outs which are not available in a timely manner. This necessitates the need to utilize clinical suspicion in conjunction with previously mentioned, more readily available labs to guide intervention. Urinalysis via microscopy and Woods lamp fluorescence are neither sensitive nor specific for ethylene glycol toxicity.[11] CT or MRI brain imaging may be considered in methanol toxicity with CNS symptoms.[3,4]

Treatment

Ensure patients are protecting their airway, breathing, and have adequate circulation. Due to the sedative nature of alcohols, respiratory depression or coma may necessitate intubation and mechanical ventilation. IV crystalloid fluids are typically required secondary to vomiting, dehydration, and vasodilation. IV sodium bicarbonate may be considered for immediate, life-threatening metabolic acidosis in patients with an arterial pH of less than 7.3.[3-5] GI decontamination is not recommended for toxic alcohol ingestions given the rapid absorption and minimal potential for benefit while increasing risk of vomiting and leading to charcoal aspiration and pneumonitis. Initial labs should include a basic metabolic panel, serum ethanol level, serum acetaminophen level, serum salicylate level, serum osmolality, and arterial blood gas. The management of isopropanol ingestions remains symptomatic with supportive care, thus further discussion will focus on methanol and ethylene glycol.

The mainstay of therapy for methanol and ethylene glycol ingestions is ADH blockade using fomepizole (4-MP) or ethanol. Ethanol remains the only option in many parts of the world; however, in the United States, 4-MP is more widely used. A prospective study in the United Kingdom indicated no difference in outcomes between ethanol and 4-MP ADH blockade, however the authors noted a higher frequency of adverse effects (16/131 vs. 2/125; $p < 0.001$) and therapeutic errors, lack of monitoring, or inappropriate use (45/131 vs. 6/125; $p < 0.0001$) with ethanol.[13] 4-MP is a competitive ADH antagonist initially approved in 1997 for ethylene glycol toxicity and in 2000 for methanol toxicity. ADH has more than 1,000 times higher affinity for 4-MP than toxic alcohols.[9,14] Given its extensive safety profile, it remains the antidote of choice in the United States. Additionally, unless patients are critically ill, use of 4-MP does not necessitate a routine ICU level of care, whereas the observation and laboratory monitoring required for ethanol infusions can often only be achieved in the ICU.[6,15–17]

Proposed indications ADH blockade for methanol or ethylene glycol include a documented plasma methanol or ethylene glycol concentration of greater than 20 mg/dL, documented recent history of ingestion of toxic amounts of methanol or ethylene glycol with an osmolal gap of greater than 10 mOsm/L, or two out of three of the following: arterial pH less than 7.3, serum bicarbonate level less than 20 mmol/L, osmolal gap greater than 10 mOsm/L, or oxalate crystalluria (if concerned for ethylene glycol).[4,5,15] High enough clinical suspicion for a toxic alcohol ingestion alone may warrant ADH blockade initially while waiting for laboratory data to return. This would likely be the scenario described in the case vignette. The patient is significantly altered and found near an empty bottle of an ethylene glycol-containing product. The goal of ADH blockade is to prevent further formation of the acid metabolites which will cause the end organ toxicity. ADH blockade is not an antidote for any acid metabolites that have already been formed. If the patient concurrently ingested ethanol, 4-MP need not be administered until the serum ethanol concentration falls to near 100 mg/dL or a decline in serum bicarbonate is observed. In the case described above, this would be something to take into consideration because the patient likely co-ingested ethanol and ethylene glycol. A serum ethanol level may need to be assessed prior to initiation of 4-MP. ADH blockade is never indicated for an isolated isopropanol ingestion. The mainstay of therapy remains symptomatic and supportive care.[3]

The initial 4-MP dose is 15 mg/kg IV once followed by 10 mg/kg IV every 12 hours for 48 hours. If therapy is continued beyond 48 hours, the dose must be increased back to 15 mg/kg IV every 12 hours. There are no contraindications other than known hypersensitivity to the drug and no known drug interactions. If patients are to undergo dialysis, the frequency of administration during dialysis must be increased to every 4 hours for intermittent hemodialysis and every 8 hours for continuous renal replacement therapy (CRRT).[9,18,19] The generally accepted and most conservative endpoint of therapy is a plasma methanol or ethylene glycol concentration of less than 20 mg/dL.[3–6,15,16]

If 4-MP is not readily available, ethanol should be utilized for ADH blockade with the same indications as 4-MP.[4,5,15] Ethanol should be administered to maintain a serum ethanol concentration of greater than 100 mg/dL to prevent toxic alcohol metabolism by ADH. A typical loading dose of 0.8 g/kg orally followed by 80–130 mg/kg/hr, which should be administered to ethanol naïve patients. Typically, a 40% ethanol solution such as vodka can be utilized. Serial ethanol levels should be drawn every 1–2 hours in addition to frequent monitoring of blood glucose and electrolytes. In ethanol-tolerant patients, the dose can be increased to 100–150 mg/kg/hr. When undergoing dialysis, 250–350 mg/kg/hr should be administered.[3] The same therapeutic endpoints should be utilized as those with 4-MP. The efficacy of ADH blockade with ethanol followed by hemodialysis has been documented in numerous case reports and case series, including several mass-outbreaks of methanol toxicity.[20,21]

In cases of severe methanol or ethylene glycol toxicity, hemodialysis can be utilized as a definitive therapy, eliminating both the parent compound and toxic metabolites in addition to correcting the acidemia. The Extracorporeal Treatments in Poisoning (EXTRIP) workgroup has published guidelines for implementation of intermittent hemodialysis or CRRT in methanol toxicity. Indications are shown in Box 3.1. Intermittent hemodialysis is preferred when feasible, and dialysis should be continued with ADH blockade until serum methanol concentrations are less than 20 mg/dL.[22] EXTRIP recommendations for ethylene glycol toxicity are currently in progress.[1] Current American Academy of Clinical Toxicology (AACT) Guidelines recommend hemodialysis be considered for clinical deterioration despite adequate supportive care, significant metabolic acidosis (pH <7.25), and renal failure or electrolyte imbalances. In the absence of a clinical indication, hemodialysis is not recommended based on a serum ethylene glycol level when 4-MP is utilized.[5]

---

[1] While the EXTRIP recommendations for ethylene glycol were in progress during preparation of this text, they have since been published and are available at: https://www.extrip-workgroup.org/ethylene-glycol

Adjunctive medications can be considered after primary interventions have been implemented. These adjunctive medications may aid in the elimination of the metabolites formed from toxic alcohols. If methanol toxicity is of concern, folic acid supplementation can enhance the metabolism of formic acid and has been shown to decrease the half-life of formic acid. It is recommended in addition to ADH blockade and hemodialysis given its safety profile. IV folic acid can be administered at 1 mg/kg (up to 50 mg) every 4–6 hours until any acidosis has resolved and methanol concentrations are less than 20 mg/dL.[3,4] Thiamine, pyridoxine, and magnesium may be considered at standard doses for ethylene glycol toxicity, all of which enhance elimination via nontoxic metabolites. There are no studies proving better outcomes, but there is minimal risk with administration and therefore these cofactors should be considered after primary interventions have been made. Additionally, patients with a history of alcohol use disorder may be malnourished and have depleted stores of these vitamins and minerals. Patients with ethylene glycol toxicity also develop hypocalcemia from the formation of calcium oxalate. Calcium should only be repleted if they are exhibiting symptomatic hypocalcemia due to the risk of further calcium oxalate precipitation.[3,5]

Other Toxic Alcohols

Propylene glycol is used as an alternative to ethylene glycol commercially and as an excipient in many pharmaceuticals such as IV phenytoin, IV diazepam, IV phenobarbital, and IV lorazepam. It is metabolized by ADH to lactaldehyde and subsequently by ALDH to lactate and pyruvate. Exposure may occur via ingestion or iatrogenically via medication administration. Massive exposures may cause lactic acidosis, hypoglycemia, seizures, and coma, however the mild lactic acidosis from propylene glycol is typically well tolerated. ADH blockade is not indicated, however dialysis may be required in cases of severe acidemia.[3,9,10]

Diethylene glycol is a solvent similar in physiochemical properties to propylene glycol. It is commonly found in brake fluid and has unfortunately been implicated in several mass poisonings when it was inadvertently included as a medication. It can cause severe nephrotoxicity and neurotoxicity.[23] Patients typically present with GI complaints and intoxication. This devolves into metabolic acidosis and oliguria or anuria with acute kidney injury (AKI) within 1–3 days. Finally, within days following the onset of AKI, neurotoxicity can develop in the form of encephalopathy, coma, and eventual death. Management with 4-MP and dialysis is indicated in similar fashion to methanol and ethylene glycol toxicity.[3,9,10,23,24]

CASE CONCLUSION

The patient's mental status continues to decline and he is intubated for airway protection. Labs are notable for a pH of 7.0 and osmolar gap of 40 mOsm/L. Fomepizole is administered along with thiamine, pyridoxine, and magnesium. Nephrology is consulted for emergent hemodialysis. He is continued on fomepizole and receives another 4 hours of hemodialysis the following day, after which time he is able to be extubated. Fomepizole is discontinued after 48 hours when a sendout ethylene glycol level from after the second round of dialysis results as 18 mg/dL. He suffers significant acute kidney injury but eventually makes a full recovery.

- End-organ toxicity from toxic alcohol ingestions is secondary to the metabolites produced via pathways similar to ethanol.
- The hallmark clinical effect overall is metabolic acidosis; methanol toxicity also exhibits retinal and neurotoxicity, while ethylene glycol toxicity also exhibits nephrotoxicity.
- In lieu of methanol and ethylene glycol levels, the anion gap and osmol gap may clue a provider in on a potential toxic alcohol exposure.
- A basic metabolic panel, measured serum osmolality, and ethanol level should be sent on the same blood draw; toxic alcohol levels are unlikely to acutely guide clinical management.
- Alcohol dehydrogenase (ADH) blockade should be accomplished with 4-MP and is reasonable to initiate with clinical suspicion. This is the primary therapy that should be focused on initially before considering adjunctive medications.
- Definitive management with hemodialysis may be indicated based on severity of illness; this may warrant an early consult with nephrology.

Further Reading

Fenves AZ, Emmett M. Approach to patients with high anion gap metabolic acidosis: core curriculum 2021. *Am J Kidney Dis.* Oct 2021;78(4):590–600.

Lao YE, Vartdal T, Froeyshov S, et al. Fomepizole dosing during continuous renal replacement therapy: An observational study. *Clin Toxicol (Phila).* Sep 29 2021:1–7.

McMartin K, Jacobsen D, Hovda KE. Antidotes for poisoning by alcohols that form toxic metabolites. *Br J Clin Pharmacol.* Mar 2016;81(3):505–515.

References

1. Ng PCY, Long BJ, Davis WT, Sessions DJ, Koyfman A. Toxic alcohol diagnosis and management: an emergency medicine review. *Intern Emerg Med.* Apr 2018;13(3):375–383. doi:10.1007/s11739-018-1799-9
2. Gummin DD, Mowry JB, Beuhler MC, et al. 2020 Annual report of the American Association of Poison Control Centers' National Poison Data System (NPDS): 38th annual report. *Clin Toxicol (Phila).* Dec 2021;59(12):1282–1501. doi:10.1080/15563650.2021.1989785

3. Nelson LS Howland MA, Lewin NA, Smith SW, Goldfrank LR, Hoffman RS. *Goldfrank's toxicologic emergencies.* 11th ed. New York: McGraw-Hill; 2019.

4. Barceloux DG, Bond GR, Krenzelok EP, Cooper H, Vale JA, American Academy of Clinical Toxicology ad hoc committee on the treatment guidelines for methanol poisoning. American Academy of Clinical Toxicology practice guidelines on the treatment of methanol poisoning. *J Toxicol Clin Toxicol.* 2002;40(4):415–446. doi:10.1081/clt-120006745

5. Barceloux DG, Krenzelok EP, Olson K, Watson W. American Academy of Clinical Toxicology practice guidelines on the treatment of ethylene glycol poisoning: ad hoc committee. *J Toxicol Clin Toxicol.* 1999;37(5):537–60. doi:10.1081/clt-100102445

6. Brent J, McMartin K, Phillips S, Aaron C, Kulig K, Methylpyrazole for Toxic Alcohols Study Group. Fomepizole for the treatment of methanol poisoning. *N Engl J Med.* Feb 8 2001;344(6):424–429. doi:10.1056/NEJM200102083440605

7. Wallgren H. Relative intoxicating effects on rats of ethyl, propyl and butyl alcohols. *Acta Pharmacol Toxicol (Copenh).* 1960;16:217–222. doi:10.1111/j.1600-0773.1960.tb01205.x

8. Pohanka M. Toxicology and the biological role of methanol and ethanol: current view. *Biomed Pap Med Fac Univ Palacky Olomouc Czech Repub.* Mar 2016;160(1):54–63. doi:10.5507/bp.2015.023

9. McMartin K, Jacobsen D, Hovda KE. Antidotes for poisoning by alcohols that form toxic metabolites. *Br J Clin Pharmacol.* Mar 2016;81(3):505–515. doi:10.1111/bcp.12824

10. Ross JA, Borek HA, Holstege CP. Toxic alcohols. *Crit Care Clin.* Jul 2021;37(3):643–656. doi:10.1016/j.ccc.2021.03.009

11. Kraut JA. Diagnosis of toxic alcohols: limitations of present methods. *Clin Toxicol (Phila).* 2015;53(7):589–595. doi:10.3109/15563650.2015.1056880

12. Hoffman RS, Smilkstein MJ, Howland MA, Goldfrank LR. Osmol gaps revisited: normal values and limitations. *J Toxicol Clin Toxicol.* 1993;31(1):81–93. doi:10.3109/15563659309000375

13. Thanacoody RH, Gilfillan C, Bradberry SM, et al. Management of poisoning with ethylene glycol and methanol in the UK: a prospective study conducted by the National Poisons Information Service (NPIS). *Clin Toxicol (Phila).* 2016;54(2):134–140. doi:10.3109/15563650.2015.1116044

14. Li TK, Theorell H. Human liver alcohol dehydrogenase: inhibition by pyrazole and pyrazole analogs. *Acta Chem Scand.* 1969;23(3):892–902. doi:10.3891/acta.chem.scand.23-0892

15. Brent J. Fomepizole for ethylene glycol and methanol poisoning. *N Engl J Med.* May 21 2009;360(21):2216–2223. doi:10.1056/NEJMct0806112

16. Brent J, McMartin K, Phillips S, et al. Fomepizole for the treatment of ethylene glycol poisoning. Methylpyrazole for Toxic Alcohols Study Group. *N Engl J Med.* Mar 18 1999;340(11):832–838. doi:10.1056/NEJM199903183401102

17. Rasamison R, Besson H, Berleur MP, Schicchi A, Megarbane B. Analysis of fomepizole safety based on a 16-year post-marketing experience in France. *Clin Toxicol (Phila)*. Jul 2020;58(7):742–747. doi:10.1080/15563650.2019.1676899

18. Fomepizole. Micromedex (electronic version). Merative USA; 2021. Accessed March 10, 2022. https://www.micromedexsolutions.com

19. Lao YE, Vartdal T, Froeyshov S, et al. Fomepizole dosing during continuous renal replacement therapy: an observational study. *Clin Toxicol (Phila)*. Sep 29 2021;60(4):451–457. doi:10.1080/15563650.2021.1980581

20. Hassanian-Moghaddam H, Nikfarjam A, Mirafzal A, et al. Methanol mass poisoning in Iran: role of case finding in outbreak management. *J Public Health (Oxf)*. Jun 2015;37(2):354–359. doi:10.1093/pubmed/fdu038

21. Rulisek J, Balik M, Polak F, et al. Cost-effectiveness of hospital treatment and outcomes of acute methanol poisoning during the Czech Republic mass poisoning outbreak. *J Crit Care*. Jun 2017;39:190–198. doi:10.1016/j.jcrc.2017.03.001

22. Roberts DM, Yates C, Megarbane B, et al. Recommendations for the role of extracorporeal treatments in the management of acute methanol poisoning: a systematic review and consensus statement. *Crit Care Med*. Feb 2015;43(2):461–472. doi:10.1097/CCM.0000000000000708

23. Jamison CN, Dayton RD, Latimer B, McKinney MP, Mitchell HG, McMartin KE. Diethylene glycol produces nephrotoxic and neurotoxic effects in female rats. *Clin Toxicol (Phila)*. Mar 2022;60(3):324–331. doi:10.1080/15563650.2021.1953049

24. Cervantes CE, Chu A, Heller D, Lemont M. Early dialysis in a rare case of combined toxic alcohols ingestion. *CEN Case Rep*. Feb 2020;9(1):11–14. doi:10.1007/s13730-019-00417-0

4 Unrelenting Insulin Release: Sulfonylurea/Meglitinide Overdose

Matthew Sheneman, Brian P. Murray, and Joseph E. Carpenter

Case Presentation

On an early Saturday morning, you are working a shift in a rural community Emergency Department when you get a call from EMS, "8 minutes out, 4-year-old boy coming in after not waking up from his nap." EMS states that, earlier this morning, the patient was put down for his nap early by grandma because he seemed more tired than usual. His grandmother didn't think anything of it, but after napping for double the amount of time he usually does, she went to check on him. At the scene, his grandmother stated, "I tried waking him by first saying his name louder and louder, then by rubbing his shoulder hard, when he didn't wake up I knew something was wrong, so I called 911." EMS checked the patient's point-of-care (POC) glucose at the scene and discovered it was 15 mg/dL. IV access was established by the paramedic, and the patient was given an IV bolus of dextrose. After a second check enroute to hospital, POC glucose

was still 32 mg/dL. His vital signs are heart rate
100 beats/min, respiratory rate 20 breaths/min,
blood pressure 95/65 mm Hg, and SpO$_2$ 98% on
room air. The patient's glucose in the ED is 28 mg/dL
and another dextrose bolus of 5 mL/kg of D10W is
administered.

What Do You Do Now?

DISCUSSION

Background

Sulfonylureas are the oldest class of oral antidiabetic medications and one of the classes that can lead to hypoglycemia. In fact, the most common adverse effect of these medications is hypoglycemia. Sulfonylureas have a narrow therapeutic window, and inadvertent hypoglycemia is common. Overdose, whether intentional or unintentional, can have severe and life-threatening toxicity due to persistent hypoglycemia. In adults aged 65 years and older, oral hypoglycemic agents are among the four most common medications associated with emergency hospitalizations.[1,2]

Sulfonylureas are categorized by their generation, with the second-generation medications possessing higher potency, fewer adverse effects, and fewer drug–drug interaction. First-generation sulfonylureas include chlorpropamide, tolbutamide, tolazamide, and acetohexamide. The second-generation sulfonylureas include glipizide, glyburide, gliclazide, and glimepiride.

Meglitinides are another class of oral antidiabetic medications that has similar mechanism of action to sulfonylureas; they have a weaker binding affinity to, and faster dissociation from, the adenosine triphosphate (ATP)-sensitive K-channels on the pancreatic beta-cell, causing a shorter half-life. Meglitinides include repaglinide and nateglinide.

Sulfonylureas and meglitinides are two of the many kinds of medications that can potentially be fatal after a single pill ingestion by pediatric patients. In 2020, the poison control centers received more than 2.2 million calls for accidental overdoses; 47% of those occurred in children younger than 6 years. Most pediatric accidental ingestions occur from personal care products and analgesics; however, sulfonylureas are the second most severe in terms of morbidity and mortality due to the profound and prolonged effects of hypoglycemia.[2]

Toxicology and Pathophysiology

Glucose is a 6-carbon structure that is the primary source of energy for much of tissues in the human body. It is essential for fueling both aerobic and anaerobic cellular respiration. Once glucose is absorbed into the body, it travels through the bloodstream to energy-requiring tissues. When glucose concentrations rise within the pancreatic beta-cells, insulin is released. Pancreatic beta-cells "sense" this increase of glucose through increased uptake of glucose into the cells through GLUT-2 transporters. The increased intracellular glucose ultimately leads to increased ATP production within the beta-cell which inhibits ATP-sensitive K-channels, preventing the influx of potassium into the cell. This leads to cell membrane depolarization, which causes voltage-dependent L-type Ca^{2+} channels to open, allowing for the influx of calcium ions into the cell. This results in calcium-dependent calcium release from the endoplasmic reticulum and causes the exocytosis of preformed insulin vesicles.

Sulfonylureas act to increase the release of insulin by binding to a subunit of the ATP-sensitive K-channels on plasma membranes of pancreatic beta-cells, inhibiting potassium efflux out of the beta cells independent of endogenous glucose. This results in the release of insulin in excess of what would have been released by the blood glucose concentration alone.[3] Insulin release generally peaks between 4 and 8 hours after sulfonylurea ingestion, although particular agents have varying half-lives, which can be on the order of several days in overdose. Since sulfonylureas do not inhibit glucose's ability to induce insulin, further increasing serum glucose will compound any overdose of the sulfonylurea by further increasing insulin release and may subsequently lead to further hypoglycemia.

These medications are largely metabolized by the liver and are eliminated renally as both the parent compound and somewhat active metabolites. Therefore patients may experience hypoglycemia when continuing their usual sulfonylurea dose in the setting of acute kidney injury due to impaired clearance.

Workup and Diagnosis

In all cases of altered mental status, a rapid POC glucose should be one of the first laboratory tests obtained. Signs and symptoms of hypoglycemia are nonspecific and can include tachycardia, tremor, diaphoresis, confusion, agitation, seizure-like activity, stroke-like symptoms, or even coma. Patients with a history of prior hypoglycemic episodes and those on beta-blockers may not manifest typical symptoms despite a low serum glucose, making the clinical diagnosis more difficult. When a patient has recurrent hypoglycemia after administration of dextrose and initial correction of the hypoglycemia, clinicians should have a high degree of suspicion for sulfo-nylurea or meglitinide toxicity.

Clinicians should seek information from family and/or friends regarding xenobiotics that the patient may have accessed, particularly any prescription medications kept in the house.

In addition to serial monitoring of POC blood glucose, serum chemistry should be obtained in all cases of known or suspected sulfonylurea toxicity. Elevated creatinine and blood urea nitrogen (BUN) could indicate impaired clearance of sulfonylureas leading to toxicity.

Treatment

If the patient presents early, approximately within 1 hour of ingestion, then active charcoal can be administered to a patient who is alert, oriented, and protecting their airway. The first definitive treatment in any patient with hypoglycemia is supplemental dextrose, indicated in all cases of hypoglycemia (<60 mg/dL). The dosing of dextrose for adults is 25–50 g of D50W or D25W IV, which can be repeated if needed [4-7]. The pediatric dosing for dextrose is either D25W or D10W bolus IV of 2–4 mL/kg or 5–10 mL/kg, respectively.[4-7] In the setting of sulfonylurea exposure, dextrose administration may stimulate additional insulin release, leading to subsequent hypoglycemia. If this occurs, octreotide is indicated.

Octreotide is the antidote of choice for sulfonylurea and meglitinide toxicity because it antagonizes the action of these agents. Sulfonylureas act by placing the pancreatic beta cells in overdrive, causing secretion of insulin.[7] Octreotide counteracts this by closing L-type voltage-gated calcium channels on pancreatic beta-islet cells, inhibiting the influx of calcium, which ultimately inhibits the secretion of insulin.[4] Octreotide can be administered either by 50 mcg subcutaneous injection or 25 mcg/hr IV and can be given every 6 hours for a up to of 24 hours. After discontinuation patients should be monitored for an additional 24 hours to assure no further episodes of hypoglycemia. This is particularly important in pediatric patients who are more prone to episodes of hypoglycemia than adults, and who may be less able to verbalize early symptoms of hypoglycemia.

If continual hypoglycemic events occur despite octreotide and boluses of dextrose, an IV infusion of D5W or D10W can be administered and titrated to effect to maintain glucose in a normal range. Typically, one would start adults at D10W infusion at 100 mL/hr with POC glucose checks at least hourly. The pediatric dose for dextrose infusion is D10W at 5 mL/kg or D5W at 10 mL/kg given IV.[4-7]

Last, disposition of these patients should always err on the side of caution since there is a high risk of the patient having prolonged toxicity. Any patients who become hypoglycemic warrant observation for 24 hours. All children with a known or suspected sulfonylurea ingestion should be observed for at least 24 hours, even in the absence of hypoglycemia, due to the concern for delayed onset. Adults with a suspected sulfonylurea overdose should be observed at least 8–12 hours with regular monitoring of blood glucose, longer if they are suspected to have ingested a sustained-release preparation.

CASE CONCLUSION

Revisiting the case presentation, the 4-year-old boy was started on an infusion of D5W. After further history-taking from grandmother, she stated that she did see that her pill bottle of glyburide was open when she found him. Patient was given octreotide in the ED and admitted to the pediatric ICU where his blood glucose levels stabilized. He was discharged 3 days later.

KEY POINTS TO REMEMBER

- Recurrent hypoglycemia even after dextrose bolus should lead to high suspicion that sulfonylurea/meglitinide toxicity is present.
- Activated charcoal can be used if patient presents within 1–4 hours of ingestion.
- Glucose can paradoxically make sulfonylurea toxicity worse.
- Octreotide is the antidote to sulfonylurea overdose.
- Patients admitted on octreotide require 24-hour observation *after* the octreotide has been discontinued.

Further Reading

Akhter MS, Uppal P. Toxicity of metformin and hypoglycemic therapies. *Adv Chronic Kidney Dis*. 2020 Jan 1;27(1):18–30.

Klein-Schwartz W, Stassinos GL, Isbister GK. Treatment of sulfonylurea and insulin overdose. *Br J Clin Pharmacol*. 2016 Mar;81(3):496–504.

McLaughlin SA, Crandall CS, McKinney PE. Octreotide: An antidote for sulfonylurea-induced hypoglycemia. *Ann Emerg Med*. 2000 Aug 1;36(2):133–138.

Zafar S, Mahali LP, Ahsan H. Role of octreotide in sulfonylurea-induced hypoglycemia. *J Endocrine Soc*. 2021 May 3;5(Suppl 1):A396.

References

1. Hantzidiamantis PJ, Lappin SL. Physiology, glucose. PubMed. 2022. Accessed March 15, 2022. https://www.ncbi.nlm.nih.gov/books/NBK545201/#_NBK545 201_pubdet_

2. Euwema MS, Swanson TJ. Deadly Single Dose Agents. Nih.gov. August 3, 2021. Accessed March 25, 2022. https://www.ncbi.nlm.nih.gov/books/NBK441849/ #:~:text=Beta%2Dblockers%20%2D%20metoprolol%2C%20labetalol

3. Klein-Schwartz W, Stassinos GL, Isbister GK. Treatment of sulfonylurea and insulin overdose. *Br J Clin Pharmacol*. 2016;81(3):496–504. doi:10.1111/bcp.12822

4. Gonzalez RR, Zweig S, Rao J, Block R, Greene LW. Octreotide therapy for recurrent refractory hypoglycemia due to sulfonylurea in diabetes-related kidney failure. *Endocr Pract*. 2007;13(4):417–423. doi:10.4158/EP.13.4.417

5. Harrigan RA, Nathan MS, Beattie P. Oral agents for the treatment of type 2 diabetes mellitus: Pharmacology, toxicity, and treatment. *Ann Emerg Med*. 2001;38(1):68–78. doi:10.1067/mem.2001.114314

6. Rowden AK, Fasano CJ. Emergency management of oral hypoglycemic drug toxicity. Emerg Med Clin *North Am*. 2007;25(2):347–356. doi:10.1016/ j.emc.2007.02.010

7. McLaughlin SA, Crandall CS, McKinney PE. Octreotide: An antidote for sulfonylurea-induced hypoglycemia. *Ann Emerg Med*. 2000;36(2):133–138. doi:10.1067/mem.2000.108183

5 Some Like It Hot: Management of Toxic Hyperthermia

Nicholas Titelbaum and Brent Morgan

Case Presentation

A 36-year-old man with no past medical history presents to the ED by EMS with a chief complaint of altered mental status. He reportedly took 0.4 g of mushrooms, 2 tablets of MDMA, and 1 stamp of LSD at a party and became confused and agitated. 911 was called, and EMS found him altered and combative, requiring physical restraints. In the ED, he did not follow commands and was unable to provide additional history. Initial vital signs are heart rate 182 beats/min, blood pressure 127/100 mm Hg, respiratory rate 30 breaths/min, temperature 108.3°F (42.4°C), and SpO$_2$ 83% on room air. On exam you find him to be shaking, minimally responsive, and combative. His pupils are dilated and minimally responsive to light. Mucous membranes are moist. His lungs are clear to auscultation bilaterally, and he is tachypneic. His abdomen has increased bowel sounds. He has a Glasgow Coma Scale (GCS) of 12, tremors, and clonus in the bilateral lower extremities. His skin is warm and diaphoretic.

What Do You Do Now?

DISCUSSION

Background

The patient in this clinical vignette presents with altered mental status, tachycardia, and profound hyperthermia after a polysubstance ingestion. An altered patient with hyperthermia (T > 00.4 °F or 38 °C) is a medically challenging presentation for emergency medicine providers. The differential is broad, with many possible nontoxicologic etiologies such as infectious processes, exertional heat stroke, and thyrotoxicosis. The differential of toxic hyperthermia is itself extensive, and obtaining a thorough history is important for determining the underlying cause of the patient's presentation. However, obtaining a history from such altered patients is likely to prove challenging, and an effort should be made to obtain collateral history from friends or family if possible.

Accurate temperature measurements are essential for not only recognizing toxic hyperthermia, but also for monitoring response to treatment. While the most common ways to check temperature in the ED include oral, axillary, temporal artery, or tympanic membrane measurements, these methods may yield inaccurate and inconsistent readings. The most accurate assessment and gold standard for assessing temperature in an agitated patient is rectally.[1-3]

If unrecognized or untreated, toxic hyperthermia can result in systemic effects damaging multiple organs. The potential complications include but are not limited to rhabdomyolysis, renal injury, liver failure, cardiac failure, hypotension, acute respiratory distress syndrome (ARDS), coagulopathy, cerebral edema, and death.[4-6]

Many drugs and toxins can produce hyperthermia. Several toxidromes, including neuroleptic malignant syndrome, serotonin toxicity, malignant hyperthermia, sympathomimetic toxicity, anticholinergic toxicity, and withdrawal from sedative-hypnotics can result in life-threatening hyperthermia. Additionally, any drug or toxin that uncouples the electron transport chain can produce hyperthermia.

The 2019 Annual Report of the American Association of Poison Control Centers' National Poison Data System (NPDS) demonstrates the potential of hyperthermia-inducing agents to cause mortality. Hyperthermia-inducing agents such as stimulants, street drugs, selective serotonin reuptake inhibitors (SSRIs), serotonin norepinephrine reuptake inhibitors (SNRIs), acetylsalicylic acid, and tricyclic antidepressants (TCAs) were among the 25 substances associated with the largest number of fatalities (see Table 5.1).[7]

Toxicology and Pathophysiology

Humans are endotherms, capable of producing body heat and regulating body temperature. Heat production is primarily produced by metabolic processes. Under normal physiologic conditions, the heat-sensitive neurons of the hypothalamus provide thermoregulation.[8] Toxicologic agents can produce hyperthermia by increasing the production of heat or by impairing the body's ability to dissipate heat. We focus here the discussion on six types of toxic hyperthermia: serotonin toxicity, neuroleptic malignant syndrome (NMS), sympathomimetic toxicity, anticholinergic toxicity, malignant hyperthermia, and uncouplers of oxidative phosphorylation.

Serotonin toxicity is caused by excessive stimulation of serotonin receptors, and toxicity most often occurs in people taking multiple serotonergic agents.[9] Xenobiotics with serotonergic effects include serotonin reuptake inhibitors, monoamine oxidase inhibitors, tramadol, fentanyl, meperidine, linezolid, St. John's wort (*Hypericum perforatum*), and many others.[10] Onset is rapid, often occurring within 6 hours of administration of serotonergic agents.[11] Excessive serotonergic stimulation of the autonomic nervous system may result in hyperthermia and tachycardia, while CNS effects include confusion and agitation. Increased serotonergic tone can also lead to neuromuscular excitation, which may manifest clinically as ocular clonus, myoclonus, hyperreflexia, or rigidity. The neuromuscular effects are often most pronounced in the lower extremities.[12]

NMS results from an abrupt reduction in central dopamine transmission in the hypothalamus and basal ganglia. Reduced dopaminergic transmission in the hypothalamus leads to impaired thermoregulation and autonomic instability, while "lead pipe" muscle rigidity and tremor are caused by basal ganglia-mediated effects.[13,14] NMS can be caused by any D_2 receptor antagonist including any antipsychotic, with the highest incidence occurring with haloperidol.[15] NMS is gradual in onset, typically occurring within 2 weeks of initiation of an antipsychotic, but it can occur after prolonged antipsychotic use, typically in the setting of a dose increase or a physical illness such as pneumonia.[16] The clinical course of NMS may fluctuate, with dramatic

TABLE 5.1 Hyperthermia-inducing agents

	Serotonin toxicity	Neuroleptic malignant syndrome (NMS)	Sympathomimetic toxicity	Anticholinergic toxicity	Malignant hyperthermia	Oxidative phosphorylation uncouplers
Inciting agents	Serotonin reuptake inhibitors, monoamine oxidase inhibitors, tramadol, fentanyl, meperidine, linezolid, St. John's wort (*Hypercium perforatum*)	Antipsychotics	**Direct:** Norepinephrine, phenylephrine, ergot alkaloids, albuterol, dobutamine, epinephrine, terbutaline **Indirect:** Amphetamine, cocaine, methylphenidate **Direct and Indirect:** Dopamine, ephedrine, phenylpropanolamine **Norepinephrine reuptake inhibition:** Bupropion, cyclic antidepressants, diphenhydramine, tramadol **Monoamine oxidase Inhibitors**	Atropine, H1 ant histamines, oxybutynin, dicyclomine, nightshade (*Atropa belladonna*), Jimson weed (*Datura stromonium*), Angel's trumpet (*Brugmansia and Datura*)	Volatile anesthetics, depolarizing muscle relaxants, severe exertion	Dinitrophenol, salicylates, phenoxy herbicides

Clinical features	Rapid onset (*Compare with NMS*) Clonus, ocular clonus, hypertonia, hyperreflexia, agitation, diaphoresis	Gradual onset, waxes and wanes (*Compare with serotonin toxicity*). "Lead pipe" rigidity, autonomic instability, altered mental status, diaphoresis	Diaphoresis, increased bowel sounds (*Compare with anticholinergic*)	Anhidrosis, absent/decreased bowel sounds, urinary retention (*Compare with sympathomimetic*)	Rigidity, hypermetabolic state	–
Notable laboratory findings	–	Low iron	–	–	Rise in end tidal CO2	Salicylate level
Management	Cooling, benzodiazepines. Cyproheptadine (efficacy unclear)	Cooling, benzodiazepines, dantrolene, bromocriptine	Cooling, benzodiazepines	Cooling, benzodiazepines. Physostigmine (if no QRS widening)	Dantrolene, cooling, benzodiazepines	Cooling, benzodiazepines

waxing and waning of symptoms potentially occurring over several hours. Risk factors for the development of NMS include young age, male gender, dehydration, the use of high-potency antipsychotics, depot preparations, rapid antipsychotic dose increases, the use of multiple antipsychotics, and co-treatment with lithium.[17,18] Parkinsonian-hyperpyrexia syndrome is a clinically indistinguishable condition occurring in patients with Parkinson disease who abruptly discontinue or change dopamine agonist therapy.[14]

Sympathomimetic toxicity results from xenobiotics that increase activity of the adrenergic nervous system. There are several mechanisms by which sympathomimetic agents may result in clinical effects or toxicity. Direct-acting sympathomimetic xenobiotics include α-adrenergic receptor agonists such as norepinephrine, phenylephrine, and ergot alkaloids as well as beta-adrenergic receptor agonists including albuterol, dobutamine, epinephrine, and terbutaline.[19] Indirect-acting sympathomimetics such as amphetamine, cocaine, and methylphenidate result in increased release of norepinephrine at the nerve endings.[19] Certain xenobiotics such as dopamine, ephedrine, and phenylpropanolamine are both direct- and indirect-acting. Xenobiotics that inhibit the reuptake of norepinephrine increase synaptic concentrations of norepinephrine, which also produces sympathomimetic effects.[20] Norepinephrine reuptake inhibitors include bupropion, cyclic antidepressants, diphenhydramine, and tramadol. Monoamine oxidase inhibitors (MAOIs) inhibit the degradation of monoamines, resulting in increased cytoplasmic norepinephrine and increased release of norepinephrine at the synapse.[21] The hyperthermia of sympathomimetic toxicity is caused by central dysregulation in the hypothalamus and increased heat production.[22] Other signs and symptoms of sympathomimetic toxicity include agitation, psychosis, seizures, mydriasis, diaphoresis, hypertension, tachycardia, and rhabdomyolysis.

Anticholinergic toxicity occurs when xenobiotics antagonize muscarinic receptors or reduce cholinergic transmission. In the CNS, muscarinic blockade results in effects such as confusion, agitation, and hallucinations. The peripheral effects of anticholinergic toxicity include mydriasis, anhidrosis, tachycardia, and urinary retention. Hyperthermia results from the impaired ability to lose heat due to anhidrosis as well as from central dysregulation in the hypothalamus.[23] Anticholinergic agents include atropine, H₁ antihistamines, oxybutynin, dicyclomine, and belladonna alkaloids found in plants such as nightshade (*Atropa belladonna*), Jimson weed (*Datura stramonium*), and Angel's trumpet (*Brugmansia* and *Datura*) (Figure 5.1).[24]

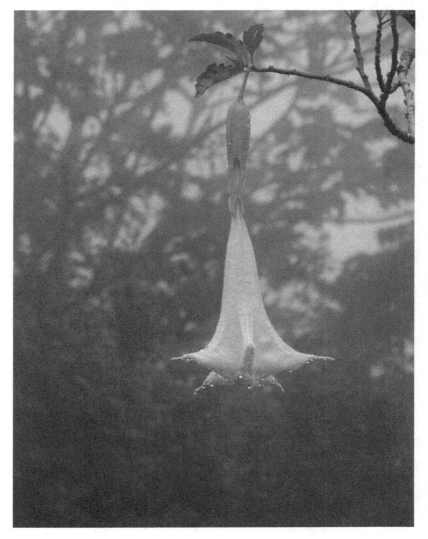

FIGURE 5.1 Angel's trumpet (*Brugmansia*), a plant containing belladonna alkaloids that can cause anticholinergic toxicity.

Photo by Nicholas Titelbaum, MD.

Malignant hyperthermia is a rare disorder caused by congenital distur- bance of calcium regulation in skeletal and cardiac muscle. Uncontrolled calcium release from skeletal muscle sarcoplasmic reticulum occurs when a patient with the disorder is exposed to volatile anesthetics such as hal- othane, depolarizing muscle relaxants such as succinylcholine, or, rarely, severe exertion.[25] Patients develop severe muscle rigidity and hyperthermia due to hypermetabolism in the skeletal muscle. Hyperthermia is not al- ways present and may develop later than other signs and symptoms. The hypermetabolic state also results in increased cardiac output, tachycardia, rhabdomyolysis, hyperkalemia, metabolic lactic acidosis, and disseminated intravascular coagulopathy.[25]

Oxidative phosphorylation uncouplers allow protons to cross the inner mitochondrial membrane into the mitochondrial matrix, dissipating the proton gradient that drives the electron transport chain's production of adenosine triphosphate (ATP) by ATP synthase. However, electrons con- tinue to flow down the electron transport chain to reduce oxygen, producing energy that is unable to be coupled to ATP synthesis and released as heat. Toxicity can manifest as hyperthermia and metabolic acidosis. Xenobiotics that uncouple oxidative phosphorylation are generally lipophilic, weak acids able to carry hydrogen ions across membranes.[26] Examples of uncoupling xenobiotics include dinitrophenol, salicylates, and phenoxy herbicides.

Workup and Diagnosis

There is significant overlap in the presentation of toxic hyperthermia eti- ologies. Therefore, obtaining a thorough medical history, which includes a medication and recreational drug history, is essential for timely and accu- rate diagnosis. Temperature should be measured accurately and monitored frequently, with a rectal temperature serving as the gold standard.

Although not necessarily helpful in making a precise diagnosis, sev- eral lab and testing modalities may be helpful in the workup of patients presenting with toxic hyperthermia. A complete blood count (CBC) can identify leukocytosis or thrombocytopenia. A complete metabolic panel (CMP) can demonstrate electrolyte abnormalities, abnormal kidney func- tion, evidence of hepatic injury, and the presence of an anion gap. A lactic acid level should also be obtained. An elevated creatine kinase (CK) level may indicate rhabdomyolysis. A blood gas can help identify the presence and severity of an acidosis. Checking a partial thromboplastin time (PTT), prothrombin time (PT), and INR may reveal a concurrent coagulopathy. As salicylates can cause hyperthermia in toxicity, a salicylate level should be obtained. If concerned for other potential ingestions, acetaminophen and ethanol levels should be obtained. An ECG should also be obtained to look for interval changes, dysrhythmias, and evidence of ischemia. A chest X-ray can be obtained if the patient is hypoxic or if there is concern for the development of ARDS. A CT brain may be helpful in patients presenting with altered mental status and may assist with the diagnosis of cerebral edema.

No diagnostic test exists to determine if a patient is experiencing serotonin toxicity. Several clinical criteria exist for making the diagnosis of serotonin syndrome, but the Hunter Serotonin Toxicity Criteria has been found to correlate best with the diagnosis of serotonin toxicity.[27,28] Per the Hunter Serotonin Toxicity Criteria, clinical findings that suggest serotonin toxicity in the setting of taking a serotonergic xenobiotic include spontaneous clonus; inducible or ocular clonus with agitation, diaphoresis, or hypertonia and temperature greater than 38°C (100.4°F); or tremor and hyperreflexia.[27]

Similarly, no universal criteria exist to diagnose NMS, although several criteria have been proposed. The *Diagnostic and Statistical Manual of Mental Disorders* (DSM-5) outlines important clinical features to make the diagnosis of NMS based on consensus recommendations.[29] NMS is suggested when the patient develops consistent symptoms within 72 hours of exposure to a dopamine agonist. Suggestive symptoms include rigidity, hyperthermia (>38.0°C measured at least 2 times orally), and diaphoresis. Other possible findings include autonomic symptoms such as tachycardia, hypertonia, sialorrhea, urinary incontinence, pallor, tachypnea, and dyspnea; mental status changes such as delirium, stupor, or coma; motor symptoms such as tremor, akinesia, dystonia, myoclonus, trismus, dysarthria, and dysphagia; and laboratory findings such as leukocytosis, elevated creatinine kinase (CK), elevated myoglobin, elevated catecholamines, elevated creatinine, decreased iron, metabolic acidosis, and hypoxia.[29] The symptoms must not be due to another substance or neurological or other general medical condition.

Sympathomimetic and anticholinergic toxicities are also both diagnosed by history and clinical presentation. While symptoms such as hyperthermia, tachycardia, agitation, and confusion may be seen in both toxicities, sympathomimetic toxicity is associated with diaphoresis and increased bowel sounds. In contrast, patients experiencing anticholinergic toxicity typically have anhidrosis, absent or decreased bowel sounds, and urinary retention.

The earliest sign of malignant hyperthermia is a rise in end tidal CO_2 following administration of a volatile anesthetic or a depolarizing muscle relaxant. The rise in end tidal CO_2 may be followed by muscular rigidity, a hypermetabolic state, and hyperthermia. Although not of acute clinical utility, people with a family history of malignant hyperthermia or a possible previous episode of malignant hyperthermia can undergo confirmatory testing. Muscle biopsy is considered the gold standard for diagnosis but is only performed at a few centers.[30] Genetic testing for the most frequent mutations leading to malignant hyperthermia can also be considered and may be more widely available.[30,31]

The diagnosis of oxidative phosphorylation uncoupler toxicity causing hyperthermia is also based on history and clinical presentation. Hyperthermia caused by salicylate toxicity may be suggested by an elevated salicylate level, however testing is not readily available for other uncouplers of oxidative phosphorylation.

Treatment

The most important interventions in the management of toxic hyperthermia are cessation of the offending xenobiotic and rapid, aggressive cooling. Ice water immersion is the most effective means to rapidly cool a patient. Studies demonstrate that ice water immersion provides more rapid cooling than evaporative cooling methods.[32-34] Bladder irrigation does not provide enough cooling to treat patients with severe hyperthermia. Temperature should be continuously measured using a rectal, or esophageal, probe, and IV access should be obtained. If an ice water immersion tub is not available, a body-bag can be used. Alternatively, two body bags can be used, with the ice water poured in between the bags, which will keep the patient dry while still providing much of the cooling benefit from an ice water immersion. Patients should be removed from ice water immersion once their core temperature reaches 38.3–38.8°C (101–102°F), but their core temperatures should continue to be measured because rebound hyperthermia may occur.

Benzodiazepines are effective for the management of agitation, seizures, and shivering that may occur during cooling. Hypotension should be managed with IV fluids and should improve as patients are cooled. Antipyretics have no role in the management of toxic hyperthermia as the thermoregulatory centers are not the cause of the elevated body temperatures.

Cooling and benzodiazepines are the primary modalities for management of serotonin toxicity. When there is a concern for serotonin toxicity but incomplete response to aggressive cooling and benzodiazepines, cyproheptadine can be considered. Cyproheptadine is a nonselective serotonin antagonist with some reports of being beneficial in humans, although its true efficacy is unclear.[35,36]

Similarly, cooling and benzodiazepines are the first-line measures for the management of NMS. The utility of dantrolene and bromocriptine in NMS is poorly studied. Dantrolene is an inhibitor of ryanodine receptor type 1 calcium-dependent calcium release channels, reducing the calcium released from the sarcoplasmic reticulum and theoretically reducing body temperature and muscle rigidity. Dantrolene used as a sole therapeutic agent may increase mortality associated with NMS. Bromocriptine is a centrally acting dopamine agonist that may be helpful in the management of moderate to severe NMS by reversing antipsychotic-induced D_2 receptor antagonism. However, the administration of bromocriptine or other dopaminergic agents may worsen the patient's underlying psychiatric illness. When medications are used to treat NMS, they should be tapered slowly to minimize the recurrence of NMS. Electroconvulsive therapy (ECT) can be considered for refractory cases of NMS, however evidence for its use is weak. Once symptoms have resolved, and after a period of 2 weeks, an alternative antipsychotic can be cautiously initiated.

The mainstay of managing patients with sympathomimetic and anticholinergic toxicities includes aggressive cooling, benzodiazepines, and supportive care. For patients experiencing anticholinergic toxicity with a normal QRS duration on ECG, physostigmine can be considered. Physostigmine reversibly inhibits acetylcholinesterase, thereby increasing the concentration of acetylcholine and reversing the central and peripheral effects of anticholinergic toxicity. Physostigmine's cholinergic effects may decrease cardiac output or lead to impaired cardiac conduction, so its use should be avoided in patients with QRS widening. When administering physostigmine, the patient should be placed on continuous cardiac monitoring, and atropine should be available at bedside in case excess cholinergic effects result.

Malignant hyperthermia should be managed by rapid cooling, cessation of the offending agent, and immediate administration of dantrolene. By reducing calcium release from the sarcoplasmic reticulum in skeletal muscle, dantrolene can rapidly reverse malignant hyperthermia's signs and symptoms. The use of dantrolene has reduced the mortality of malignant hyperthermia from 64% to less than 5%.[37,38] While most efficacious if administered rapidly after acute malignant hyperthermia, dantrolene can still improve outcomes if given hours to days later. When dantrolene is used, calcium channel blockers must be avoided because coadministration can lead to hyperkalemia and hypotension.[39]

The management of hyperthermia caused by uncouplers of oxidative phosphorylation also includes aggressive cooling, benzodiazepines, and supportive care. For the specific management of salicylate toxicity, please see Chapter 2.

Long-Term Concerns

People who develop an acute episode of malignant hyperthermia should avoid all causative agents. Because malignant hyperthermia is a genetic condition, family members should also be informed and may need evaluation. In people taking antipsychotic medications who develop NMS, an alternative antipsychotic can be cautiously initiated 2 weeks after symptoms resolve.

CASE CONCLUSION

Ice bags are placed on the patient, and cold fluids are infused intravenously. However, the patient's hypoxia worsens and his heart rate slows. He goes into cardiac arrest one hour after presenting to the ED. Return of spontaneous circulation is achieved with CPR and epinephrine, after which the patient is intubated and started on vasopressors. His lab work demonstrates lactic acidosis, coagulopathy, hypoglycemia, and multiorgan injury. A foley catheter is placed and his bladder is irrigated with cold saline, but he remains hyperthermic. He is admitted to the intensive care unit (ICU) and dies 14 hours after presenting to the hospital.

KEY POINTS TO REMEMBER

- The differential diagnosis for toxic hyperthermia is broad, and there are several mechanisms by which xenobiotics can cause hyperthermia.
- Diagnosing specific causes of toxic hyperthermia requires a thorough history and attention to a patient's medications.
- The mainstay of management for toxic hyperthermia includes rapid cooling, benzodiazepines, supportive care, and avoidance of the offending agent.
- Dantrolene is an antidote for malignant hyperthermia that should be administered as soon as malignant hyperthermia is suspected.
- The gold standard for monitoring temperature is with a non-glass rectal probe.

Further Reading

Foong AL, Grindrod KA, Patel T, Kellar J. Demystifying serotonin syndrome (or serotonin toxicity). *Can Fam Physician.* 2018;64(10):720–727.

Hopkins PM, Girard T, Dalay S, et al. Malignant hyperthermia 2020: guidelines from the Association of Anaesthetists. *Anaesthesia.* 2021;76:655–664.

Hymczak H, Gołąb A, Mendrala K, et al. Core temperature measurement-principles of correct measurement, problems, and complications. *Int J Environ Res Public Health.* 2021;18:106060.

Ware MR, Feller DB, Hall KL. Neuroleptic malignant syndrome: diagnosis and management. *Prim Care Companion CNS Disord.* 2018;20:17r02185.

References

1. Hymczak H, Gołąb A, Mendrala K, et al. Core temperature measurement-principles of correct measurement, problems, and complications. *Int J Environ Res Public Health.* 2021;18:106060.
2. Mogensen CB, Wittenhoff L, Fruerhøj G, Hansen S. Forehead or ear temperature measurement cannot replace rectal measurements, except for screening purposes. *BMC Pediatr.* 2018;18:15.

3. Niven DJ, Laupland KB, Steflox HT. Accuracy of peripheral thermometers for estimating temperature. *Ann Intern Med* 2016;165:73–74.

4. Hadad E, Weinbroum AA, Ben-Abraham R. Drug-induced hyperthermia and muscle rigidity: a practical approach. *Eur J Emerg Med.* 2003;10:149–154.

5. Tulapurkar ME, Almutairy EA, Shah NG, et al. Febrile-range hyperthermia modifies endothelial and neutrophilic functions to promote extravasation. *Am J Respir Cell Mol Biol.* 2012;46:807–814.

6. Walter EJ, Carraretto M. The neurological and cognitive consequences of hyperthermia. *Crit Care.* 2016;20:199.

7. Gummin DD, Mowry JB, Beuhler MC, et al. 2019 Annual report of the American Association of Poison Control Centers' National Poison Data System (NPDS): 37th annual report. *Clin Toxicol (Phila).* 2020;58:1360–1541.

8. Tan CL, Knight ZA. Regulation of body temperature by the nervous system. *Neuron.* 2018;98:31–48.

9. Woytowish MR, Maynor LM. Clinical relevance of linezolid-associated serotonin toxicity. *Ann Pharmacother.* 2013;47:388–397.

10. Foong A, Grindrod KA, Patel T, Kellar J. Demystifying serotonin syndrome (or serotonin toxicity). *Can Fam Physician.* 2018;64:720–727.

11. Simon LV, Keenaghan M. Serotonin syndrome. StatPearls. 2021. Accessed January 15, 2022. https://www.ncbi.nlm.nih.gov/books/NBK482377/

12. Isbister GK, Buckley NA, Whyte IM. Serotonin toxicity: a practical approach to diagnosis and treatment. *Med J Austr.* 2007;187:361–365.

13. Gillman PK. Neuroleptic malignant syndrome: mechanisms, interactions, and causality. *Mov Disord.* 2010;25:1780–1790.

14. Gibb WRG, Griffith DNW. Levodopa withdrawal syndrome identical to neuroleptic malignant syndrome. *Postgrad Med.* 1986;62:59–60.

15. Strawn JR, Keck PE, Caroff SN. Neuroleptic malignant syndrome: answers to 6 tough questions. *Curr Psychiatr.* 2008;7:95–101.

16. Ananth J, Parameswaran S, Gunatilake S, Burgoyne K, Sidhom T. Neuroleptic malignant syndrome and atypical antipsychotic drugs. *J Clin Psychiatry.* 2004;65:464–470.

17. Ware MR, Feller DB, Hall KL. Neuroleptic malignant syndrome: diagnosis and management. *Prim Care Companion CNS Disord.* 2018;20:17r02185.

18. Joseph JK, Thomas K. Lithium toxicity: a risk factor for neuroleptic malignant syndrome. *J Assoc Physicians India.* 1991;39:572–573.

19. Farzam K, Kidron A, Lakhkar AD. Adrenergic drugs. StatPearls. 2021. Accessed January 15, 2022. https://www.ncbi.nlm.nih.gov/books/NBK534230/

20. Modell JG, Tandon R, Beresford TP. (1989) Dopaminergic activity of the antimuscarinic antiparkinsonian agents. *J Clin Psychopharmacol.* 1989;9:347–351.

21. Finberg JPM. Update on the pharmacology of selective inhibitors of MAO-A and MAO-B: focus on modulation of CNS monoamine neurotransmitter release. *Pharmacol Ther.* 2014;143:133–152.

22. Jamshidi N, Dawson A. The hot patient: acute drug-induced hyperthermia. *Aust Prescr.* 2019;42:24–28.

23. Walter E, Carraretto M. Drug-induced hyperthermia in critical care. *J Intensive Care Soc.* 2015;16:306–311.

24. Soulaidopoulos S, Sinakos E, Dimopoulou D, Vettas C, Cholongitas E, Garyfallos A. Anticholinergic syndrome induced by toxic plants. *World J Emerg Med.* 2017;8:297–301.

25. Hopkins PM, Girard T, Dalay S, et al. Malignant hyperthermia 2020: guidelines from the association of anaesthetists. *Anaesthesia.* 2021;76:655–664.

26. Terada H. Uncouplers of oxidative phosphorylation. *Environ Health Perspect.* 1990;87:213–218.

27. Dunkley EJC, Isbister GK, Sibbritt D, Dawson AH, Whyte IM. The Hunter Serotonin Toxicity Criteria: simple and accurate diagnostic decision rules for serotonin toxicity. *QJM.* 2003;96:635–642.

28. Ables AZ, Nagubilli R. Prevention, recognition, and management of serotonin syndrome. *Am Fam Physician.* 2010;81:1139–1142.

29. American Psychiatric Association. *Diagnostic and Statistical Manual of Mental Disorders.* 5th ed. (DSM-5). American Psychiatric Association; 2013.

30. Ellinas H, Albrecht MA. Malignant hyperthermia update. *Anesthesiol Clin.* 2020;38:165–181.

31. Girard T, Trevers S, Voronkov E, Siegemund M, Urwyler A. Molecular genetic testing for malignant hyperthermia susceptibility. *Anesthesiology.* 2004;100:1076–1080.

32. Clements JM, Casa DJ, Knight JC, et al. (2002) Ice-water immersion and cold-water immersion provide similar cooling rates in runners with exercise-induced hyperthermia. *J Athl Train.* 2002;37:146–150.

33. Laskowski LK, Landry A, Vassallo SU, Hoffman RS. (2015) Ice water submersion for rapid cooling in severe drug-induced hyperthermia. *Clin Toxicol.* 2015;53:181–184.

34. Smith JE. (2005) Cooling methods used in the treatment of exertional heat illness. *Br J Sports Med.* 2005;39:503–507.

35. Lappin RI, Auchincloss EL. Treatment of the serotonin syndrome with cyproheptadine. *N Engl J Med.* 1994;331:1021–1022.

36. Graudins A, Stearman A, Chan B. Treatment of the serotonin syndrome with cyproheptadine *J Emerg Med.* 1998;16:615–619.

37. Britt BA, Kalow W. Malignant hyperthermia: a statistical review. *Can Anaesth Soc J.* 1970;17:293–315.

38. Rosenberg H, Davis M, James D, Pollock N, Stowell K. (2007) Malignant hyperthermia. *Orphanet J Rare Dis.* 2007;2:21.

39. Yoganathan T, Casthely PA, Lamprou M. Dantrolene-induced hyperkalemia in a patient treated with diltiazem and metoprolol. *J Cardiothoracic Anesth.* 1988;2:363–364.

6 Neuroleptic Malignant Syndrome Versus Serotonin Syndrome

Jasmine Gentry and Katie Lippert

Case Presentation

You are working at your local small-town ER when an 18-year-old woman comes in via EMS with report of a suicide attempt. Family members are trying to figure out what the patient may have ingested. EMS reports that the patient was agitated and combative on initial assessment. Initial vitals are reported as blood pressure 165/80 mm Hg, heart rate 120 beats/min, temperature 102.2°F/39°C, respiratory rate 18 breaths/min, oxygen saturation: 98% on room air. IV access was obtained; no other interventions were performed en route to the ER. Upon arrival to the ER, she is clearly agitated and is difficult to redirect. She has mydriatic pupils to 7 mm bilaterally, and you note that she has inducible clonus in her lower extremities. As you are evaluating the patient, she begins to seize. Blood glucose is 85 mg/dL. You immediately give 4 mg of Ativan IV. At that time, the family calls to report that the mother's bottle of fluoxetine (Prozac) is empty and was just refilled yesterday for a 3-month supply. They also report that they found cocaine in her room but are unaware of her using drugs previously.

What Do You Do Now?

DISCUSSION

Background

Serotonin syndrome and neuroleptic malignant syndrome (NMS) encompass a spectrum of disorders related to the use of psychotropic drugs. At its core, serotonin syndrome results from the augmentation of serotonin in the brain, while NMS is the outcome of severely diminished dopamine neurotransmission. What is often challenging in distinguishing the two is their overlapping features. Both syndromes present with altered mentation such as agitation and/or encephalopathy, autonomic dysfunction, and hyperthermia. Both are life-threatening medical emergencies. Focus then remains on several key differentiating factors, including symptom onset, relationship to drug dosage, reflexes, and offending drugs.

Toxicology and Pathophysiology

Serotonin Syndrome

Drug interaction of the serotonin receptor is complex, with seven known receptor classes, each with many subtypes. However, 5-HT1A and 5-HT2A are the most important with respect to the development of serotonin syndrome. Selective serotonin reuptake inhibitors (SSRIs) are commonly used to treat depression, modulating serotonin along with norepinephrine neurotransmission. By preventing the serotonin transporter from removing serotonin from the synaptic junction, excess of the neurotransmitter remains available for continued drug-receptor interaction.[1] Serotonergic drugs are found in many other drug classes, for example in monoamine oxidase inhibitors (MAOIs), tricyclic antidepressants (TCAs), sympathomimetic stimulants, piperidine derivative medications such as meperidine and fentanyl, triptans, and antibiotics such as linezolid.[1] Their effects are not limited to the inhibition of reuptake channels, but rather encompass the enhancement of serotonin synthesis and release, inhibition of its breakdown, or direct agonistic actions on the serotonin receptor itself.

Serotonin toxicity and its syndromic presentation result from excessive stimulation of the serotonin 5-HT1A and 5-HT2A receptors. This exists on a spectrum of symptom severity, which increases in a dose-related fashion.[1–3]

Although, the dosage at which toxicity will occur is not consistent between different patients, a typical patient is one who has either overdosed on a single or few agents, had a recent dosage change to a medication they have been on, or had a new addition of a serotonergic drug in the setting of existing medications with serotonergic effects.[1] It is this increase in the exposure amount of serotonin within the median raphe nucleus of the brainstem that is the precipitating factor in the development of serotonin syndrome, as well as the progression from mild to severe toxicity. Symptoms that are unique to serotonin syndrome, and not seen in NMS, include mydriasis, hyperreflexia that is more pronounced in the lower extremities, myoclonus, tachycardia, hypertension, and GI upset.[1] Hypertension specifically is twice as common as hypotension.[1] Symptoms may begin abruptly with exposure to threshold-exceeding doses of serotonin.[1,3] Case reports document these effects within hours to days following initiation of new medications or increases in dosages of current regimens.[3] It is important to note that SSRIs differ from other serotonergic medications in their limited interactions on electrolyte signaling channels within the cardiac membrane. Specifically, they have little effect on calcium, sodium, or potassium channels. Exceptions to this include citalopram, escitalopram, fluoxetine, and venlafaxine which have shown to have rare QTc prolonging effects.[2]

Neuroleptic Malignant Syndrome

While many drugs are precipitants of serotonin syndrome, NMS is unique in that the offending drugs are almost exclusively restricted to the antipsychotic class of medications.[1,4] These drugs were developed for the treatment of schizophrenia.[1] The dopamine hypothesis posits that the positive symptoms of schizophrenia, specifically hallucinations, delusions, thought alterations, and movement changes, are due, in part, to excess signaling in the mesolimbic and mesocortical dopamine pathways.[4] The five subtypes of the dopamine receptor (D_1–D_5) are found in various parts of the brain; however, the D_2 is the primary receptor implicated in the manifestation of schizophrenia symptoms and the target of antipsychotic medical treatment.[4] The first-generation antipsychotics, also known as *typical antipsychotics*, were the first drugs used in the treatment of schizophrenia. While they made headway in the treatment of positive symptoms of schizophrenia, they have little to no effect on the negative symptoms, manifesting as anhedonia, mutism, and catatonia.[4] This class of medications is further subdivided into their affinity for the D_2 receptor and designated as either low-potency (thioridazine and chlorpromazine) or high-potency (haloperidol). The second-generation of antipsychotics, the *atypical antipsychotics*, are newer drugs that can treat both the positive and negative symptoms of schizophrenia. These drugs have effects at muscarinic, H_1 histamine, and alpha-adrenergic receptors. NMS has been associated with all generations of antipsychotics in the literature.[4]

NMS is understood to be due to a reduction in dopamine transmission centrally due to antagonistic effects at the D_2 receptor.[1] Leading evidence suggests this antagonism is concentrated in the striatum, hypothalamus, and mesocortex. This results in four primary symptoms: altered mental status, muscular rigidity (also called "lead pipe rigidity"), hyperthermia, and autonomic dysfunction.[1,4] This tetrad typically develops insidiously over the course of 3–4 days. Low dopamine signaling in the striatum and hypothalamus causes a dysregulation in the body's ability to maintain a homeostatic temperature. Coupled with increased muscle tone. this impairment in thermoregulation presents as hyperthermia with core temperature that can reach as high as 106°F/41°C. Muscle rigidity and tremors can exacerbate the hyperthermia as it raises the body's temperature even further, making this a life-threatening emergency. Autonomic dysfunction manifests as hypertension, blood pressure fluctuations, diaphoresis, and urinary incontinence. The characteristic "lead pipe rigidity" is a classic clinical finding in which passive movement of the affected limb is met with a smooth, steady resistance against the direction of force applied. It is not limited to the extremities, but presents diffusely through all the musculature of the body, including skeletal and smooth muscles.[4] Case reports show involvement of the muscles of the oropharynx presenting as dysphagia and even the smooth muscles of the saliva glands with hypersalivation.[4]

What is unique about NMS is that the relationship between dose and precipitation of symptoms is idiosyncratic. Reports of NMS have been made with the initiation of a single medication dose, while other cases reflect symptoms after years of stable therapy.[5] A further differentiating feature distinguishing NMS from serotonin syndrome is the timeline of presenting symptoms. While serotonin syndrome typically presents after exposure, neuroleptic malignant syndrome occurs gradually, and may wax and wane over several days.[1]

One important consideration is that patients on dopaminergic medications, such as patients with Parkinson's syndrome, may present with a syndrome similar to NMS, *parkinsonian-hyperpyrexia syndrome*.[6] These individuals are managed long-term with the dopamine agonists, carbidopa-levodopa, and adjuncts such as bromocriptine and amantadine.[6] Acute withdrawal from their dopaminergic medications results in a clinical presentation that is nearly identical to NMS.[1,6]

The morbidity and mortality of both syndromes is attributed to hyperthermia.[1] As a shared feature, hyperthermia is mediated by autonomic dysregulation in serotonin syndrome and centrally and peripherally in NMS. Sustained core body temperatures above 106°F/41°C are clinically associated with protein denaturation and ensuing rhabdomyolysis.[1,4] The inevitable lactic acid accumulation further exacerbates existing metabolic acidosis, and end-organ effects are seen with declining renal function, steep inclines in transaminases that correlate with ischemic liver injury, and disseminated intravascular coagulopathy, leading to a vicious rapid decompensation and eventual death.[1,4,5]

Workup and Diagnosis

In the workup of both syndromes, the establishment of peripheral IV access, cardiac monitoring, and core temperature measurement is key. Addressing impairments in airway, breathing, and circulation is critical, and there should be a low threshold for intubation in both syndromes. Pure SSRI overdoses surprisingly have limited toxicity and infrequently present with seizures and serotonin syndrome.[1] Care must then be paid to the possibility of a polysubstance overdose with other serotonergic drugs such as cocaine, hallucinogens, and amphetamines as these patients have higher complication rates.[1] Routine laboratory studies should be drawn including a complete blood count; comprehensive metabolic panel; and creatine phosphokinase, serum ethanol, acetaminophen, and salicylate levels, as well as a urine drug screen. In the absence of a clear exposure history, given the hyperthermia and altered mental status, patients may undergo CT of the head without contrast and a lumbar puncture with cerebrospinal fluid analysis to assess for CNS and infectious-related etiologies. In serotonin syndrome, laboratory studies are expected to be unremarkable, with possible metabolic acidosis and rhabdomyolysis in severe cases of hyperthermia and muscle rigidity.[1] It is possible to see hyponatremia due to an SSRI-induced syndrome of inappropriate antidiuretic hormone secretion (SIADH) effect.[7] In NMS, routine labs may reveal rhabdomyolysis with renal impairment, electrolyte disturbances with ensuing cardiac arrhythmias, hepatic failure, and iron deficiency anemia.[1,4] Seizures in these patients is often due to hyperthermia, and patients often are toxic and septic-appearing.[4]

Serotonin syndrome is a clinical diagnosis and there is no confirmatory test to aid in the diagnosis.[1] Therefore, the diagnosis of serotonin syndrome is one of exclusion. The Hunter Serotonin Toxicity Criteria are reported to be 84% sensitive and 97% specific and are based on the presence of neuromuscular and autonomic dysregulation findings. The criteria follow.[8]

In the presence of a known ingestion of a serotonergic drug, serotonin toxicity exists if any of the following are present:

- Spontaneous myoclonus
- Inducible clonus *plus* agitation or diaphoresis
- Ocular clonus *plus* agitation or diaphoresis
- Tremor *plus* hyperreflexia
- Hypertonia *plus* temperature above 100.4°F/38°C plus ocular clonus or inducible clonus

NMS is also a clinical diagnosis, made by the recognition of the culprit drug as a causative agent and the clinical presentation of four key symptoms of hyperthermia, rigidity, mental status changes, and autonomic instability.[4,5] Unfortunately, no clinical rule or guideline has been established to aid in the diagnosis of NMS. The *Delphi method* is an international consensus that presents positive clinical and laboratory findings as well as the exclusion of alternative causes, but it has yet to be fully validated for use in the clinical setting.[9] The DSM-5 classification of NMS is as follows[10]:

A. Major criteria (all required)
  1. Exposure to a dopamine blocking agent
  2. Severe muscle rigidity
  3. Hyperthermia

B. Other criteria (at least of two of the following)

    4. Diaphoresis

    5. Dysphagia

    6. Tremor

    7. Incontinence

    8. Altered level of consciousness

    9. Mutism

   10. Tachycardia

   11. Elevated or labile blood pressure

   12. Leukocytosis

   13. Increased creatine phosphokinase

Treatment

For serotonin toxicity, discontinuation of all agents is paramount. Supportive care, including aggressive cooling measures, is then started. As patients with serotonin syndrome may present with agitation and seizures, benzodiazepines are first line, followed by barbiturates, which may be more sedating.[1] Although rare, QT prolongation may occur within select SSRIs such as citalopram, escitalopram, or fluoxetine, and with selective serotonin norepinephrine reuptake inhibitors (SNRIs) such as venlafaxine, and tricyclic antidepressants.[2] In such cases, prompt determination of the hemodynamic stability of the patient is necessary; this is done by assessing level of consciousness and vitals. Unstable patients with hemodynamic instability and/or who are pulseless require immediate electrical cardioversion, and advanced cardiac life support (ACLS) should be initiated for subsequent cardiac arrest. Stable patients should be treated medically with a 1–2 g bolus of IV magnesium sulfate as first-line therapy. This may be repeated in boluses up to a total of 4 g per hour, then transitioned to a continuous infusion.

Cyproheptadine is a serotonin receptor antagonist that can be used in the treatment of serotonin syndrome. It has been shown to prevent the development of serotonin syndrome in animal models when subjects are pretreated with cyproheptadine, but its benefit in acutely toxic patients is questionable. It may decrease symptomatology but has not been proved to decrease mortality or shorten the duration of toxicity. It is indicated for patients with mild to moderate serotonin syndrome as an adjunctive medication. It can be given at an initial dose of 4–8 mg PO, and then is repeated every 2 hours if no initial response. Cyproheptadine treatment should be terminated after 16 mg if no response is noted. It is only available in an oral formulation, but can be crushed and given through a nasogastric, orogastric, or percutaneous feeding tube.

The literature has mixed data on the use of other anti-serotonergic agents such as methysergide, and dopamine agonists such as bromocriptine have no role.[1,4] When muscle rigidity is present, the use of paralytic agents to abate the muscle contraction and prevent further hyperthermia is indicated and is useful in the treatment and prevention of life-threatening hyperthermia secondary to excessive muscle contraction.[2]

Physicians must be vigilant for rhabdomyolysis and metabolic acidosis in patients with muscle rigidity in the presence of hyperthermia. All patients require admission to the hospital for further observation with expected improvement within 24 hours. ICU admission is indicated in severe cases, including patients who are intubated, require rigorous anti-epileptic therapy and sedation, or in cases of significant polysubstance ingestions. Benzodiazepines are the first-line agents used for seizures, and further escalations to barbiturates and propofol should be second- and third-line respectively. Patients requiring airway protection with endotracheal intubation should undergo rapid-sequence intubation with a non-depolarizing neuromuscular blocking agent for paralysis. This is due in part to succinylcholine's ability to precipitate malignant hyperthermia in genetically predisposed individuals. In such a patient who already is hyperthermic due to serotonin syndrome, this can result in a drastic and uncontrolled increase in skeletal muscle oxidative metabolism, leading to a further increase in body temperature, worse complications, and high mortality. Typically, serotonin syndrome persists for about 24 hours after discontinuation of the offending agent but may persist for several days in rare instances.

Patients presenting with NMS undergo a similar treatment process. Discontinuation of the offending agent followed by early and aggressive resuscitation with fluids and rapid cooling can be life-saving. First-line therapy for agitation and muscle contraction consists of gamma-aminobutyric acid (GABA) agonist medications including benzodiazepines, barbiturates, and propofol for severe cases; this therapy further aids in the cooling process as it prevents further temperature increases.[1,4] Dopamine-directed therapy with bromocriptine, carbidopa/levodopa, and amantadine may be utilized. Most cases resolve within 2 weeks; however, patients may be hospitalized for several weeks depending on the presence of severe sequelae such as renal failure, cardiac involvement, or intensive care utilization. Fluid hydration is critical as insensible losses will be increased from the hyperthermia and diaphoresis. Cases involving injectable depot formulations of antipsychotic medications may result in protracted toxicity because it is not possible to stop the offending medication. Increased mortality has been shown in patients with subsequent renal impairment and concomitant alcohol use.[1]

Long-Term Concerns

As prior episodes of serotonin syndrome and NMS are risk factors for subsequent events, care and consideration must be made in the decision to restart possibly offending agents. Often patients require long-term antidepressant or antipsychotic therapy, making this decision critical and one that necessitates shared decision-making. A suggested approach in the prevention of NMS includes a waiting period of 2 weeks following resolution of symptoms, preference for lower potency antipsychotic agents, avoidance of lithium or dehydration, and careful monitoring for symptoms.[1]

CASE CONCLUSION

Following administration of 4 mg lorazepam the patient had termination of her seizure. A full physical exam was performed and most notable for a young female who is altered and post-ictal, and only responsive to pain. The patient was diaphoretic, with brisk lower extremity reflexes including > 10 beats of clonus in the ankles. ECG showed sinus tachycardia with narrow QRS complexes, normal QTc intervals, and no ischemic changes. Chest X-ray and head CT were normal. Labs were notable for an elevated CPK of 10,000 U/L and a creatinine of 1.3 mg/dl, indicative of acute rhabdomyolysis and acute kidney injury. After two additional seizures and the patient was intubated and placed on fentanyl and midazolam infusions. IV fluids and external cooling measures were initiated, and the patient was admitted to the medical intensive care unit with a diagnosis of serotonin syndrome. On the second day of admission, she was extubated, and was ultimately transferred to a psychiatric facility after a four day stay.

- Increased muscle tone is more pronounced in the lower extremities in serotonin syndrome.
- In neuroleptic malignant syndrome (NMS), the onset of hyperthermia is often delayed, with fevers ranging from 39°C to 42°C.
- The diffuse muscle "lead pipe rigidity" in NMS can be manifested as trouble swallowing (dysphagia) and excess secretion of saliva (sialorrhea), increasing the risk that these patients may not be able to tolerate secretions and protect the airway.
- For both serotonin toxicity and NMS, the mainstays of treatment are discontinuing the offending agent(s), rapid cooling, and control of agitation with gamma-aminobutyric acid (GABA) agonists.

Further Reading

Juurlink DN. Chapter 67: Antipsychotics. In: Nelson L, Hoffman R, Howland MA, Lewin N, Goldfrank L, Smith SW, eds. *Goldfrank's Toxicologic Emergencies*, 11th ed. McGraw-Hill Education; 2019:1032–1044.

Levine M, LoVecchio F. Chapter 180: Antipsychotics. In: Tintinalli J, ed. Tintinalli's *Emergency Medicine*, 8th ed. McGraw Hill; 2016:1231–1232.

LoVecchio F, Mattison E. Atypical and serotonergic antidepressants. In: Tintinalli J, ed. *Tintinalli's Emergency Medicine*, 8th ed. McGraw Hill; 2016:1219–1224.

Stork CM. Chapter 69: Serotonin reuptake inhibitors and atypical antidepressants. In: Nelson L, Hoffman R, Howland MA, Lewin N, Goldfrank L, Smith SW, eds. *Goldfrank's Toxicologic Emergencies*, 11th ed. McGraw-Hill Education; 2019:1054–1064.

References

1. Perry PJ, Wilborn CA. Serotonin syndrome vs neuroleptic malignant syndrome: a contrast of causes, diagnoses, and management. *Ann Clin Psychiatry*. 2012;24(2):155–162.
2. Funk KA, Bostwick JR. A comparison of the risk of QT prolongation among SSRIs. *Ann Pharmacother*. 2013;47(10):1330–1341. doi:10.1177/1060028013501994
3. Liu Y, Yang H, He F, et al. An atypical case of serotonin syndrome with normal dose of selective serotonin inhibitors. *Medicine*. May 2019;98(19):e15554.

4. Marsden CD, Jenner P. The pathophysiology of extrapyramidal side effects of neuroleptic drugs. *Psychol Med*. 1980;10:55–72. [PubMed: 6104342]

5. Nimmagadda SR, Ryan DH, Atkin SL. Neuroleptic malignant syndrome after venlafaxine. *Lancet*. 2000;355(9221):2165. doi:10.1016/s0140-6736(05)72791-4

6. Newman EJ, Grosset DG, Kennedy PGE. The Parkinsonism hyperpyrexia syndrome. *Neurocrit Care*. 2009;10:136–140. [PubMed: 18712508]

7. Arinzon ZH, Lehman YA, Fidelman ZG, Krasnyansky II. Delayed recurrent SIADH associated with SSRIs. *Ann Pharmacother*. 2002;36(7–8):1175–1177. doi:10.1345/aph.1A337

8. Dunkley EJC, Isbister GK, Sibbritt D, Dawson AH, Whyte IM. The Hunter Serotonin Toxicity Criteria: simple and accurate diagnostic decision rules for serotonin toxicity. *QJM*. 2003;96(9):635–642. doi:10.1093/qjmed/hcg109

9. Gurrera RJ, Caroff SN, Cohen A, et al. An international consensus study of neuroleptic malignant syndrome diagnostic criteria using the Delphi method. *J Clin Psychiatr*. 2011;72:1222–1228.

10. Widiger TA. *Diagnostic and Statistical Manual of Mental Disorders (DSM)*. Oxford University Press; 2022.

7 To Chelate or Not to Chelate: When Too Much Iron Is Too Much

T. Christy Hallett

Case Presentation

A 2-year-old boy with no significant past medical history presents to the ED with vomiting and recent ingestion of his mother's iron pills. Last week, the patient's mother was placed on oral ferrous sulfate for iron deficiency anemia. She left her son in a playpen to shower and returned to find him next to her nightstand with an empty prescription container. She estimates that about 20 pills of 325 milligrams were left. The ingestion happened approximately 2.5 hours ago. The patient has had three episodes of nonbilious nonbloody emesis. On examination, he is fussy and tachycardic with a distended diffusely tender abdomen and large melanotic stool in his diaper. Vital signs are temperature 99.7°F/37.6°C, heart rate 155 beats/min, respiratory rate 18 breaths/min, blood pressure 84/58 mm Hg, and SpO_2 98% on room air. He weighs 14 kg.

What Do You Do Now?

DISCUSSION

Background

Iron ingestions are now rare but in the 1990s they were one of the leading causes of calls to poison centers for pediatric poisonings in the United States. Changes in packaging and mass media campaigns increased awareness of the dangers of iron-containing prenatal vitamins in the latter part of the decade, which vastly reduced unintentional pediatric iron ingestions.[1]

Iron is an essential element in life processes. It can undergo the acceptance and donation of an electron from its ferric (Fe^{2+}) and ferrous states (Fe^{3+}), respectively. Elemental iron is protein-bound and found in myoglobin, hemoglobin, and cytochrome enzymes. Iron is absorbed through the GI tract, and free iron ions in the body are quickly bound to transferrin which transports iron to other body regions to carry out vital processes such as hematopoiesis. Iron can be stored as ferritin in the liver and heart. The body cannot excrete iron directly and relies on the GI tract to regulate iron absorption.

Iron supplementation is available as iron salts and nonionic preparations. Ferrous sulfate, ferrous gluconate, and ferrous fumarate salts differ in the amount of elemental iron per milligram of medication (see Table 7.1).

TABLE 7.1 **Common oral iron formulations and their elemental iron content**

Formulation	Elemental iron (%)
Ionic	
Ferrous chloride	28
Ferrous fumarate	33
Ferrous gluconate	12
Ferrous lactate	19
Ferrous sulfate	20
Nonionic	
Carbonyl iron	98
Polysaccharide iron	46

Adapted from Goldfrank's Toxicologic Emergencies, 11th edition.

Nonionic forms such as carbonyl iron and polysaccharide iron are considered safer due to limited GI absorption rates. Parenteral forms of iron are available. Iatrogenic overdoses generally have good outcomes.[2]

Toxicology and Pathophysiology

Iron overdoses cause free radical formation and direct cellular damage to the GI tract. The breakdown in the gastric mucosa allows iron to freely move down the concentration gradient from gut to blood without impedance. Excess iron is transported to accumulate in the brain, liver, and other tissues. High tissue levels may inhibit oxidative phosphorylation, causing a high anion gap metabolic acidosis. Patients are unlikely to develop symptoms with ingestions of less than 20 mg/kg of elemental iron. The lethal dose is ingestion of more than 60 mg/kg of elemental iron.

Iron toxicity occurs in five stages. The stages can arise at different points in the post-ingestion course depending on the severity of the ingestion. The first stage is primarily due to direct damage to the GI epithelium and marked by nausea, vomiting, diarrhea, and diffuse abdominal pain. In extreme cases, epithelial damage can lead to ulceration, hematemesis, bowel infarction and necrosis, GI hemorrhage, and significant volume loss resulting in hemodynamic instability. If no GI symptoms occur in the first 6 hours of iron ingestion, toxicity is unlikely. The second stage typically occurs 6–24 hours after ingestion and is referred to as the "latent" phase. Although GI symptoms resolve during this phase, cellular toxicity is still ongoing. The patient may be lethargic, tachycardic, or have metabolic acidosis. During this phase, the clinician must maintain vigilance as relatively asymptomatic patients may be critically ill. The third phase is considered the "shock" phase. In massive ingestions of more than 60 mg/kg of elemental iron, this phase may appear within the first few hours post-ingestion. For ingestions of approximately 40 mg/kg of elemental iron, this phase may appear 12–24 hours post-ingestion. This phase is caused by hypovolemia, decreased cardiac output, and vasodilation leading to poor tissue perfusion and lactic acidosis. Iron-induced coagulopathy worsens bleeding and furthers hypovolemia. The fourth phase is marked by liver failure and occurs in the first few days due to oxidative damage to the hepatic endothelial cells. Upon biopsy, there will be periportal necrosis. The fifth phase is rare but is characterized by gastric obstruction and strictures and happens 2–8 weeks after ingestion.

Workup and Diagnosis

The type and amount of iron ingested are significant factors to consider first. Assess the formulation ingested and amount, if known, to determine the amount of elemental iron ingested per kilogram of the patient's weight. Any patient suspected to have ingested more than 20 mg/kg of elemental iron, an unknown amount, or with GI symptoms warrants further evaluation. Most common iron supplementation forms found prescribed and over the counter are ferrous sulfate and ferrous fumarate. Over-the-counter supplementations iron can be the singleton supplement or found in multivitamins. The label will show which ferrous salt is used. In the pediatric case described, the patient ingested more than 90 mg/kg of elemental iron and was exhibiting GI symptoms.

Iron-containing pills may be radiopaque on abdominal X-ray; however a negative X-ray does not exclude significant iron ingestion. Iron pill fragments seen on abdominal X-ray can help guide GI decontamination via whole-bowel irrigation. The workup should include serum iron level 4–6 hours post-ingestion when peak serum concentrations occur for suspected iron overdoses. Peak serum concentrations of 300–500 mcg/dL typically have GI toxicity with limited systemic toxicity. Levels of greater than 500 mcg/dL often cause systemic symptoms including shock and lethargy. Metabolic acidosis with increased lactate and leukocytosis of greater than 15,000/mm^3 and hyperglycemia of greater than 150 mg/dL can be seen after overdose; however, these are unreliable and should not be used to rule in or out a significant overdose.

Treatment

Treatment of an iron ingestion includes initial stabilization of the patient. Many patients will be hypovolemic from GI fluid losses, requiring IV fluid resuscitation. Serum iron, complete blood count, arterial or venous blood gas with lactate, and serum electrolytes with liver function tests should be drawn along with an abdominal X-ray. GI decontamination may be considered after stabilization. Iron is not adsorbed by activated charcoal. The preferred method to limit iron absorption is via whole-bowel irrigation with nasogastric or orogastric tube placement and polyethylene glycol administration at large volume rates (500 mL/hr for pediatric patients and 1–2 L/hr for adults). The rate can start low and gradually increase to the targeted rate as tolerated. Surgical or endoscopic removal of concretions or pharmacobezoars has been reported in patients with massive ingestions and those with retained tablets despite whole-bowel irrigation.[3]

Chelation therapy is indicated in iron overdoses with persistent vomiting, shock-like symptoms with metabolic acidosis, lethargy, or serum iron levels of greater than 500 mcg/dL.[4] IV deferoxamine chelates iron not bound to transferrin form ferrioamine, which is renally eliminated. Urine will turn a reddish-brown hue, often described as *vin rose*. Management should not be directed by the presence of this coloration. Treatment is given intravenously starting at 5 mg/kg/hr and gradually increased to a goal of 15 mg/kg/hr. Typically, hypotension is the rate-limiting factor.

Adverse side effects of deferoxamine include pulmonary edema after prolonged infusion, injection site reactions, and infections. Patients on deferoxamine are at risk of *Yersinia enterocolica* sepsis because the deferoxamine-iron complex acts as a siderophore and promotes the growth of the bacteria.[3] Typically, deferoxamine infusions are limited to 24 hours to prevent pulmonary symptoms but are potentially necessary for extreme iron overdoses.

Hemodialysis does not play a role in the enhanced elimination of iron; however, exchange transfusion has been used in massive iron overdoses in the pediatric population.

Long-Term Concerns

Most patients with iron overdoses will not have long-term effects if they present early and are treated appropriately. Patients with massive overdoses who present late and survive may require surgical interventions for gastric outlet obstruction and strictures.

CASE CONCLUSION

The patient was immediately taken to the resuscitation bay and IV access obtained. He was given a normal saline bolus, which improved his tachycardia. His venous blood gas returned with pH 7.10, bicarbonate 10 mEq/L, lactate 4.2 mmol/L, and glucose of 252 mg/mL. Abdominal X-ray showed multiple radiopaque pills and fragments with no evidence of pneumoperitoneum. A nasogastric tube was placed and continuous polyethylene glycol was started at 250 mL/hr. The remaining labs were significant for a leukocytosis of 18,000, metabolic acidosis with bicarbonate of 8 mEq/mL, anion gap of 20, mild transaminitis with AST and ALT of 152 and 110 units/L; his serum iron level at approximately 3 hours post ingestion was 531 mcg/dL. IV deferoxamine infusion was initiated at 70 mg/hr and the patient was admitted to the pediatric ICU (PICU). In the PICU, the patient's blood pressure was monitored closely with an arterial line and deferoxamine infusion was increased to 210 mg/hr. The rate of the polyethylene glycol was also increased to 500 ml/hr. Serial abdominal x-rays showed improving pill burden. The patient was on IV deferoxamine for a total of 24 hours and serum iron levels were down-trending toward a normal range. A diet was restarted on hospital day 2 and the patient was discharged on hospital day 4.

KEY POINTS TO REMEMBER

- A patient who does not develop GI symptoms within the first 6 hours is not likely to have any iron toxicity.
- Iron toxicity occurs in five stages: GI, latent, shock and metabolic acidosis, hepatotoxicity, and gastric outlet obstruction.
- Workup of a patient with suspected iron overdose includes stabilization, calculation of elemental iron ingested, and obtaining peak serum iron levels 4–6 hours post-ingestion along with other supporting labs.
- Deferoxamine is a chelator used in the treatment of iron overdoses. Indications include persistent vomiting, hemodynamic instability, metabolic acidosis, lethargy, or serum iron level of greater than 500 mcg/dL.
- Adverse effects of deferoxamine include acute respiratory distress syndrome (ARDS) and *Yersinia enterocolitica* sepsis.

Further Reading

Halil H, Tuygun N, Polat E, Karacan CD. Minimum ingested iron cut-off triggering serious iron toxicity in children. *Pediatr Int*. 2019;61(5):444–448. doi:10.1111/ped.13834

Yu D, Giffen MA Jr. Suicidal iron overdose: A case report and review of literature. *J Forensic Sci.* 2021;66(4):1564–1569. doi:10.1111/1556-4029.14701

Yuen HW, Becker W. Iron toxicity. StatPearls [Internet]. 2021. Accessed: December 10, 2021. https://www.ncbi.nlm.nih.gov/books/NBK459224/

References

1. Bateman DN, Eagling V, Sandilands EA, et al. Iron overdose epidemiology, clinical features and iron concentration-effect relationships: the UK experience 2008–2017. *Clin Toxicol (Phila).* 2018;56(11):1098–1106. doi:10.1080/15563650.2018.1455978

2. Biary R, Li L, Hoffman RS. Intravenous iron overdose: treat the patient not the number. *Toxicol Commun.* 2019;3(1):37–39. doi:10.1080/24734306.2019.1615731

3. Nelson L, Hoffman R, Howland MA, Lewin N, Goldfrank L, Smith SW. *Goldfrank's Toxicologic Emergencies.* 11th ed. McGraw-Hill Education; 2019.

4. Olson KR, Benowitz NL, Blanc PD, Clark RF, Wu AHB. *Poisoning and Drug Overdose.* 7th ed. McGraw-Hill; 2017.

8 How Low Can You Go? Beta-Blocker and Calcium Channel Blocker Overdoses

Michael Frein and Jessica Zhen

Case Presentation

You are working in the ED when an 18-year-old woman arrives for attempted suicide by ingestion. Per EMS report they were called by the patient's friend after she told them that she had just taken a whole bottle of one of her parents' prescription medications. On scene, two bottles of medications are found: metoprolol succinate 25 mg and diltiazem 120 mg.

On arrival she is found to be alert and oriented but complains of feeling lightheaded. She states that she took almost a full bottle of only one of these medications about 1–2 hours prior with the intent of killing herself; however, she cannot remember which medication she took. Both bottles appear empty. Her initial vital signs are a heart rate 45 beats/min, blood pressure 78/40 mm Hg, respiratory rate 20 breaths/min, SpO_2 98% on room air, temperature of 98.6°F/37°C. On exam she is pale and diaphoretic, lungs are clear to auscultation. Point-of-care (POC) glucose is 190 mg/dL and her ECG demonstrates sinus bradycardia at 42 bpm with a first-degree AV block and a QRS segment less than 100 ms.

What Do You Do Now?

Given the history and initial vital signs:

Which of the medications did she take?
What clues differentiates between beta-blocker (BB) and calcium channel blocker (CCB) ingestion?
What interventions need to be done immediately?
What is the course and potential complications of BB and CCB toxicity?

DISCUSSION

Background

CCBs and BBs are some of the most prescribed antihypertensive medications. They are used to treat a variety of common conditions including hypertension, angina, anxiety, arrhythmias, and Raynaud's phenomenon. However, they are not benign medications. Based on the 2019 Annual Report of the American Association of Poison Control Centers' National Poison Data System (NPDS), CCBs and BBs rank sixth and seventh, respectively, for categories associated with the largest number of fatalities. Additionally, cardiovascular drugs rank fourth in terms of categories of xenobiotics most frequently involved in adult (>20 years) exposures.[1]

Managing CCB and BB overdose can be quite challenging, particularly if there is limited history on presentation or uncertainty of an ingestion. Additional diagnoses to consider in an undifferentiated hypotensive and/or bradycardic patient include but are not limited to:

Medication induced: CCB/BB, digoxin, cholinergic/organophosphate agents, alpha blockade (prazosin), central alpha-2 agonist (clonidine, guanfacine), opioids
Cardiac: Myocardial infarction, sick sinus syndrome
Neurologic/reflex-mediated: Increased intracranial pressure, intraabdominal hemorrhage, vasovagal response
Metabolic: Hyperkalemia, hypothermia, hypothyroidism/myxedema coma
Infectious: Lyme disease, syphilis, Chagas disease

Depending on the timing of ingestion and presentation, GI decontamination should be considered, but caution should be taken with the potential for vomiting and subsequent aspiration which can lead to charcoal pneumonitis. As with any critical patient or those with the potential to deteriorate, addressing the ABCs should be performed first. It is imperative to think about early airway control while the patient is still hemodynamically stable. Similarly, early central access and even arterial line placement may be considered in patients for whom there is a concern for rapid decompensation. If stable, and timing allows, or while preparing the more invasive therapies, additional treatments can be trialed in the short term to optimize hemodynamics. Such considerations include fluid boluses, IV calcium, glucagon, atropine, or methylene blue. Additionally, if extracorporeal membrane oxygenation (ECMO) capabilities are available in your area, early consultation for venous-arterial ECMO to bridge the patient until their body can clear the drug is recommended in severe presentations.

Toxicology and Pathophysiology

Calcium Channel Blockers

CCBs directly inhibit L-type calcium channels found on smooth muscle in the myocardium, vasculature, and GI tract, as well as in pancreatic islet cells. Nondihydropyridine (NDHP) CCBs (diltiazem, verapamil) block calcium channels in both the heart and vasculature but have a greater effect on cardiac function. This leads to early myocardial depression, hypotension, and bradycardia.[2] They are typically used in the treatment of hypertension, stable angina, and cardiac arrhythmias. Dihyrdopyridine (DHP) CCBs (those ending in -dipine) act selectively on calcium channels in smooth musculature of blood vessels to promote vasodilation causing hypotension and reflex tachycardia. They are typically used in the treatment of hypertension and stable angina. However, at high doses, they lose this selectivity and exhibit increased cardiac effects leading to myocardial depression and bradycardia.[2]

CCB cardiac effects	CCB peripheral effects
Negative chronotropy (rate of contraction)	Vasodilation (DHPs > NDHPs)
Negative inotropy (strength of contraction)	
Negative dromotropy (speed of conduction)	Inhibits insulin release
Negative bathmotropy (myocardial excitability)	GI smooth muscle relaxation

Beta-Blockers

Cardiac myocytes contain an abundance of beta-1 and, to a lesser extent, beta-2 adrenergic receptors. Catecholamines normally bind to these receptors and initiate a signal cascade that increases cyclic adenosine monophosphate (cAMP) and activates protein kinase A, which phosphorylates several targets, ultimately increasing the amount of calcium in the sarcoplasmic reticulum to be used for the muscle contraction. BBs prevent this catecholamine-induced cascade thereby indirectly lowering calcium influx into the myocyte and resulting in reduced inotropy and chronotropy, with almost no effect on peripheral vasculature,[2] although after a large overdose, BBs can result in a vasodilatory effect.

B_1 blockade: cardiac effects	B_2 blockade: peripheral effects
Negative chronotropy (rate of contraction)	Vascular smooth muscle contraction
Negative inotropy (strength of contraction)	Decreased glycogenolysis
Negative dromotropy (speed of conduction)	Decreased gluconeogenesis
Negative bathmotropy (myocardial excitability)	Bronchospasm

Through different mechanisms, CCBs and BBs ultimately alter calcium concentrations within the cardiac myocytes to exert their intended effects: slowing heart rate (chronotropy), lowering the force of contraction (inotropy), decreasing conduction through AV node (dromotropy), and decreasing myocardial excitability and action potential threshold (bathmotropy). Therefore, the general clinical presentation for both CCB and BB overdose is similar, with a toxidrome defined by bradycardia, hypotension, and a combined cardiogenic and vasodilatory shock in addition to general symptoms of nausea, vomiting, altered/depressed mental status, and possible seizures (particularly with propranolol due to the addition of sodium channel blockade and the ability to readily cross the blood–brain barrier) and coma. After an ingestion of one of these agents, when which agent ingested is not known, evaluating the peripheral effects may help distinguish the agent. CCBs act on the L-type calcium channels in pancreatic islet cells inhibiting insulin release, which leads to hyperglycemia and reduced utilization of glucose in cardiac myocytes.[2,3] Conversely, BBs act on beta-2 receptors on the liver and downregulate gluconeogenesis and glycogenolysis, which typically results in euglycemia in adults but can precipitate hypoglycemia in children.

CCB toxicity	BB toxicity
Bradycardia	Bradycardia (most common presenting)
Hypotension	Hypotension
Heart blocks and failure	Ventricular dysrhythmias
Decreased mental status	Decreased mental status
Hyperglycemia	Euglycemia/hypoglycemia (children)

The onset of symptoms depends on the formulation, dosage, amount, and specific drugs ingested; however, in most immediate-release formulations symptom onset is typically within 6–8 hours. Extended-release formulations, particularly after amlodipine overdoses, symptoms can develop up to 24 hours from time of ingestion.[3]

Special Considerations

Propranolol and labetalol: Block cardiac sodium channels, which may lead to widening of the QRS segment and monomorphic ventricular tachycardia. The ECG may show evidence of a Brugada pattern. Additionally, propranolol is lipophilic, allowing it more easily enter the brain and cause altered mental status and seizures.[4]

Sotalol: Blocks cardiac potassium channels, which may lead to significant QTc segment prolongation and ventricular dysrhythmias. It has a longer half-life compared to other common BBs and CCBs.[5]

Workup and Diagnosis

In any suspected ingestion, obtaining a detailed history from the patient, EMS, and individuals present is extremely important. There should be a strong focus on medication history including prescriptions, over-the-counter medications, and access to others' medications. Co-ingestions, particularly acetaminophen and salicylates, should always be suspected and evaluated for. The number and dosage of pills ingested, extended-release versus immediate-release, and time of ingestion should be sought. Even if an ingestion is suspected, in a patient with hypotension and bradycardia, other toxicologic and nontoxicologic diagnoses, as previously mentioned, must still be considered. Therefore, the workup should reflect these alternative diagnoses as well as elucidating potential adverse consequences of the ingestion. In general, a broad workup is indicated.

Recommended laboratory analysis should include a POC glucose; complete metabolic panel; magnesium; phosphorus; complete blood count with differential; thyroid stimulating hormone with reflex free T4; acetaminophen, salicylate, and ethanol levels; urinalysis; urine drug screen; digoxin level as appropriate; and urine pregnancy based on relevance. Of note, serum calcium is often normal in CCB overdose; it is the intracellular calcium in the myocardium and smooth muscle that causes the toxicity.

POC ultrasound (POCUS) is an easy bedside tool for rapid evaluation of a patient with hypotension and bradycardia. Performing a rapid US for shock and hypotension (RUSH) exam can help to rule out a number of problems and can aid in the differentiation between cardiac failure and vasodilation. This delineation allows for quicker initiation of interventions, particularly vasopressors, that will benefit the patient most because treatments are based on hemodynamic status.

Serial ECGs

- Bradycardia
- Various heart blocks (AVB more with Verapamil)
- Dysrhythmias
- Wide QRS, tall R waves in aVR, Brugada pattern (propranolol)
- Prolonged QTc (sotalol)

Treatment

As with any critical patient or those with the potential to decompensate, addressing immediate life threats and the ABCs is crucial. Basic first-line interventions can be utilized for both mild to moderate overdoses and, in severe cases, while more invasive treatments are being prepared for. In general, anyone with symptomatic bradycardia can and should be given atropine with the consideration for cardiac pacing if unsuccessful. There is little risk to either of these, however studies have shown difficulty obtaining capture with pacing owing in part to the negative bathmotropy of both the CCB and BBs. Theoretically this makes sense because cardiac dysfunction in CCB/BB overdose is a myocardial rather than conduction problem. If the patient is truly hypotensive, it is likely due to pump failure or vasodilation rather than hypovolemia, however, administering an IV fluid bolus, especially in undifferentiated shock, will cause little harm and can be a temporizing measure. POCUS can help clarify the source of hypotension and help determine the best vasopressors to use (i.e., pressors with more alpha vs. beta agonism). Extensive fluid resuscitation can potentially cause fluid overload and cardiac depression. If the patient presents within 1–2 hours after ingestion, GI decontamination should be considered with activated charcoal and possibly whole-bowel irrigation, especially with extended-release formulations and massive ingestions.[6] Performing both is not recommended, and the local poison center can help determine which may be more beneficial.

Other therapies that are generally recommended based on potential benefit and low likelihood of harm are IV calcium and glucagon administration. Calcium administration can help to improve the hypotension by increasing intracellular calcium levels.[7] It has shown benefits in animal studies but has yielded inconsistent results in human studies.[8] Glucagon improves inotropy by increasing myocardial intracellular cAMP by activating adenyl cyclase directly, thereby bypassing beta-blockade. Although it is thought of as a BB antidote, it may still be effective in CCB overdose, particularly for the NDHPs.[7] If glucagon works, a constant infusion can be initiated. Of note, glucagon is quite expensive and there may be supply limitations in smaller facilities. If the patient has a good response to glucagon, milrinone may be another option because it works similarly by increasing cAMP levels. It is preferred for use in refractory isolated bradycardia (poor cardiac contractility as opposed to vasodilation) because it can cause vasodilation and worsen hypotension.[3]

In severe cases or with active clinical deterioration, more aggressive measures are likely necessary to combat or circumvent the CCB/BB effects. With significant hypotension and shock, vasopressors are necessary to maintain adequate mean arterial pressures and should be initiated as early adjunct treatment. They can be titrated and adjusted based on clinical response to other treatments. In BB overdose, the seemingly preferred agent is epinephrine, versus norepinephrine in CCB toxicity. This is likely due to NDHP CCBs having more of a vasodilation effect that is countered by norepinephrine vasoconstriction. If one is more accessible or more familiar, that may be the deciding factor, and both will stabilize the blood pressure. A common approach to pressors is starting with norepinephrine and, if needed, adding epinephrine second-line and finally dobutamine versus phenylephrine third-line depending on POCUS. Of note, very high infusion doses may be necessary; this will exceed "max dose protocols" to overcome the profound receptor antagonists with the goal of normal physiology. With such extreme doses, the risk for arrhythmias also increases and continuous monitoring is essential. Invasive hemodynamic monitoring is encouraged, including arterial lines, echocardiography, and pulmonary artery catheters to better assess and tailor hemodynamic interventions. Using the lowest effective dose and frequently titrating based on this monitoring and the effects of other treatments is key to vasopressor use in these toxicities.

In a patient with cardiogenic shock, hyperinsulinemia euglycemia (high-dose insulin and glucose) therapy should be considered. Under normal conditions, myocytes preferentially utilize fatty acids for energy; however, under stressed conditions myocytes rely on glucose metabolism as their primary source of energy. Therefore, insulin increases inotropy via metabolic support by promoting glucose utilization by myocytes during shock. Furthermore, in CCB toxicity, there is an insulin deficiency, and insulin infusion will directly counter this issue and improve glucose uptake and utilization by the myocytes. This therapy should be initiated with the support and guidance of clinical pharmacy as doses are exceedingly high, take time to prepare, and can take up to 60 minutes to have an effect. Therefore, it should be initiated as early as possible in severe cases and in conjunction with vasopressors. As this therapy can be continued for days, it is important to understand and monitor for electrolyte derangements—most notably hypokalemia as insulin shifts potassium into cells—but it can also cause hypomagnesemia and hypophosphatemia so frequent labs are necessary.[9] Electrolyte repletion should be done cautiously due to mainly hypokalemia being mainly from intracellular shifts. Additionally, owning to the large doses of insulin, hypoglycemia is of great concern. Frequent—every 15 minutes initially, then every 30 minutes once a stable effective infusion rate of insulin has been achieved—POC blood glucoses should be checked, and an infusion of D25 or D50 should be initiated concurrently with the insulin. Last, all medications should be prepared using the highest concentrations available because these patients are receiving a lot of excess fluids through these high-dose infusions and can become fluid overloaded.

If all therapies fail to improve hemodynamics, a few final treatments can be attempted. IV lipid emulsion therapy has several postulated mechanisms of action that could be beneficial in BB and CCB toxicity. It is thought to act as a lipid sink, surrounding the xenobiotic so it cannot bind to its receptor and thus rendering it ineffective. It also provides a fatty acid energy source that myocytes can utilize. Potentially, it also acts as a shuttle, encapsulating the agent and transporting it to liver and/or kidney for metabolism. Overall, while well-known for local anesthetic systemic toxicity, it has weaker evidence for use in other xenobiotics, although there are multiple case reports that report benefit after BB and CCB overdoses. There are many potential adverse reactions, including pancreatitis, acute lung injury, interference with laboratory analysis, negatively affecting ECMO machines, and negatively affecting the efficacy of vasopressors as well as other therapies and the potential for worsening toxicity by increasing absorption of lipophilic toxins from the GI tract.[10] Therefore, this treatment should be utilized in consultation with a toxicologist or poison control. Methylene blue is not routinely used but can be considered as a last resort in refractory vasodilatory shock. Evidence is limited to a small number of case reports that have shown efficacy.[11,12] It works by inhibiting nitric oxide synthase and guanylate cyclase to decrease cyclic guanosine monophosphate (cGMP) production and is thought to aid in blood pressure support because CCBs increase nitric oxide synthesis. Serotonin syndrome can occur, and patients should be closely monitored. In patients with G6PD deficiency, there is a risk of hemolytic anemia. Finally, veno-arterial ECMO should be considered, if available, in cases of refractory cardiogenic shock with no improvement to the above therapies or in prolonged cardiopulmonary resuscitation and cardiac arrest.

Some Special Considerations Regarding Therapies

- The pharmacy should be alerted early to assist with multiple drips and to concentrate infusions as much as possible to help mitigate volume overload.

- Hemodialysis works well for hydrophilic toxins (which have a low volume of distribution); it will only be effective for nadolol, sotalol, timolol, and atenolol.
- BBs with sodium channel blockade properties (propranolol, acebutolol, carvedilol) can cause QRS widening and lead to ventricular arrhythmias. If seen on ECG or monitor, this should be treated with IV bicarbonate, similar to tricyclic antidepressant-associated cardiotoxicity.
- Sotalol has potassium channel blockade properties which can cause prolonged QTc and torsade de pointes. Ensure that electrolytes, particularly potassium and magnesium, are optimized.
- Whole-bowel irrigation can be performed in severe ingestions and those of long-acting formulations.

Treatment	Dose	Mechanism/Notes
Activated charcoal	1 g/kg (max 50 g) × 1	If presenting within 1–2 hours of ingestion
Atropine	Adults: 0.5–1 mg IV q2–3 min (max 3 g)	For symptomatic bradycardia
Pacing	Transcutaneous vs. transvenous	
IV fluids	20 cc/kg	Crystalloid
Norepinephrine	Adults: 0.05 mcg/kg/min to start. Recommend rapid titration to effect.	Preferred first line vasopressor Titrate to mean arterial pressure (MAP) of 65 mm Hg Very high doses often necessary; up to 150 mcg/min have been reported in the literature

Treatment	Dose	Mechanism/Notes
Epinephrine	Adults: 0.05 mcg// kg/min to start. Recommend rapid titration to effect.	Possibly better effect in BB toxicity Titrate to MAP of 60 mm Hg Very high doses often necessary; up to 100 mcg/min have been reported in the literature
IV calcium	Gluconate: bolus 3 g Chloride: bolus 1 g q5min, drip 10–50 mg/kg/hr	CaCl requires central venous access but is preferred. Aim for 14 mg/dL Ca level but can go as high as 15–20 if tolerated well. Avoid if digoxin toxicity is possible.
IV glucagon	Bolus: 5 mg q10min × 2 Drip: 5 mg/hr	Can cause severe nausea and vomiting so pretreat with antiemetic and be cautious with aspiration. If bolus is effective, initiate the drip.
High-dose insulin	1 U/kg bolus 0.5–1 U/kg/hr (max 10 U/kg/hr)	Titrate to correct hypotension

Treatment	Dose	Mechanism/Notes
Dextrose	1-amp D50 with insulin bolus	Titrate to avoid hypoglycemia
	1 mL/kg/hr D50W concurrently with insulin infusion	Target glucose 125–250 mg/dL
		Glucose checks q15min until stability maintained, then q30min
IV lipid emulsion	1.5 mL/kg bolus of 20% lipid	Infusion rate can be increased if blood pressure drops.
	0.25 mL/kg/min infusion (max dose 12 mL/kg)	Generally continued for 30–60 minutes.
Methylene blue	2 mg/kg bolus over 15 mins	
	1 mg/kg/hr infusion	

Long-Term Concerns

As discussed above, there are many options when treating severe CCB and BB overdoses. It is important to be aware of the adverse effects of each of these interventions and how these therapies might interfere with one another. Very close electrolyte monitoring is extremely important in a few of these therapies, particularly hyperinsulinemia euglycemia therapy, and repeated IV calcium administration. Nursing staff and others assisting in caring for these patients must be aware of these concerns and the importance of strict electrolyte monitoring.

If the patient experiences significant or refractory shock from their overdose it is quite possible to have inadequate perfusion to vital organs. Acute kidney injury or failure and bowel ischemia are potential complications.

In terms of disposition, all symptomatic BB or CCB ingestions and any sotalol or extended-release formulation ingestions should be admitted for observation. Asymptomatic ingestions of immediate-release preparations can be observed in the ED for 4–6 hours.

If the patient recovers from the overdose, no long-term sequelae are expected, unless the patient experienced an anoxic brain injury from cardiac arrest.

CASE CONCLUSION

Based on the lab work obtained revealing hyperglycemia, you have suspicion that the patient took her bottle of diltiazem. Although you consider activated charcoal given the recent ingestion, the patient develops significant nausea shortly after arrival and with her unstable vital signs, you elect not administer charcoal to avoid aspiration. As nursing staff places 2 large bore IVs, an IV fluid bolus is started. The patient receives multiple doses of IV calcium gluconate and atropine with only transient improvements in her hypotension and bradycardia. Given the persistent shock state, a central venous catheter is placed and patient is started on a norepinephrine drip. The patient is quickly titrated up to the maximum dose of norepinephrine. Due to the refractory shock, a second vasopressor, epinephrine, is started. In conjunction with poison control, the decision is made to initiate hyperinsulinemia euglycemia therapy. The patients hemodynamics stabilize and she is admitted to the ICU for close hemodynamic and laboratory monitoring.

KEY POINTS TO REMEMBER

- Although the patient may be hemodynamically stable on arrival, clinical decompensation can be precipitous, especially based on the timing and magnitude of the ingestion. Gaining early central access and predicting the need for airway intervention before it becomes crash is crucial.
- Involve support services as soon as possible: poison control center, clinical pharmacist, ICU, social services/psychiatry.
- Keep a broad differential for patients presenting with bradycardia and hypotension, always inquiring about

pharmacologic causes. Common toxicological differentials for hypotension and bradycardia include CCB and BB overdose, clonidine, opioids, cholinergics, and digoxin.
- Certain CCBs and BBs have unique characteristics or cause certain symptoms/findings:
  - Propranolol is extremely neurotoxic due to it being lipophilic and freely crossing the blood–brain barrier, quickly causing seizures and coma. It also has sodium channel blockade properties, which stabilizes the membrane and causes QRS widening and dysrhythmias.
  - A single pill of many of these agents can kill a child.
  - Hemodialysis is ineffective in any CCB overdose and most BBs, only helpful with nadolol, sotalol, and atenolol.
  - Sotalol prolongs the QT due to potassium channel blockade, leading to fatal dysrhythmias.

Further Reading

https://toxandhound.com/toxhound/sneak-in/—Physiologic Effects of Cardiac Toxicity in Calcium channel and beta blocker toxicity
https://toxandhound.com/toxhound/hdi-vs-pressor/—High Dose Insulin versus Vasopressors in Calcium channel and beta blocker toxicity
https://toxandhound.com/toxhound/cocaine-beta-blockers-dogmalysis-wont-hunt/ —Dogmas of Calcium channel and beta blocker toxicity

References
1. Gummin DD, Mowry JB, Beuhler MC, et al. 2019 Annual report of the American Association of Poison Control Centers' National Poison Data System (NPDS): 37th annual report. Clin Toxicol (Phila). 2020 Dec;58(12):1360–1541.
2. DeWitt CR, Waksman JC. Pharmacology, pathophysiology and management of calcium channel blocker and beta-blocker toxicity. Toxicol Rev. 2004;23(4):223–238. doi:10.2165/00139709-200423040-00003.
3. Graudins A, Lee HM, Druda D. Calcium channel antagonist and beta-blocker overdose: antidotes and adjunct therapies. Br J Clin Pharmacol. 2016 Mar;81(3):453–461. doi:10.1111/bcp.12763
4. Rennyson SL, Littmann L. Brugada-pattern electrocardiogram in propranolol intoxication. Am J Emerg Med. 2010 Feb;28(2):256.e7–256.e8. doi:10.1016/j.ajem.2009.05.020

5. Khalid MM, Galuska MA, Hamilton RJ. Beta-blocker toxicity [Updated 2021 Jul 26]. StatPearls [Internet]. 2021. https://www.ncbi.nlm.nih.gov/books/NBK448097/. Accessed 06/30/2022.

6. Thanacoody R, Caravati EM, Troutman B, et al. Position paper update: whole bowel irrigation for gastrointestinal decontamination of overdose patients. *Clin Toxicol (Phila)*. 2015 Jan;53(1):5–12. doi:10.3109/15563650.2014.989326. Epub 2014 Dec 16.

7. Chakraborty RK, Hamilton RJ. Calcium channel blocker toxicity [Updated 2021 Jul 25].StatPearls [Internet]. 2021. https://www.ncbi.nlm.nih.gov/books/NBK537147/. Accessed 06/30/2022.

8. St-Onge M, Dubé PA, Gosselin S, et al. Treatment for calcium channel blocker poisoning: a systematic review. *Clin Toxicol (Phila)*. 2014;52:(9)926–944.

9. Krenz JR, Kaakeh Y. An overview of hyperinsulinemic-euglycemic therapy in calcium channel blocker and β-blocker overdose. *Pharmacotherapy*. 2018 Nov;38(11):1130–1142. doi:10.1002/phar.2177

10. Cao D, Heard K, Foran M, Koyfman A. Intravenous lipid emulsion in the emergency department: a systematic review of recent literature. *Journal of Emerg Med*. 2015;48(3)387–397.

11. Ahmed S, Barnes S. Hemodynamic improvement using methylene blue after calcium channel blocker overdose. *World J Emerg Med*. 2019;10(1):55–58. doi:10.5847/wjem.j.1920-8642.2019.01.009

12. Saha BK, Bonnier A, Chong W. Rapid reversal of vasoplegia with methylene blue in calcium channel blocker poisoning. *Afr J Emerg Med*. 2020;10(4):284–287. doi:10.1016/j.afjem.2020.06.014

9 Vitamins That Kill: Vitamin A and D Overdoses

Stephanie Hon

Case Presentation

A 19-year-old woman presented to the ED with a history of increasing abdominal pain and thirst over the past 2–3 weeks. She reported intermittent bloating and a 15-kg weight gain over a 6-month period. Her past medical history included severe cystic acne. Historically, she had taken isotretinoin, which successfully treated her acne; however, the patient began self-treatment 8 months ago with vitamin A/D, purchased online, to maintain her clear skin. Each capsule contained retinyl palmitate of 10,000 IU and vitamin D_3 as cholecalciferol 400 IU. Her diet recently also consisted of heavy consumption of carrots, carrot juice, and sweet potatoes. On examination, she had rough, dry skin along with yellow-orange discoloration of both hands and feet. Her abdomen was distended and slightly firm. Laboratory investigations revealed bilirubin 10 ug/dL, alkaline phosphatase 308 U/L, ALT 107, AST 78 U/L. Her creatinine was elevated at 2.0 mg/dL, and she had slight hypercalcemia with serum Ca^{2+} at 12 mg/dL. CT scan showed an enlarged liver with moderate-volume ascites without splenomegaly.

What Do You Do Now?

DISCUSSION

Background

Vitamins are considered essential micronutrients that organisms need for proper metabolism and growth. They cannot be synthesized within organisms in sufficient quantities necessary for metabolism and therefore must be obtained via diet. Vitamins are already present in some foods naturally, but most processed foods are often fortified with essential vitamins. Although most people do not need to take vitamin supplements as long as they eat a healthy, balanced diet, an increasing number of patients self-treat with unregulated supplements and medications purchased over-the-counter (OTC) or online. Vitamin supplement use has increased over time in the United States, about 10% every 10–15 years according to the National Health and Nutrition Examination Survey (NHANES). Many individuals share mistaken beliefs that vitamin preparations provide extra health benefits if they are ingested in qualities greater than the recommended dietary allowances (RDA). The most commonly used OTC vitamin preparations generally do not exceed 100% of the RDA, but excessive vitamin intake is more likely to occur in users who also take single vitamin supplements or in individuals taking supplements who also eat a healthy diet that includes fortified foods and beverages (Table 9.1). Some vitamins, mostly those that are fat soluble, are associated with toxicities and adverse effects when ingested in very large doses chronically.[1]

Vitamins A and D are considered essential fat-soluble vitamins. Vitamin A is involved in the maintenance of normal immune, visual, and reproductive function, while Vitamin D provides more hormone-like function in the prevention and treatment of rickets, osteomalacia, and osteoporosis, and the treatment of hypoparathyroidism. Unlike the water-soluble vitamins, the fat-soluble vitamins tend to accumulate in the body [2]. The RDA for vitamin A in adults 19 years and older is 900 mcg retinol activity equivalents (RAE) for men (3,000 IU) and 700 mcg RAE for women (2,333 IU). Oral vitamin A toxicity can be acute or chronic due to oral ingestion over a longer duration. Severe adverse effects of chronic vitamin A toxicity include liver toxicity, renal toxicity, CNS toxicity, changes to skin texture and color, and teratogenicity. For most patients who discontinue the vitamin, the symptoms gradually reverse and complete recovery is the norm unless damage to the nerves and brain have already occurred.[3]

Vitamin A is present in two forms. Preformed vitamin A as retinol is derived from retinyl esters, its storage form, in animal sources of food. Provitamin A carotenoids are vitamin A precursors and are found in plants. Among the carotenoids, beta-carotene is most efficiently made into retinol. The term "vitamin A" was classically only used to refer to the compound retinol. Currently, it is used to describe all retinoids, compounds chemically related to retinol that exhibit the biological activity of retinol. Retinol can be converted in the body to the retinoids, retinal, and retinoic acid. Synthetic retinoids have been developed via chemical modification of naturally occurring retinoids, often for a specific therapeutic purpose. Vitamin A activity is expressed in RAEs. One RAE corresponds to 1 mcg of retinol or 3.33 IU of vitamin A activity as retinol. One RAE also corresponds to 12 mcg of beta-carotene. Supplements of vitamin A can contain 10,000–50,000 IU per unit dose. Fish-liver oils may contain more than 180,000 IU/g.[4]

Vitamin D plays a vital role in maintaining healthy bones and calcium levels. A lack of vitamin D leads to hypocalcemia and defects in bone mineralization. Although rare, too much vitamin D can result in life-threatening hypercalcemia. Vitamin D toxicity should always be considered as a differential diagnosis in patients with hypercalcemia.[1] A recommended daily intake of vitamin D involves 600–800 IU/d depending on age. Several international guidelines often refer to serum 25(OH)D concentrations of more than 150 ng/mL posing a significant risk of vitamin D toxicity; individuals prescribed high doses of vitamin D should be regularly monitored.[5]

Vitamin D is a dietary supplement used for the prevention and/or treatment of deficiency syndromes. Vitamin D is the name given to both ergocalciferol (vitamin D_2) and cholecalciferol (vitamin D_3). Vitamin D can also be thought of as a hormone precursor that can be manufactured by the body. It is the only vitamin synthesized by the conversion of 7-dehydrocholesterol to cholecalciferol by exposure to sunlight or shortwave ultraviolet light. Supplements of cholecalciferol can contain 400–5,000 IU per unit dose, while ergocalciferol supplements can contain 400–50,000 IU per unit dose.[1,5]

Toxicology and Pathophysiology

Vitamin A

Ingestion is the most common route of exposure. Available forms include capsules, tablets, topical preparations, and intramuscular solutions. Animal livers are rich in vitamin A.[6] Due to their diet of fish and seals, polar bear livers contain the highest levels of vitamin A compared to any other animal. It has been known since the 19th century that the ingestion of polar bear and seal liver may be toxic for humans; the first human case of vitamin A toxicity after eating large amounts of polar bear liver was first reported in 1943. In a paper the same year, Moore Rodahl described several instances from other past researchers, explorers, and expeditions (1596, 1861, 1856, 1897, 1913) in which people ate polar bear liver and became very ill. Rodahl went on an expedition in 1939 to get specimens of polar bear and/or seal liver to identify what the actual "toxic substance" was. They fed the livers to rats, and one died.[7]

Vitamin A is readily absorbed from the intestine as retinyl esters and depends on bile and fat for optimal absorption. Peak serum levels are reached 4 hours after ingestion of a therapeutic dose. The vitamin is distributed to the general circulation via the lymph and thoracic ducts. Ninety percent of vitamin A is stored in the liver, sequestered by Ito cells, from which it is mobilized as the free alcohol, retinol. Ninety-five percent is carried bound to plasma proteins, the retinol-binding protein. Vitamin A undergoes hepatic metabolism as a first-order process and is excreted via the feces and urine. Beta-carotene is converted to retinol in the wall of the small intestine. Retinol can be converted into retinoic acid and excreted into the bile and feces. The elimination half-life of retinol may range from 2 to 9 hours; however, the half-life of vitamin A is about 12 days.[1]

The exact mechanism leading to toxicity is not known. Both acute and chronic toxicity may occur.[6] Chronic retinoid toxicity may stimulate bone resorption and inhibit formation, contributing to osteoporosis and hip fractures. Etretinate specifically has been linked to renal dysfunction characterized by elevated creatinine levels.[8] Cholesterol levels, specifically LDL, serum transaminases, and triglycerides, have been found to be elevated in patients using bexarotene, isotretinoin, and acitretin. These elevations typically occur 2–8 weeks after initiation of therapy with normalization over another 2–4 weeks. Cases describing fibrotic liver damage, hepatic stellate cell activation, and acute hemorrhagic pancreatitis have also been reported.[6,9]

Alcohol abuse, viral hepatitis, some medications and the presence of other liver diseases may accelerate liver damage, which can be fatal. In a large series of 41 patients with chronic vitamin A liver toxicity, cirrhosis was present in 17 patients. Cirrhotic and noncirrhotic portal hypertension with ascites and hydrothorax may be also present.[10] Teratogenic risks are significantly associated with isotretinoin and often involve malformations of the face (cleft lip/palate), heart (transposition of the great vessels), and CNS (microcephaly, hydrocephalus). Neural crest cell toxicity is thought to be the mechanism.[4]

Acute toxicity is uncommon in adults. However, vitamin A ingestions of greater than 1 million IU in adults and greater than 300,000 IU in children have resulted in the development of increased intracranial pressure (symptoms described include headache, dizziness, vomiting, visual changes, and bulging fontanel in infants). The most common adverse effect of topical retinoids is skin irritation, notably erythema and peeling. Acute ingestions of greater than 12,000 IU per kilogram are also considered toxic.[1]

Toxicity is more frequently seen with chronic ingestion of high doses of 25,000–50,000 IU per day. Vitamin A toxicity in children develops following chronic ingestion of 4–10 times the recommended daily allowance for weeks to months. Malnutrition and individual tolerance may also be factors in predisposition to toxicity.[3] Signs and symptoms of toxicity include vomiting, anorexia, agitation, fatigue, double vision, headache, bone pain, alopecia, skin lesions, increased intracranial pressure, hypothyroidism, and papilledema. Hepatic toxicity typically requires months or years of daily high doses of vitamin A. Risk factors for vitamin A toxicity are age, body weight, and renal insufficiency.[6] The hypercalcemia caused by chronic vitamin A ingestion is explained through the up-regulation of osteoclasts by retinol metabolites.[8] There are no known cases of vitamin A toxicity associated with beta-carotene ingestion.[1,6]

Individuals should be advised not to ingest more than the recommended maximum amount of supplemental vitamin A during pregnancy due to teratogenicity being a major concern. Because topical forms of vitamin A (i.e., tretinoin) can cause severe birth defects, miscarriage, or premature births, women are advised to use two effective forms of birth control beginning 1 month before starting the topical vitamin A and will need to continue at least 1 month after the last dose. Frequent pregnancy tests before and during treatment are also highly recommended. Unless the woman had no uterus or is post-hysterectomy, birth control is strongly encouraged even if ever becoming pregnant is doubted or if menopause is thought to have already occurred.[4]

Vitamin D

Vitamin D is readily absorbed from the GI tract. Cholecalciferol is metabolized in the liver to 25-hydroxycholecalciferol and then to 1,25-dihydroxycalciferol (calcitriol) in the kidney. This mobilizes stores of calcium from the bone matrix to the plasma. Cholecalciferol is stored in adipose and muscle tissue. The metabolites of vitamin D compounds are excreted primarily in bile and feces.[1]

Vitamin D is necessary for the absorption of calcium and phosphorous from the GI tract. The daily requirement is small and normally met in part by exposure to sunlight. Due to its cumulative action, dosing should be carefully controlled. Excess vitamin D in the form of 1,25-dihydroxycalciferol results in hypercalcemia and hypercalciuria due to increased calcium absorption, bone demineralization, and hyperphosphatemia.[11,16]

Any one of vitamin D's three forms (vitamin D, 25(OH)D, or 1,25(OH)2D) may lead to vitamin D toxicity. Acute toxicity is rarely reported. The current "no observed adverse effect level," or tolerable upper intake dose, was conservatively set at 2,000 IU per day; however, infants have reportedly tolerated up to 60,000–100,000 IU per kilogram acutely without ill effect. Chronic toxicity in children has been reported to occur in doses of greater than 5,000 IU per day given for several weeks (>75,000 IU per day in adults). Common symptoms of toxicity include nausea, flatulence, and diarrhea. Other nonspecific symptoms reported include altered mental status, muscle weakness, fatigue, and bone pain. Renal failure may also occur due to precipitation of calcium in the kidneys. Hypercalcemia is characteristic of vitamin D toxicity. Vitamin D serum levels may be useful, as well as serum calcium and alkaline phosphatase levels.[5]

Workup and Diagnosis

It is suggested that a thorough drug history be taken for all patients who are being investigated for abnormal liver function and/or electrolyte abnormalities, and vitamin A and D at any dose should be considered a possible cause for deranged liver function and calcium abnormalities, respectively. Patients consuming vitamin A supplements should be aware of the toxic effect of vitamin A overdose, and physicians should recognize this entity in the differential diagnosis of chronic liver diseases.[1] It is important that the risks of seemingly innocuous vitamins are highlighted to both patients and medical professionals.

For suspected vitamin A toxicities, plasma vitamin A concentrations may be helpful in diagnosis but are not clinically useful in treatment and are not available at most institutions. The reference range for vitamin A is 20–60 mcg/dL, and a toxic level is higher than 60–100 mcg/dL.[12] Serum aminotransferase level, bilirubin, INR, and calcium concentrations should be evaluated in patients with chronic overdose. Other common labs for evaluation may also include electrolytes, thyroid panel, and beta-hCG for women who are of childbearing age. Lumbar puncture may be necessary to confirm the diagnosis of benign intracranial hypertension and relieve symptoms. Ultrasound and CT imaging of the liver and liver cell biopsy may be beneficial to assess extent of liver damage.[6] For serum carotene, the normal range is 50–300 mcg/dL. Hypercarotenemia is reported among people who take carotene nutrient supplements and can result in xanthoderma, a yellow to orange-yellow macular discoloration of the skin. Often, this yellowing of the skin can be mistaken for hyperbilirubinemia. True hyperbilirubinemia is differentiated from hypercarotenemia by the presence of scleral icterus in patients with hyperbilirubinemia.[13] The skin discoloration seen in hypercarotenemia can also be removed by wiping the skin with an alcohol swab.

For suspected vitamin D toxicities, monitor vital signs and mental status closely. Consider obtaining an ECG to evaluate for prolonged PR interval, shortened QT interval, and flattened T waves. Serum calcium and phosphate concentrations are mandatory and should be monitored closely along with renal function. Plasma concentrations of 25-hydroxyvitamin (25(OH)D) are generally elevated with vitamin D toxicity and can confirm the diagnosis but are often not considered useful to guide therapy.[5]

Skeletal and hand radiography may be considered to assess calcifications in chronic vitamin A and vitamin D toxicity.[1]

Treatment

Vitamin A

In massive acute overdose, decontamination is advised with activated charcoal or gastric lavage in extremely large overdoses. Plasma vitamin A levels can aid in diagnosis but are not clinically useful in treatment. Upon discovery of a potential overdose, exposure to vitamin A should be immediately discontinued. Young children should be monitored for symptoms of increased intracranial pressure. Elevated intracranial pressure should be treated with mannitol, dexamethasone, furosemide, acetazolamide, and hyperventilation as needed. Acute cases may require admission with close monitoring. The hypotension needs to be managed with fluids, and the hypercalcemia may require calcitonin and corticosteroids. Vital signs and fluid and electrolyte status should be monitored closely. In rare cases, lumbar puncture with drainage of CSF may be required to alleviate symptoms. A statin or fibrate may be considered to treat retinoid-induced hyperlipidemia. Artificial tears and/or lubricating eye drops can be considered for dry eyes. In general, vitamin A toxicity often resolves itself spontaneously within days to weeks following withdrawal of vitamin A. The pigmentation of carotenemia usually disappears with the omission of carrots from the diet.[1,6]

Vitamin D

Exposure to all forms of vitamin D should be stopped. Toxicity from vitamin D is often hard to manage partly due to the long half-life and high lipid solubility in the liver, muscles, and fat. Hypercalcemia due to a vitamin D overdose theoretically can last up to 18 months after the administration of vitamin D is discontinued.[14]

Treatment should be supportive and symptomatic. Hypercalcemia treatment should include a low-calcium diet and prednisone, as necessary. Other therapies may also include loop diuretics, and the administration of isotonic sodium chloride solution to correct dehydration and restore kidney function is recommended. Antiresorptive therapy with use of calcitonin or

TABLE 9.1 **Vitamin content of foods**

Food	Portion	Vitamin A content per portion[a]
Turkey liver	100 gm	~75,000 IU
Sweet potato	Medium	~22,000 IU
Paprika	7 gm	~3,700 IU
Carrot	Medium	~10,200 IU
Spinach	100 gm	~9,400 IU
Lettuce	100 gm	~7,500 IU
Cantaloupe	100 gm	~3,400 IU
Carrot juice	8 oz	~50,000 IU
V8 vegetable juice	8 oz	~2,000 IU

Food	Portion	Vitamin D content per portion[b]
Wild salmon	100 gm	~600–1,000 IU as vitamin D_3
Fish-farmed salmon	100 gm	~100–250 IU as vitamin D_3
Canned sardine	100 gm	~300 IU as vitamin D_3
Canned mackerel	100 gm	~250 IU as vitamin D_3
Canned tuna	100 gm	~230 IU as vitamin D_3
Cod liver oil	5 mL	~400–1,000 IU as vitamin D_3
Egg yolk	1 unit	~20 IU as vitamin D_3
Fresh mushroom	100 gm	~100 IU as vitamin D_2
Sun dried mushroom	100 gm	~1,600 IU as vitamin D_2

[a]Goldberg JS. Monitoring maternal beta carotene and retinol consumption may decrease the incidence of neurodevelopmental disorders in offspring. *Clin Med Insights Reprod Health*. 2011 Dec 19;6:1–8. doi:10.4137/CMRH.S8372. PMID: 24453512; PMCID: PMC3888066.
[b]Maeda SS, Borba VZ, Camargo MB, Silva DM, Borges JL, Bandeira F, Lazaretti-Castro M; Brazilian Society of Endocrinology and Metabology (SBEM). Recommendations of the Brazilian Society of Endocrinology and Metabology (SBEM) for the diagnosis and treatment of hypovitaminosis D. *Arq Bras Endocrinol Metabol*. 2014 Jul;58(5):411–33. doi:10.1590/0004-2730000003388. PMID: 25166032.

bisphosphonates can be useful in severe cases in which hypercalcemia is the result of suspected increased osteoclastic bone resorption.[15,16] Other therapies aimed to either decrease concentrations of vitamin D or minimize metabolites have been proposed including phenobarbital, ketoconazole, hydrochloroquine, and CYP450 inducers such as rifampin.[11]

CASE CONCLUSION

Doppler ultrasound showed normal flow in the three hepatic veins and in the portal vein. Liver biopsy demonstrated enlarged, clear stellate cells in the hepatic sinusoids; the stellate cells also contain fat vacuoles, consistent with hypervitaminosis A. The patient was treated with IV hydration and corticosteroids and advised to discontinue supplement use and modify her diet to reduce vitamin A and D intake. Her symptoms significantly improved, and she was discharged on hospital day 7.

KEY POINTS TO REMEMBER

- Vitamin A is a fat-soluble vitamin found in chicken liver, fish, egg yolk, and vegetables, specifically in carrots. Supplements of vitamin A can contain 10,000–50,000 IU per unit dose. Fish-liver oils may contain more than 180,000 IU/g.
- When ingested acutely in overdose, vitamin A can cause pseudotumor cerebri. However, toxicity with vitamin A is most commonly associated with chronic ingestion of more than 25,000 IU/day by children and 50,000 IU/day in adults.
- Signs and symptoms of vitamin A toxicity include nausea, vomiting, abdominal pain, anorexia, fatigue, diplopia, headache, bone pain, alopecia, skin lesions, cheilosis, and signs of papilledema. Laboratory abnormalities include elevated liver transaminases, bilirubin, and calcium.
- Vitamin D is a fat-soluble vitamin. It is used for the prevention and treatment of rickets, osteomalacia, osteoporosis, and the treatment of hypoparathyroidism. Vitamin D is found in many dietary supplements and also commonly found in fortified foods such as cheese, milk, and bread.

- Vitamin D regulates calcium homeostasis via interactions with the intestines and bones.
- Toxicity is mild after acute overdose. Although rare, more severe toxicity occasionally develops after chronic ingestion of large vitamin D amounts. Symptoms of concern include hypercalcemia, seizures, and cardiac dysrhythmias.
- Treatment of chronic A and D vitamin toxicity involves discontinuing the supplements and supportively treating hypercalcemia and hepatoxicity.

Further Reading

Bendich A, Langseth L. Safety of vitamin A. *Am J Clin Nutr.* 1989 Feb 1;49(2):358–371.
Penniston KL, Tanumihardjo SA. The acute and chronic toxic effects of vitamin A. *Am J Clin Nutr.* 2006 Feb 1;83(2):191–201.
Taylor PN, Davies JS. A review of the growing risk of vitamin D toxicity from inappropriate practice. *Br J Clin Pharmacol.* 2018 Jun;84(6):1121–7.

References

1. Ginsburg BY. Vitamins. In: Nelson LS, Howland MA, Lewin NA, et al., eds. *Goldfrank's Toxicologic Emergencies.* 11th ed. McGraw-Hill Education; 2019:654-668.
2. Granado-Lorencio F, Rubio E, Blanco-Navarro I, Pérez-Sacristán B, Rodríguez-Pena R, García López FJ. Hypercalcemia, hypervitaminosis A and 3-epi-25-OH-D3 levels after consumption of an "over the counter" vitamin D remedy: a case report. *Food Chem Toxicol.* 2012;50(6):2106–2108. doi:10.1016/j.fct.2012.03.001
3. Hathcock JN, Hattan DG, Jenkins MY. Evaluation of vitamin A toxicity. *Am J Clin Nutr* 1990;52:183–202.
4. Goldsmith LA, Bolognia JL, Callen JP, et al., American Academy of Dermatology. American Academy of Dermatology Consensus Conference on the safe and optimal use of isotretinoin: summary and recommendations. *J Am Acad Dermatol.* 2004 Jun;50(6): 900–6.
5. Asif A, Farooq N. Vitamin D Toxicity. [Updated 2023 May 24]. In: StatPearls [Internet]. Treasure Island (FL): StatPearls Publishing; 2023 Jan-. Available from: https://www.ncbi.nlm.nih.gov/books/NBK557876/
6. Olson JM, Ameer MA, Goyal A. Vitamin A Toxicity. [Updated 2023 May 14]. In: StatPearls [Internet]. Treasure Island (FL): StatPearls Publishing; 2023 Jan-. Available from: https://www.ncbi.nlm.nih.gov/books/NBK532916/
7. Rodahl K, Moore T. The vitamin A content and toxicity of bear and seal liver. *Biochem J.* 1943 Jul;37(2):166.

8. Beijer C, Planken EV. Hypercalciëmie door chronisch vitamine-A-gebruik bij een bejaarde patiënte met nierinsufficiëntie [Hypercalcemia due to chronic vitamin A use by an elderly patient with renal insufficiency]. *Ned Tijdschr Geneeskd.* 2001;145(2):90–93.

9. Bioulac-Sage P, Quinton A, Saric J, Grimaud JA, Mourey MS, Balabaud C. Chance discovery of hepatic fibrosis in patient with asymptomatic hypervitaminosis A. *Arch Pathol Lab Med.* 1988 May;*112*(5):505–509.

10. LiverTox: Clinical and Research Information on Drug-Induced Liver Injury [Internet]. Bethesda (MD): National Institute of Diabetes and Digestive and Kidney Diseases; 2012-. Vitamin A. [Updated 2020 Nov 4]. Available from: https://www.ncbi.nlm.nih.gov/books/NBK548165/

11. Marcinowska-Suchowierska E, Kupisz-Urbańska M, Łukaszkiewicz J, Płudowski P, Jones G. (2018). Vitamin D toxicity-a clinical perspective. *Front Endocrinol.* 2018;9:550. https://doi.org/10.3389/fendo.2018.00550

12. National Institute of Health. (2022). *Vitamin A and Carotenoids.* U.S. Department of Health and Human Services. https://ods.od.nih.gov/factsheets/Vitamina-HealthProfessional/

13. Stack KM, Churchwell MA, Skinner RB Jr. Xanthoderma: case report and differential diagnosis. *Cutis.* 1988 Feb;*41*(2):100–102. PMID: 3345684.

14. Conti G, Chirico V, Lacquaniti A, et al. Vitamin D intoxication in two brothers: be careful with dietary supplements. *J Pediatr Endocrinol Metab.* 2014; 27(7–8): 763–767.

15. Feige J, Salmhofer H, Hecker C, et al. Life-threatening Vitamin D intoxication due to intake of ultra-high doses in multiple sclerosis: a note of caution. *Mult Scler.* 2019; 25(9):1326–1328.

16. Bell DA, Crooke MJ, Hay N, et al. Prolonged vitamin D intoxication: presentation, pathogenesis and progress. *Intern Med J.* 2013;*43*(10):1148–1150.

10 Rats Hate This Stuff: Potent Long-Acting Vitamin K Antagonists

Reena Underiner and Jonathan de Olano

Case Presentation

A 37-year-old man with past medical history of depression comes to the ED after ingesting ethanol and an unknown substance. He states that he ate something from a carton in his garage. On arrival, he appears intoxicated but is otherwise asymptomatic and has no complaints. He has normal vital signs and an unremarkable exam. Screening bloodwork includes a complete blood count (CBC), complete metabolic panel (CMP), prothrombin time (PT)/INR and partial thromboplastin time (PTT), all of which are unremarkable. His ECG is unremarkable, and acetaminophen and salicylate levels are negative. His ethanol level is 152 mg/dL. The patient is observed for 8 hours in the ED. His repeat labs are unremarkable, he has normal hemodynamics and is clinically sober. The patient is cleared by psychiatry and discharged home.

A week later, he returns to the ED, now complaining of hematuria, gingival bleeding, and bruising throughout his extremities. He denies starting new medications or ingesting any substances since he was last seen in the ED. On physical examination, his vital signs are blood pressure 110/90 mm Hg, heart rate 138 beats/min, respiratory rate 22 breaths/min, temperature 98.4°F/36.9°C; O_2 saturation 98% on room air. He appears anxious, pale, and in mild distress. His pupils are equal, round, and reactive, and his extraocular movements are intact. There is mild gingival bleeding. Skin is dry and pale appearing, with a slight delay in cap refill. Heart sounds are tachycardic with a regular rhythm, and lungs are clear to auscultation. Abdomen examination reveals multiple areas of ecchymosis over the abdomen and flank, but otherwise is soft, nontender, non-distended, and has normal bowel sounds throughout. His skin demonstrates multiple areas of ecchymosis in different stages of healing over his abdomen, flank, and extremities, and these are mildly tender to palpation. A digital rectal exam demonstrates dark-colored stools.

On further history, the patient admits to an intentional ingestion of an unknown quantity of rat poison, brodifacoum, that he had in his garage a week earlier.

What Do You Do Now?

DISCUSSION

Background

The coagulation cascade is a model that illustrates how the body prevents blood loss and inappropriate clotting. After tissue injury, the coagulation cascade is initiated to obtain hemostasis. This involves the activation of a series of clotting factors which ultimately leads to the formation of a stable fibrin clot. Within this traditional model, intrinsic and extrinsic pathways begin the coagulation cascade, which involves the activation of different factors. The intrinsic pathway is activated by trauma inside the vascular system exposing endothelial collagen, leading to activation of factor XII. Furthermore, the intrinsic pathway involves clotting factors VIII, IX, and XI. The extrinsic pathway, on the other hand, is activated through the release of tissue factors after being externally damaged. It involves clotting factors III and VII. Both the intrinsic and extrinsic pathways result in the formation of factor X, which then initiates the common pathway, activating factors II and XIII and leading to clot formation. A decrease in any coagulation factors within each pathway, either inherited or acquired, can lead to impaired coagulation. Multiple classes of xenobiotics are used specifically for the purpose of anticoagulation. Vitamin K antagonists (VKA), such as warfarin, impair the activation of factors II, VII, IX, and X, leading to anticoagulation effects.

Superwarfarins are a class of VKA xenobiotics that have an increased potency and prolonged effects relative to warfarin. As the name suggests, superwarfarins are derived from warfarin, but are significantly more potent, with most estimated to be approximately 100 times the potency of warfarin.[1] They were initially developed as a rodenticide after it was discovered that rodents had developed a resistance to warfarin.[2] The most common superwarfarins include bromadiolone and brodifacoum, which can be found in varying concentrations within commonly found rodenticides (Figure 10.1). Other common long-acting VKAs used as rodenticides include chlorophacinone, diphacinone, difenacoum, difethialone, and flocoumafen. These rodenticides can exist in either solid bait or liquid forms, with the liquid forms having higher concentrations of superwarfarins.[3] Ingestions of superwarfarins are relatively uncommon, with 10,413 exposures reported to the National Poison Data System

Warfarin:

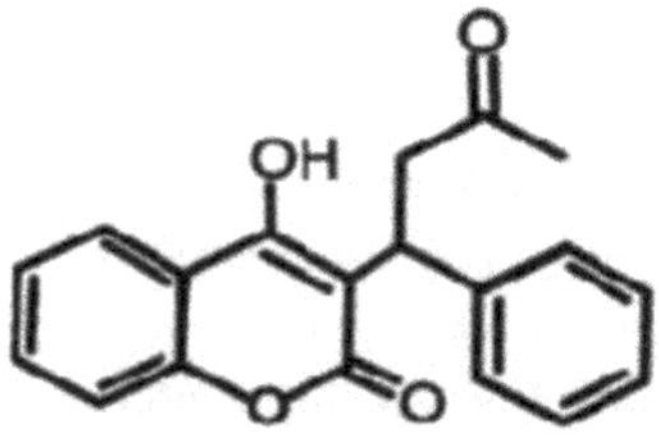

Brodifacoum:

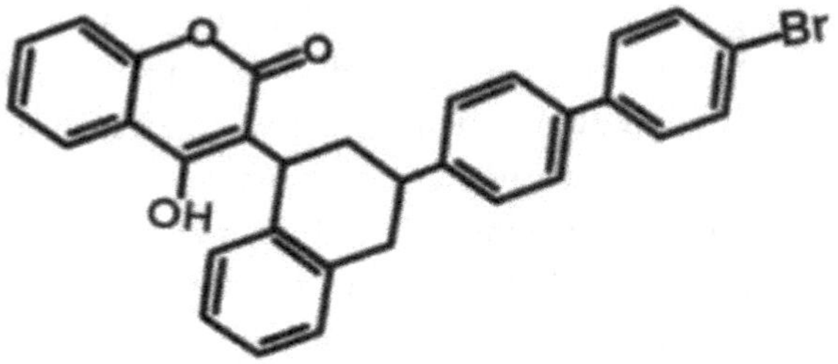

Bromadiolone:

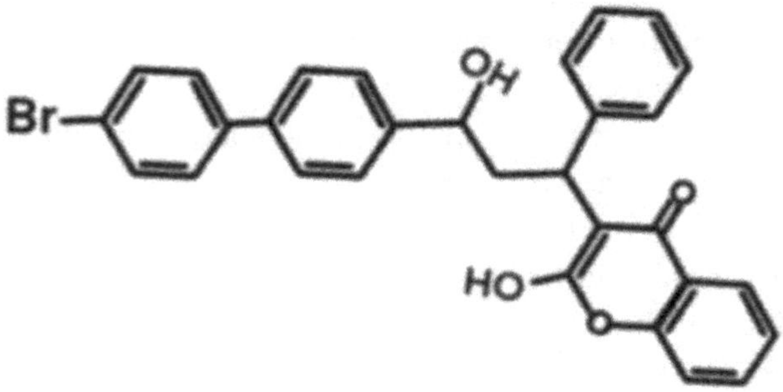

FIGURE 10.1 Chemical structures of warfarin, bromadiolone, and brodifacoum.

Illustration by Rahel Gizaw.

over a 25-year period and roughly 2,750 patients treated annually.[4] Most exposures occur by exploratory and unintentional ingestions in children under age 6.[4] In adults, however, ingestions are typically intentional and often occur in the setting of a suicide or homicide attempt. There have also been reported cases of ingestion in the setting of Munchausen syndrome.[5]

Occupational exposures have been reported but are less common.[6] In recent events, an outbreak of brodifacoum-laced synthetic cannabinoids in the Midwest in 2018 affected more than 300 people and resulted in at least 7 deaths.[7-9] It remains unclear how, or for what reason, these long-acting VKAs were introduced into the drug supply.

Toxicology and Pathophysiology

Warfarins and superwarfarins function as vitamin K antagonists. Specifically, they inhibit two enzymes, vitamin K epoxide reductase and vitamin K quinone reductase, which function to cycle the inactive epoxide form of vitamin K to the active hydroquinone form (Figure 10.2. By inhibiting these enzymes, warfarins prevent the activation and recycling of vitamin K, resulting in a vitamin K deficiency. This in turn results in an inability to activate vitamin K-dependent clotting factors, which include factors II, VII, IX, and X as well as anticoagulant proteins C, S, and Z.

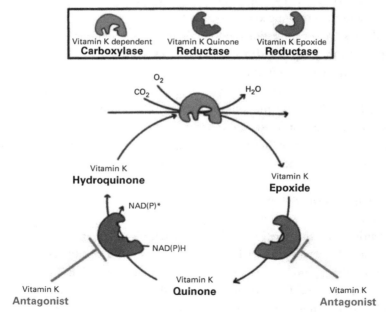

FIGURE 10.2 Vitamin K cycle.

Illustration by Rahel Gizaw.

Unlike factor Xa inhibitors or direct thrombin inhibitors, which immediately have anticoagulation effects by inhibiting a coagulation factor, VKAs block the regeneration of new factor formation. As a result, they don't have an immediate effect on coagulation because it is instead dependent on factor levels, which have half-lives ranging from 4 to 72 hours.[10] As such, initial coagulation labs obtained on the day of ingestion are usually normal, with abnormalities developing after several days when circulating functional clotting factors have been depleted. The result is a delayed effect on the INR after exposure to a VKA of approximately 15 hours, or three factor VII half-lives.[11] Similarly, clinical bleeding is also delayed, most commonly presenting 3–9 days after exposure.[4]

In addition to delayed presentations, superwarfarins can have prolonged effects over a period of weeks to months. They are bound in the liver and are suspected to undergo enterohepatic recirculation.[12] Due to their highly lipophilic nature and bulky aromatic side chains, they have a very long half-life (20–130 days for brodifacoum)[13] significantly longer than that of warfarin. Additionally, superwarfarins may undergo zero-order kinetics, leading to their prolonged elimination.[13]

Because most ingestions in children are unintentional exploratory exposures, they typically involve lower doses. As a result, children may be asymptomatic even multiple days after exposure. In adults, ingestions are commonly intentional and involve larger, more toxic doses. Because of these larger doses and the long half-life of superwarfarins, the anticoagulant effects may last for several months. Not only does this put patients at increased risk of bleeding for a prolonged period, but it also necessitates prolonged treatment over the course of months.

Workup and Diagnosis

History of the ingestion, including the substance, approximate amount, intention, and time are essential in the diagnosis of a long-acting VKA ingestion. The exact product ingested as well as the quantity can help risk stratify the approximate concentrations of superwarfarin in commercial rodenticides. The formulation should be noted, as liquid forms of rodenticides often have higher concentrations of superwarfarins as compared to the bait formulations.[14]

Due to the delayed presentation of symptoms, the date of ingestion is of particular importance. Some patients may be completely asymptomatic; this can often be the case in children with exploratory unintentional exposures. In those who are symptomatic, presentations vary widely and can include hematuria, gastrointestinal hemorrhage, hemoptysis, hemarthroses, and bruising. In one review, hematuria was found to be the most common feature.[4] Less commonly, there have been reports of patients presenting with both thrombosis and bleeding, thought to be the result of hypercoagulability from protein C and S deficiency in combination with coagulopathy from a deficiency in vitamin K-dependent factors.[15,16] In children presenting with signs of coagulopathy, consideration of nonaccidental trauma is critical and cannot be overlooked. Forensics and law enforcement may need to be involved if there is a concern for nefarious intent.

On the day of ingestion, the physical exam will likely be normal. For delayed presentations, those with small or unintentional ingestions may maintain a normal physical exam. In those who are symptomatic, signs of coagulopathy predominate. The exam may reveal purpura or ecchymosis, epistaxis, gingival bleeding, hematomas, joint effusions, and melena. Patients also may have flank or abdominal tenderness if retroperitoneal hemorrhage has occurred. Similarly, altered mental status and neurologic deficits are possible if intracranial hemorrhage has developed.

Lab tests including coagulation studies will be normal soon after ingestion. It is critical to remember that measurable coagulopathy may not develop until hours to days after ingestion when factor levels have been depleted; thus, normal coagulation labs acutely after ingestion do not rule out superwarfarin toxicity, and labs must be repeated in 2–3 days. Days after ingestion, elevations in PT/INR and PTT will develop. Superwarfarin toxicity should be considered in any patient with unexplained coagulopathy. A plasma mixing study will correct the elevation in coagulation levels. Individual coagulation factors can be measured, and vitamin K-dependent factors (Factors II, VII, IX, and X) will be reduced. Vitamin K epoxide levels should be elevated and can help differentiate a vitamin K antagonist from acquired vitamin K deficiency. Serum quantitative analysis of superwarfarin levels will confirm the diagnosis but may not be available at all institutions and often will have long turnaround times. Qualitative serum and urine superwarfarin tests are also available. Serial serum levels of superwarfarins may help determine the length of therapy.[17]

Imaging studies should be obtained on a case-by-case basis. Due to the high risk of bleeding in these patients, CT imaging to evaluate for retroperitoneal hemorrhage should be considered in those with abdominal or flank plan. A head CT may be warranted to evaluate for intracranial hemorrhage in those with headaches, seizures, decreased level of consciousness, or neurologic abnormalities. A chest X-ray should be considered in those presenting with dyspnea, as hemothorax is possible.

Treatment

Like other poisonings, the initial management in long-acting VKA ingestions after stabilization is decontamination. The goal is for activated charcoal to adsorb to the xenobiotic prior to the body absorbing it. A consensus guideline of medical toxicologists recommends patients be transported to an ED without delay to receive activated charcoal. [17] An exception is in patients with unintentional ingestions of less than 1 mg of a long-acting VKA and generally children under the age of 6 years old with unintentional exposures.[17] Yet there is still some risk in pediatric patients. A retrospective review of 10,762 brodifacoum exposures in children found 67 had evidence of coagulopathy. [18] While animal studies suggest enterohepatic recirculation of many superwarfarins, there is no evidence for efficacy of multidose activated charcoal in humans. The practice guideline also recommends against the use of ipecac syrup and gastric lavage.[17] Ipecac syrup should be avoided because it has been associated with subarachnoid hemorrhage and death in a patient with brodifacoum toxicity.[19] If there is evidence of GI bleeding, activated charcoal would be contraindicated and unlikely to be effective as VKA would have already been absorbed. Additionally, charcoal would limit direct visualization of the source of bleeding by endoscopy or colonoscopy. The role of whole-bowel irrigation is unclear in the setting of an acute superwarfarin ingestion.

In those for whom it is unclear whether a superwarfarin ingestion took place, serial PT/INR measurements can be helpful and help to guide treatment. The mainstay of treatment is high-dose vitamin K supplementation.

The dosing regimen and frequency remain unclear and are largely based on case reports. Dosing typically ranges from 50 to 200 mg, with frequencies typically BID or TID. Oral supplementation has been shown to be as effective as IV regarding 24-hour reversal.[20] IV vitamin K should be reserved for actively symptomatic patients. IV administration of vitamin K has been associated with severe anaphylactoid reactions at a rate of approximately 3 per 10,000 doses, thus the benefits must be weighed carefully against the risks.[21]

For those with critical bleeding, four-factor prothrombin complex concentrate (4F-PCC) is recommended in addition to vitamin K, as per the 2020 ACC Expert Consensus Decision Pathway for management of bleeding in patients on oral anticoagulants, which can be extrapolated to apply to this patient population.[222] If no PCC is available, fresh-frozen plasma (FFP) may be given, though higher doses may be required due to lower concentrations of clotting factors. PCC is advantageous in that it can be stored at room temperature and does not require thawing prior to administration, as compared to FFP. Multiple doses of both 4F-PCC or FFP may be required given the prolonged half-life of superwarfarins.

The duration of outpatient vitamin K supplementation will be dose- and xenobiotic-specific. A 2015 review found that treatment regimens ranged from 28 to 730 days, with an average of 168 days.[4] Return of normal INR often occurs prior to adequate clearance of the superwarfarin itself, making it difficult to assess adequate treatment. Patients are often followed outpatient with serial measurements of INR with concomitant tapering of the oral vitamin K schedule. A study by Nosal et al. has suggested that serial measurements of superwarfarin levels may help guide decisions on when to taper off the vitamin K supplementation.[14]

Due to the long half-life of superwarfarins, patients will need a prolonged course of oral vitamin K on an outpatient basis. This poses multiple challenges. First, the oral vitamin K supplements are quite expensive, with one 5 mg tablet estimated to cost up to $122. Patients are typically taking multiple pills per day for months at a time, creating a significant burden, both financial and in terms of the sheer number of pills needed. In one study in Illinois, patients were quoted costs of $24,000–34,000 per month, which can be unmanageable for many patients.[9] Additionally, the half-life of oral vitamin K is 6 hours, and adherence to a treatment schedule with multiple doses per day can be difficult. Adherence to this treatment regimen can be particularly difficult in those with psychiatric illness and those who ingested the substance in a suicide attempt.

Long-Term Concerns

For patients who had intentional ingestions of a long-acting VKA, special attention should be placed on their psychiatric stability upon discharge from the hospital. The act of not treating their coagulopathy with daily vitamin K is in effect suicidal behavior. Therefore, the patient needs careful psychiatric consideration for adherence to long-term medical management.

CASE CONCLUSION

The patient's workup on return to the ED demonstrated several abnormalities. The ECG was sinus tachycardia at 136 bpm, with normal intervals. Laboratory studies revealed hemoglobin 6.5 g/dL, white blood cell count 15,200/mcL, platelet count 435,000/μL, sodium 138 mEq/L, potassium 4.1 mEq/L, chloride 102 mEq/L, bicarbonate 20 mEq/L, blood urea nitrogen 42 mg/dL, creatinine 1.3 mg/dL, glucose 135 mg/dL, alkaline phosphate 70 IU/L, aspartate transaminase 24 IU/L, alkaline transaminase 20 IU/L, and total bilirubin 2.4 mg/dL; acetaminophen, ethanol, and salicylate levels are undetectable. Urine analysis was positive for red blood cells and gross hematuria. His INR was greater than 10, PT 132 sec, and PTT was 65 sec. A CT scan of the chest, abdomen, and pelvis was remarkable for extensive subcutaneous hematomas to the left flank and abdomen. A CT scan of the head was unremarkable.

The patient received 2 units pRBCs as well as 4F-PCC and a slow infusion of 10 mg IV vitamin K. He was then transitioned to 50 mg BID oral vitamin K. He remained inpatient until normalization of his INR and cessation of both his gross hematuria and melena. The psychiatry team was closely involved in his care while inpatient and arranged frequent outpatient follow-up with the patient to encourage compliance with his prolonged course of treatment. He was then discharged on continued oral vitamin K therapy, which was tapered over the course of 5 months.

- Patient should be referred immediately to the ED after an acute exposure of superwarfarin for activated charcoal treatment.
- Lab abnormalities indicative of coagulopathy may not develop until days after ingestion.
- Vitamin K treatment is the mainstay of treatment and will be needed for an extended period of time due to the long half-life.
- In acute critical bleeding, four-factor PCC is recommended in addition to Vitamin K.
- Careful psychiatric assessment for medication compliance should be addressed prior to discharge.

Further Reading

Caravati EM, Erdman AR, Scharman EJ, et al. Long-acting anticoagulant rodenticide poisoning: an evidence-based consensus guideline for out-of-hospital management. *Clin Toxicol (Phila)*. 2007;45(1):1–22. doi:10.1080/15563650600795487

Kelkar AH, Smith NA, Martial A, et al. An outbreak of synthetic cannabinoid-associated coagulopathy in Illinois. *New Engl J Med*. 2018;379:1216–1223.

King N and Tran MH. Long-acting anticoagulant rodenticide (superwarfarin) poisoning: a review of its historical development, epidemiology, and clinical management. *Transfus Med Review*. 2015 Oct;29(4):250–258.

References

1. Gebauer M. Synthesis and structure-activity relationships of novel warfarin derivatives. *Bioorg Med Chem*. 2007;15:2414–2420.
2. Hadler MR, Shadbolt RS. Novel 4-hydroxycoumarin anticoagulants active against resistant rats. *Nature*. 1975 Jan 24;253(5489):275–277. doi:10.1038/253275a0. PMID: 1113846
3. Australian Pesticides and Veterinary Medicines Authority. Public Chemical Registration Information System Search. https://portal.apvma.gov.au/pubcris.
4. King N, Tran MH. Long-acting anticoagulant rodenticide (superwarfarin) poisoning: a review of its historical development, epidemiology, and clinical management. *Transfus Med Review*. 2015 Oct; 29(4):250–258.
5. Chua JD, Friedenberg WR. Superwarfarin poisoning. *Arch Intern Med*. 1998 Sep 28;158(17):1929–1932. doi:10.1001/archinte.158.17.1929. PMID: 9759690.
6. Ozdemir et al. A case of superwarfarin poisoning due to repetitive occupational dermal rodenticide exposure in a worker. *Turk J Haematol*. 2016 Sep;33(3):251–253.

7. Kumar S, Bhagia G. Brodifacoum-laced synthetic marijuana toxicity: a fight against time. *Am J Case Rep*. 2020;21:e927111. Published 2020 Nov 2. doi:10.12659/AJCR.927111

8. Arepally GM, Ortel TL. Bad weed: synthetic cannabinoid-associated coagulopathy. *Blood*. 2019 Feb 28;133(9):902–905. doi:10.1182/blood-2018-11-876839. Epub 2019 Jan 17. PMID: 30655273.

9. Kelkar AH, Smith NA, Martial A, Moole H, Tarantino MD, Roberts JC. An outbreak of synthetic cannabinoid-associated coagulopathy in Illinois. *N Engl J Med*. 2018 Sep 27;379(13):1216–1223. doi:10.1056/NEJMoa1807652. PMID: 30280655.

10. Warfarin package insert: https://www.accessdata.fda.gov/drugsatfda_docs/label/2010/009218s108lbl.pdf. Accesses 2022-3-28.

11. Fihn SD, et al. The risk for and severity of bleeding complications in elderly patients treated with warfarin. *Ann Intern Med*. 1996;124:970–979. [PubMed: 8624064]

12. Lindeblad M, Lyubimov A, van Breemen R, Gierszal K, Weinberg G, Rubinstein I, Feinstein DL. The Bile Sequestrant Cholestyramine Increases Survival in a Rabbit Model of Brodifacoum Poisoning. *Toxicol Sci*. 2018 Oct 1;165(2):389–395. doi:10.1093/toxsci/kfy147. PMID: 29897553; PMCID: PMC6154278.

13. Brodifacoum (HSG 93, 1995). Inchem.org.

14. Nosal DG, van Breemen RB, Haffner JW, Rubinstein I, Feinstein DL. Brodifacoum pharmacokinetics in acute human poisoning: implications for estimating duration of vitamin K therapy. *Toxicol Commun*. 2021;5(1):69–72. doi:10.1080/24734306.2021.1887637

15. Papin F, Clarot F, Vicomte C, et al. Lethal paradoxical cerebral vein thrombosis due to suspicious anticoagulant rodenticide intoxication with chlorophacinone. *Forensic Sci Int*. 2007;166:85–90.

16. De Paula EV, Montalvao SA, Madureira PR, Jose Vieira R, Annichino-Bizzacchi JM, Ozelo MC. Simultaneous bleeding and thrombosis in superwarfarin poisoning. *Thromb Res*. 2009;123:637–639.

17. Caravati EM, Erdman AR, Scharman EJ, et al. Long-acting anticoagulant rodenticide poisoning: an evidence-based consensus guideline for out-of-hospital management. *Clin Toxicol (Phila)*. 2007;45(1):1–22. doi:10.1080/15563650600795487

18. Shepherd G, Klein-Schwartz W, Anderson BD. Acute, unintentional pediatric brodifacoum ingestions. *Pediatr Emerg Care*. 2002 Jun;18(3):174–178. doi:10.1097/00006565-200206000-00006. PMID: 12066002.

19. Kruse JA, Carlson RW. Fatal rodenticide poisoning with brodifacoum. *Ann Emerg Med*. 1992; 21:331–336.

20. Lubetsky A et al. Comparison of oral vs intravenous phytonadione (vitamin K1) in patients with excessive anticoagulation: A prospective randomized controlled study. *Arch Intern Med*. 2003 Nov 10;163:2469–2473.

21. Britt RB, Brown JN. Characterizing the severe reactions of parenteral vitamin K1. *Clin Appl Thromb Hemost.* 2018;24(1):5–12. doi:10.1177/1076029616674825
22. Guyatt GH, et al. Executive summary: antithrombotic therapy and prevention of thrombosis, 9th ed: American College of Chest Physicians Evidence-Based Clinical Practice Guidelines. *Chest.* 2012;141(2 suppl):7S–47S. [PubMed: 22315257]

11 Stuffing Is for Turkeys: Management of Illicit Drug Stuffers

Zachary Illg

Case Presentation

A 27-year-old man presents to the ED accompanied by police. Prior to arrival, he was pulled over by police for running a red light. He reports he had a few small baggies of methamphetamine in his vehicle and ingested them in haste as he was concerned the police would discover them. He became nervous following this ingestion and notified the police, who subsequently brought the patient to the ED. Upon evaluating the patient, he reports feeling anxious but is otherwise without complaints. He has a history of tobacco dependence and gastroesophageal reflux disease. Additionally, he reports smoking methamphetamine one to two times per week to help him stay awake at work. He does not take any medications regularly. His temperature is 98.9°/37.2°C F, his heart rate is 98 beats/min, and his blood pressure is 132/88 mm Hg.

What Do You Do Now?

DISCUSSION

Background

Body packing, pushing, and stuffing are methods individuals use to conceal illicit drugs internally. Doses ingested can range from one to two "hits," or doses, of the illicit substance to multiples of a lethal quantity of the substance. Body stuffing, which the patient in the vignette above performed, is the ingestion of drugs, often in small quantities and in haste, upon being taken into custody to avoid discovery by law enforcement.[1] The ingested drugs are often poorly wrapped, given the rapidity with which they are ingested. Drugs can also be inserted rectally or vaginally to conceal them from discovery, and this may be referred to as "body pushing."[2] In contrast, "body packing" is the internal concealment of large, thoughtfully packaged quantities of illicit drugs to transport them from one location to another.[1] Commonly stuffed illicit drugs include heroin, cocaine, and methamphetamine. There is limited epidemiological data regarding body stuffers, and this problem's commonality or scope is not well defined.

Toxicology and Pathophysiology

The underlying toxicologic and pathophysiologic mechanisms depend on the drug or drugs ingested by a body stuffer. As previously mentioned, opioids, cocaine, and methamphetamine are commonly stuffed xenobiotics. Opioids, such as heroin, cause CNS depression. Their main toxic effects are often a result of respiratory depression, which, if left untreated, can lead to cardiorespiratory failure and death. Cocaine and amphetamines, on the other hand, are stimulants that cause CNS excitation, often with resultant agitation and autonomic hyperactivity at toxic doses. Stimulants can lead to hyperthermia, rhabdomyolysis, and death if left untreated. The time to peak effect following the ingestion of an illicit xenobiotic is variable and depends on the xenobiotic ingested and the presence and quality of packaging. Loosely or poorly packaged xenobiotics can be anticipated to leak or rupture early in the clinical course, causing more rapid release of xenobiotics into the GI tract and systemic absorption than is usually seen with body packers. Packaging used to distribute illicit drugs includes small reclosable zipper-lock plastic bags, plastic wrap, balloons, and aluminum foil, among others.

Workup and Diagnosis

The diagnosis of the internal concealment of a xenobiotic is often based on the history and physical examination. Any patient who reports ingesting an illicit drug should be presumed to have done so and treated accordingly. The diagnosis may be further supported by clinical evidence of a xenobiotic ingestion such as hypertension and tachycardia in the setting of a sympathomimetic ingestion. However, many patients who present to the ED following the reported ingestion of an illicit drug are asymptomatic and have normal hemodynamics. Knowing the management and required duration of observation prior to discharge is of paramount importance for these individuals. Premature discharge of an asymptomatic patient who reported the ingestion of an illicit drug may lead to the delayed, out-of-hospital development of symptoms given the unpredictable kinetics of loosely or poorly packaged xenobiotics.

There is no consensus on the required duration of observation in asymptomatic body stuffers. However, multiple studies have shown that in body stuffers who present to an ED, all individuals who developed symptoms did so within 6 hours of ingestion.[3-5] It is recommended that an asymptomatic body stuffer be observed in the ED for the development of symptoms for at least 6 hours from the time of ingestion. If an individual presents with or develops symptoms during their ED stay, they should be monitored until complete resolution of their symptoms. These patients should be monitored in a setting commensurate with their symptoms, with those exhibiting severe toxicity requiring treatment in an intensive care setting. However, there remains the possibility that patients develop toxicity after the 6-hour mark. Efforts should be made to discharge the patient to an environment where they can continue to be observed by a friend or family member.

Abdominal imaging should be considered in cases of body stuffing; abdominopelvic CT without oral contrast is the preferred modality.[6] However, it should be noted that there are cases of false-negative abdominal CT imaging in body stuffers.[7-9] Thus, advanced imaging may aid in diagnosing a xenobiotic ingestion but should not be relied on to rule out an ingestion. The patient in our scenario is asymptomatic aside from reported anxiety and has stable vital signs. No specific diagnostic testing is required at this time. However, the patient requires a minimum of 6 hours of observation for the development of toxicity in the ED.

Treatment

Treatment for symptomatic body stuffers is specific to the xenobiotic ingested and is supportive in nature. Rapid body cooling and benzodiazepines may be required in the setting of a sympathomimetic toxidrome, whereas naloxone and airway monitoring may be needed for an opioid toxidrome. However, the roles of activated charcoal and whole-bowel irrigation (WBI) also need to be considered in the case of a body stuffer.

A dose of activated charcoal is recommended for most body stuffers, given its potential to adsorb the ingested xenobiotic.[10,11] It should be given as soon as possible following the ingestion, ideally upon a patient's arrival at the ED. Activated charcoal is generally safe and well-tolerated but should be withheld if the patient is uncooperative or unable to protect their airway, given the risk of aspiration and resultant pneumonitis.

There is a paucity of evidence to support the routine administration of WBI for the treatment of a body stuffer. Its theoretical benefit is decreased colonic transit time with prompt expulsion of any ingested packets. However, it is postulated that WBI may increase the solubility and absorption of the ingested xenobiotic, potentially worsening toxicity.[9–11] Additionally, the WBI solution may increase peristalsis, increasing the risk of packet rupture. WBI is not routinely recommended in the management of a body stuffer. This contrasts with the management of a body packer, where WBI is often utilized due to the large GI burden of the packed drugs and the risk of severe toxicity and mortality if a packet ruptures.

Less commonly encountered treatment modalities include endoscopy, colonoscopy, and bronchoscopy, which are uncommon scenarios and are not routinely recommended. Depending on the intervention, these should only be considered following consultation with a toxicologist and gastroenterologist or pulmonologist, depending on the location of the xenobiotic. When there is a question about the appropriate management course for a confirmed or suspected body stuffer, prompt consultation with a toxicologist or poison center should be considered.

Long-Term Concerns

There are no specific long-term sequelae anticipated due to the act of body stuffing. However, long-term effects from unrecognized toxicity and delayed treatment of various xenobiotics are a concern. For example, failure to promptly identify and treat respiratory failure with resultant hypoxia in the setting of an opioid ingestion may lead to permanent morbidity seen in the setting of hypoxic-ischemic encephalopathy.

CASE CONCLUSION

In our scenario, a dose of activated charcoal should be given to adsorb any xenobiotic that may be in the patient's GI tract. Further treatment, if necessary, will consist of symptomatic and supportive care if the patient develops signs or symptoms of methamphetamine toxicity. In the case of a body packer, management recommendations may differ, and surgical removal of drug packages is indicated if the patient exhibits symptoms of toxicity.[12] This is because the ingested packages often contain large quantities of the drug and, if ruptured, pose the risk of severe, life-threatening toxicity despite antidotal administration.

KEY POINTS TO REMEMBER

- Body stuffers ingest drugs in haste to avoid detection, often by law enforcement, while body packers internally conceal larger quantities of well-packaged drugs for transport.
- Activated charcoal is an important adjunct in the treatment of body stuffers.
- Whole-bowel irrigation has not been shown to be of benefit in the management of body stuffers and may increase the absorption of an ingested illicit xenobiotic.
- Even if initially asymptomatic, body stuffers require a minimum of 6 hours of observation before medical clearance.
- The absence of drug remnants or packaging on CT imaging does not rule out a drug ingestion.

Further Reading

Hassanian-Moghaddam H, Amraei F, Zamani N. Management recommendations for body stuffers at emergency units. *Arh Hig Rada Toksikol.* 2019;70(2):90–96. doi:10.2478/aiht-2019-70-3199

Heymann-Maier L, Trueb L, Schmidt S, et al. Emergency department management of body packers and body stuffers. *Swiss Med Wkly*. 2017;147:w14499. Published 2017 September 12. doi:10.4414/smw.2017.14499

Prosser J. Internal concealment of xenobiotics. In: Nelson LS, Howland M, Lewin NA, Smith SW, Goldfrank LR, Hoffman RS, eds. *Goldfrank's Toxicologic Emergencies*. 11th ed. McGraw-Hill.

Yamamoto T, Malavasi E, Archer JR, Dargan PI, Wood DM. Management of body stuffers presenting to the emergency department. *Eur J Emerg Med*. 2016;23(6):425–429. doi:10.1097/MEJ.0000000000000277

References

1. Heymann-Maier L, Trueb L, Schmidt S, et al. Emergency department management of body packers and body stuffers. *Swiss Med Wkly*. 2017;147:14499. Published 2017 September 12. doi:10.4414/smw.2017.14499

2. Booker RJ, Smith JE, Rodger MP. Packers, pushers and stuffers—managing patients with concealed drugs in UK emergency departments: a clinical and medicolegal review. *Emerg Med J*. 2009;26(5):316–320. doi:10.1136/emj.2008.057695

3. Yamamoto T, Malavasi E, Archer JR, Dargan PI, Wood DM. Management of body stuffers presenting to the emergency department. *Eur J Emerg Med*. 2016;23(6):425–429. doi:10.1097/MEJ.0000000000000277

4. Moreira M, Buchanan J, Heard K. Validation of a 6-hour observation period for cocaine body stuffers. *Am J Emerg Med*. 2011;29(3):299–303. doi:10.1016/j.ajem.2009.11.022

5. Jordan MT, Bryant SM, Aks SE, Wahl M. A five-year review of the medical outcome of heroin body stuffers. *J Emerg Med*. 2009;36(3):250–256. doi:10.1016/j.jemermed.2007.06.022

6. Shahnazi M, Hassanian-Moghaddam H, Gachkar L, et al. Comparison of abdominal computed tomography with and without oral contrast in diagnosis of body packers and body stuffers. *Clin Toxicol (Phila)*. 2015;53(7):596–603. doi:10.3109/15563650.2015.1054501

7. Eng JG, Aks SE, Waldron R, Marcus C, Issleib S. False-negative abdominal CT scan in a cocaine body stuffer. *Am J Emerg Med*. 1999;17(7):702–704. doi:10.1016/s0735-6757(99)90166-3

8. West PL, McKeown NJ, Hendrickson RG. Methamphetamine body stuffers: an observational case series. *Ann Emerg Med*. 2010;55(2):190–197. doi:10.1016/j.annemergmed.2009.08.005

9. Prosser J. Internal concealment of xenobiotics. In: Nelson LS, Howland M, Lewin NA, Smith SW, Goldfrank LR, Hoffman RS. Eds. *Goldfrank's Toxicologic Emergencies*. 11th ed. McGraw-Hill.

10. Hassanian-Moghaddam H, Amraei F, Zamani N. Management recommendations for body stuffers at emergency units. *Arh Hig Rada Toksikol*. 2019;70(2):90–96. doi:10.2478/aiht-2019-70-3199

11. Utecht MJ, Stone AF, McCarron MM. Heroin body packers. *J Emerg Med*. 1993;11(1):33–40. doi:10.1016/0736-4679(93)90007-t

12. Mandava N, Chang RS, Wang JH, et al. Establishment of a definitive protocol for the diagnosis and management of body packers (drug mules). *Emerg Med J*. 2011;28(2):98–101. doi:10.1136/emj.2008.059717

12 When Antidiarrheals Stop More Than Loose Bowels: Loperamide-Induced Cardiac Dysfunction

Rita Farah and Brent Morgan

Case Presentation

A 27-year-old man with no past medical history presents to the ED for generalized weakness, shortness of breath and a syncopal episode. The patient is alert and oriented. On physical exam, his skin is warm, clammy, and pale. An ECG obtained on arrival shows a sinus rhythm with high-grade atrioventricular block with a QRS of 126 ms and a QTc of 337 ms (Figure 12.1a). During the history, the patient admits to ingesting 72 tablets of 2 mg loperamide 2 days earlier and again on the day of presentation in order to treat his opioid withdrawal symptoms. Vital signs are heart rate 61 beats/min, blood pressure 133/92, respiratory rate 20 breaths/min, temperature 99°F/37.2°C, SpO_2 99% on room air. The basic metabolic panel is within normal limits: serum sodium (140 mEq/L), potassium (3.5 mEq/L), chloride (104 mmol/L), CO_2 (24 mmol/L), magnesium (2.2 mg/dL), and calcium (9.3 mg/dL). Arterial blood

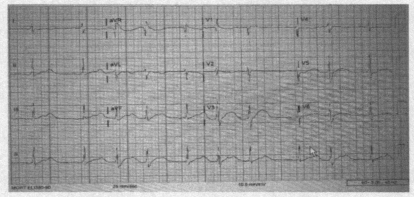

(b)

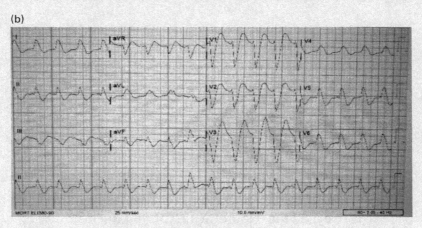

FIGURE 12.1 (A). Initial ECG showing sinus rhythm with QRS widening: heart rate of 61 bpm, QRS duration of 126 ms, QTc of 337 ms.

(B). ECG showing sustained ventricular tachycardia; HR 105 bpm, QRS duration of 201 ms, QTc of 426 ms.

gases reveal respiratory alkalosis (pH 7.53, pCO_2 26.8 mm Hg). The patient receives several hypertonic saline boluses for the prolonged QRS and is placed on continuous cardiac monitoring. He experiences several runs of ventricular tachycardia with a pulse treated with amiodarone (150 mg IV over 10 minutes) and metoprolol 2.5 mg IV (Figure 12.1b). In the third hour post-admission, the patient is experiencing several episodes of pulseless ventricular tachycardia requiring CPR. Subsequently, he arrests, requiring cardioversion and endotracheal intubation.

What Do You Do Now?

A young patient with no medical history presenting with several cardiac conduction abnormalities is a medically challenging case presentation. Obtaining a history that includes all medications, herbs, and supplements that the patient takes can reveal critical information.

DISCUSSION

Background

Loperamide is a widely used nonprescription antidiarrheal agent. It was initially classified as a Schedule V medication under the US Controlled Substances Act because of concerns of abuse related to its opioid properties.[1] However, in 1982, loperamide became an over-the-counter drug after post-marketing surveillance data demonstrated low risk for physical dependence and abuse.[1]

As early as 2005, high-dose loperamide use was mentioned in online-based forums for its euphoric effects and for the relief of opioid withdrawal symptoms.[2] During the same time frame, emerging reports on loperamide toxicity revealed its potential for misuse due to its ease of access and low cost.

Analysis of cases reported to the National Poison Data System (NPDS) between 2010 and 2015 showed a 91% increase in loperamide exposures, including eight deaths.[3] Also, from January 1, 2012 to September 30, 2018, the NPDS reported a sustained increase in the number of intentional "misuse" or "abuse" of loperamide exposures from 92 cases in 2012 to 272 cases in 2017, causing 18 deaths.[4] Furthermore, the Medical Expenditure Panel Survey data showed an incidence of cardiovascular events ranging between 2.44 and 3.46 per 100,000 prescriptions of loperamide in the United States between 2014 and 2016. In July 2016, the US Food and Drug Administration released a boxed warning about serious cardiac arrhythmias, including cardiac arrest, associated with loperamide abuse.[5]

Toxicology and Pathophysiology

Loperamide is a phenylpiperidine derivative with a chemical structure similar to meperidine (Figures 12.2a,b). It acts as a peripheral mu-opioid receptor agonist in the myenteric plexus of the large intestine, inhibiting secretion and peristalsis and increasing transit time and anal sphincter tone.[6] Also, loperamide blocks intestinal calcium channels.

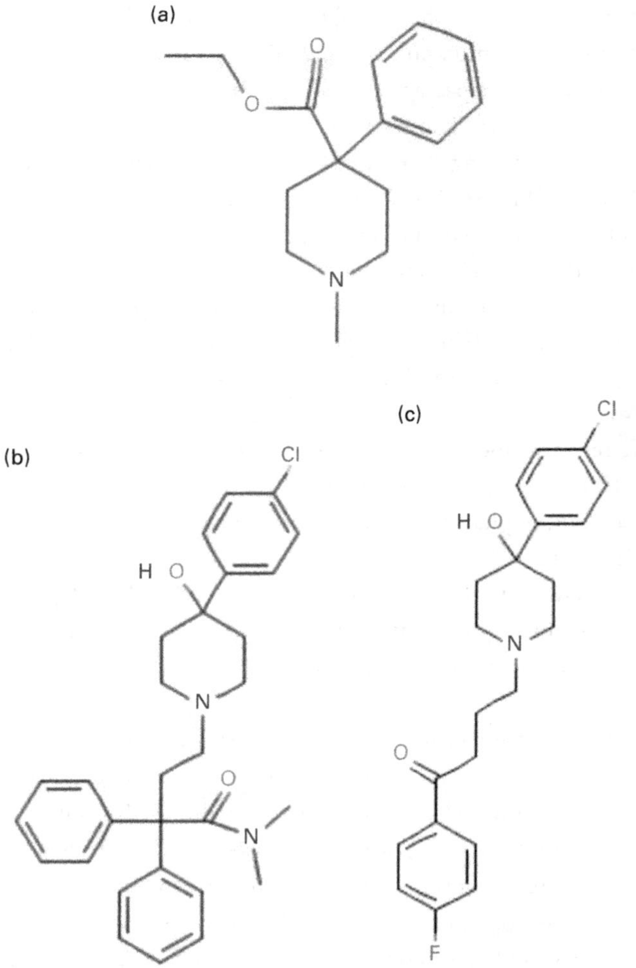

FIGURE 12.2 (A) Meperidine structure.[a] (B) Loperamide structure.[b] (C) Haloperidol structure.

[a]National Center for Biotechnology Information. PubChem Compound Summary for CID 4058, Meperidine. https://pubchem.ncbi.nlm.nih.gov/compound/Meperidine. Accessed Feb. 10, 2022.

[b]National Center for Biotechnology Information. PubChem Compound Summary for CID 3955, Loperamide. https://pubchem.ncbi.nlm.nih.gov/compound/Loperamide. Accessed Feb. 10, 2022.

[c]National Center for Biotechnology Information. PubChem Compound Summary for CID 3559, Haloperidol. https://pubchem.ncbi.nlm.nih.gov/compound/Haloperidol. Accessed Feb. 10, 2022.

Loperamide has a wide therapeutic index largely as a result of its low oral bioavailability (0.3%). It is metabolized by cytochrome P450 CYP3A4 and 2C8 to the active metabolite N-desmethyl-loperamide.[7] When taken at therapeutic doses, the pharmacokinetics of loperamide are shaped by P-glycoprotein (P-gp) efflux pumps which limit its absorption from the small intestines as well as its passage through the blood–brain barrier.[8] The half-life of loperamide is 10.8 hours, with a range of 9.1 to 14.4 hours.[6] Genetic polymorphisms resulting in reduced P-gp activity or concomitant use of lo-peramide with CYP3A4, CYP2C8, or P-gp inhibitors (Table 12.1) increase loperamide plasma concentrations and prolong its elimination half-life.[7]

Loperamide toxicokinetics are not well understood, but, at high doses, loperamide appears to saturate P-gp efflux pumps resulting in increased penetration into the CNS through the blood–brain barrier. This mech-anism explains the misuse of high-dose loperamide for the relief of opioid withdrawal symptoms as well as for recreational abuse. In this setting, the literature reports a median daily dose of 200 mg (134–400 mg), the equiv-alent of 100 tablets (67–200 tablets).[9] Drugs that can potentially interact with loperamide's pharmacodynamics and pharmacokinetics are summa-rized in Table 12.2.[10]

It is noteworthy that respiratory depression, CNS depression, and death were reported in infants following ingestion of loperamide. This is most probably due to the immaturity of the blood–brain barrier P-gp in infants.[11–12]

However, the primary toxicity of high-dose loperamide involves cardiac function. Loperamide is thought to inhibit sodium-gated cardiac channels, leading to the QRS complex widening and the cardiac delayed rectifier (hERG) potassium channel, which increases the QT interval.[13] QT pro-longation is more commonly reported,[14] and this could be explained by the higher affinity of loperamide for potassium channels compared to sodium channels. QRS and QT prolongations can lead to ventricular dysrhythmias, ventricular tachycardia, torsade de pointes, ventricular fibrillation, Brugada syndrome-like ECG changes, cardiac arrest, and death. Based on studies done on tricyclic antidepressants (TCAs), it is reasonable to define drug-induced QRS widening as a QRS of greater than 100 ms.[15] A drug-induced QTc prolongation of greater than 500 ms has been a threshold of concern for cardiac arrhythmias, most clearly torsade de pointes.

TABLE 12.1 **Drugs that can potentially interact with loperamide**

Drug class	Drug	Mechanism of interaction with loperamide
Antifungals	Itraconazole Ketoconazole[a] Fluconazole	CYP3A4 and P-gp inhibitors
Antibacterials	Clarithromycin[b] Erythromycin Ciprofloxacin	CYP3A4 inhibitors
Antidepressants	Nefazodone	CYP3A4 inhibitors
Calcium channel blocker	Diltiazem Verapamil[b]	CYP3A4 inhibitors
Class I antiarrhythmic agent	Quinidine	P-gp inhibitors
Histamine H$_2$ receptor antagonists	Cimetidine Ranitidine[c]	CYP3A4 inhibitors
Immunosuppressants	Cyclosporine	P-gp inhibitors
Antivirals (protease inhibitors)	Indinavir Nelfinavir Ritonavir[b] Saquinavir	CYP 3A4 inhibitors
Lipid-lowering	Gemgibrozil	CYP2C8 inhibitors
Antimalarial	Quinine	P-gp inhibitors
Food and supplements	Grapefruit juice Goldenseal *Panax ginseng* American ginseng *(Panax quinquefolius)* Garlic (*Allium sativum*)	CYP 3A4 inhibitors

[a] Systemic ketoconazole is classified as p-gp inhibitor.
[b] CYP3A4 and p-gp inhibitors.
[c] Weak CYP 3A4 inhibitor.

TABLE 12.2 Summary of the management plan of loperamide overdose

Management	Details
Activated charcoal	Can be given beyond the 1-hour window due to the slowing effect of loperamide on peristalsis
Naloxone	The lowest effective dose of naloxone should be used to prevent respiratory depression.
	The AACT and AAPCC loperamide position statement endorsed by the ACMT, recommends a starting dose of 0.4 mg.
	Naloxone should be titrated to maintain adequate respirations.
ACLS protocols	Applied to the management of cardiac dysrhythmias
Overdrive pacing	Transvenous electrical pacing to resolve torsade de pointes
Magnesium sulfate	2 g IV over 5–20 minutes once a perfusing rhythm is achieved
Isoproterenol	Indicated for the suppression of ventricular ectopy
Electrolytes (K^+, Mg^{2+}, Ca^{2+})	Optimizing electrolytes help preventing further QT prolongation
Sodium bicarbonate	QRS widening can be treated with a bolus of 1–2 mEq/Kg
Intravenous lipid emulsion	Reserved for severe cardiotoxicity and patients who remain severely unstable despite otherwise optimal (due to lack of good data).
Extracorporeal membrane oxygenation	Indicated for patients with cardiovascular collapse not responding to standard treatment measures.

Loperamide concentrations required to block sodium and potassium channels are not achieved with therapeutic doses (up to 16 mg/day).[16] Massive ingestion of loperamide as a single agent or pharmacokinetic manipulation by the concomitant use of P-gp and/or CYP inhibitors (Table 12.1) result in high serum levels and cardiotoxicity.[17,18]

The active metabolite N-desmethyl-loperamide appears to have a lower affinity to the (hERG)[14] potassium channel than loperamide but can achieve a much higher systemic concentration. Therefore, it is hypothesized that N-desmethyl-loperamide could be an essential contributor to loperamide-associated cardiac toxicity.

Workup and Diagnosis

Patients presenting with cardiac toxicity should be admitted and observed until resolution of toxicity; this includes obtaining an ECG and instituting continuous cardiac monitoring. Loperamide is not a part of routine drug screening. Nevertheless, high-dose loperamide should be included in the differential diagnosis of patients presenting with unexplained syncope or ECG changes such as QTc prolongation, episodes of torsade de pointes, ventricular tachycardia, or Brugada pattern, especially if opioid use disorder is suspected.[18]

Treatment

The management of loperamide toxicity is largely supportive (Table 12.2). In the setting of acute overdose and in the absence of contraindications, it is reasonable to attempt decontamination with activated charcoal.[18] Given the slowing effect of loperamide on peristalsis, the administration of activated charcoal (AC) beyond the typical 1 hour of ingestion can be considered. Wu et al. advised administering AC within 2–4 hours of an acute ingestion.[18]

In addition to airway support, naloxone may be used in patients with respiratory depression.[13] Given the possibility of opioid withdrawal, the lowest effective dose of naloxone should be used. Successful use of IV naloxone at doses of 0.01 to 0.3 mg has been described in pediatric patients.[12] The American Academy of Clinical Toxicology (AACT) and the American Association of Poison Control Centers (AAPCC) loperamide position statement endorsed by the American College of Medical Toxicology (ACMT) recommends a starting dose of 0.4 mg naloxone in patients with respiratory depression after acute overdose, with dose titration to achieve stable respiratory status.[4] Because naloxone has a shorter half-life than loperamide, a continuous naloxone infusion may be necessary, with titration to maintain adequate respirations. Vital signs and neurological and cardiopulmonary status should be observed for at least 24 hours after the last naloxone use to ensure patient does not deteriorate clinically.

Standard advanced cardiac life support protocols are applied for the management of cardiac arrhythmias. Synchronized cardioversion should be used for patients with ventricular tachycardia and hemodynamic instability, and asynchronous cardioversion should be used for patients with ventricular fibrillation or ventricular tachycardia without pulses.

Torsade de pointes that do not resolve spontaneously should be managed with asynchronous cardioversion. Magnesium (2 g) should be given intravenously over 5–20 minutes once a perfusing rhythm is achieved. In several overdose cases, torsade de pointes appeared to benefit from overdrive pacing using transvenous electrical pacing or isoproterenol to suppress ventricular ectopy and prevent recurrent dysrhythmias. Amiodarone can also be considered for patient with recurrent dysrhythmias.

Optimizing electrolytes including potassium, calcium, and magnesium aims at preventing further QT prolongation. QRS widening is treated with serum alkalinization by bolus dosing of sodium bicarbonate (1–2 mEq/Kg). Alkalinization should be continued for at least 12–24 hours after the ECG has normalized because of the redistribution of the drug from the tissue. Treating physicians should keep in mind that sodium bicarbonate can cause hypokalemia, which in turn can worsen QT prolongation. Hypokalemia occurs due to an extracellular shift of hydrogen ions with an intracellular shift of potassium ions to compensate for alkalosis. Given the risk of hypokalemia, frequent potassium monitoring is warranted, with repletion given carefully.[15]

Loperamide is lipophilic (log P = 4.77) and highly protein-bound (97%)[11]; therefore, hemodialysis is not expected to be beneficial. Although good data on the efficacy of intravenous lipid emulsion (ILE) are lacking, it is reasonable to consider ILE in patients with severe cardiotoxicity and those who remain severely unstable despite otherwise optimal care.[18] Loperamide case reports lack details on ILE dosing. Dosing recommendations are provided by the ACMT[19] and at http://www.lipidrescue.org; however, these recommendations are not specific to loperamide toxicity. It is noteworthy that loperamide is slowly eliminated in the setting of an overdose, and prolonged infusions of ILE are generally best avoided. In patients with cardiovascular collapse not responding to standard treatment measures, extracorporeal membrane oxygenation (ECMO) may be considered. Structure similarities between loperamide and haloperidol explain the dystonic reactions seen in loperamide overdoses (Figure 12.2c). Dystonic reactions can be treated with benztropine (1–4 mg IV or orally, maximum 6 mg/day) or diphenhydramine.

Long-Term Concerns

A review of 19 cases of abuse of loperamide showed that the length of stay ranged between 1 and 16 days. Follow-up done 1–2 months after the encounter revealed that patients did not sustain ECG abnormalities.[20] However, when present, the underlying opioid use disorder should be addressed, and patients should be offered medications for opioid use disorder as well as addiction therapy to reduce the recurrence of loperamide misuse and the likelihood of illicit opioid use.[18]

CASE CONCLUSION

Patient became increasingly hemodynamically unstable and was started on the following:

- IV bolus of 20% lipid emulsion at 1.5 ml/Kg over 1 minute
- Continuous infusion of 20% lipid emulsion at 0.25 ml/kg/min over 60 minutes
- Lidocaine 1 mg/kg IV bolus and then 0.03 mg/kg/min infusion
- Several boluses of hypertonic saline (100 mL) through central access line

The ventricular tachycardia ceased. Over the next 24 hours, the patient improved, was extubated without complications, and was transferred out of the ICU to a regular bed with telemetry monitoring and lidocaine infusion. Close monitoring showed a progressive improvement in ECG intervals. The lidocaine infusion was continued for 24 hours after the ECG returned to normal. On day 7, the patient was transferred to an inpatient substance use disorder treatment facility.

- At therapeutic doses of loperamide, CNS effects are minimal because of poor bioavailability of loperamide, important first-pass metabolism, and P-gp–mediated efflux out of the CNS.
- High-dose loperamide or concomitant use of loperamide with CYP 3A4, CYP 2C8 or P-gp inhibitors can lead to CNS symptoms and cardiac toxicity.
- Unexplained syncope or ECG changes, particularly QT prolongation and QRS widening in patients with a history of opioids use disorder, should lead clinicians to consider loperamide overdose in their differential diagnosis.
- The management of loperamide toxicity is largely supportive.
- When present, the underlying opioid use disorder should be addressed and patients should be offered medication-assisted opioid therapy to reduce the recurrence of loperamide abuse.

Further Reading

Eggleston W, Palmer R, Dubé PA, et al. Loperamide toxicity: recommendations for patient monitoring and management. *Clin Toxicol*. 2020;58(5):355–359. doi:10.1080/15563650.2019.1681443

Wu PE, Juurlink DN. Clinical review: loperamide toxicity. *Ann Emerg Med*. 2017;70(2):245–252. doi:10.1016/j.annemergmed.2017.04.008

References

1. Drug Enforcement Administration. Diversion control division. Accessed March 24, 2022. https://www.deadiversion.usdoj.gov/index.html
2. Daniulaityte R, Carlson R, Falck R, et al. "I just wanted to tell you that loperamide WILL WORK": A web-based study of extra-medical use of loperamide. *Drug Alcohol Depend*. 2013;130(1–3):241–244. doi:10.1016/j.drugalcdep.2012.11.003
3. Vakkalanka JP, Charlton NP, Holstege CP. Epidemiologic trends in loperamide abuse and misuse. *Ann Emerg Med*. 2017;69(1):73–78. doi:10.1016/j.annemergmed.2016.08.444
4. Eggleston W, Palmer R, Dubé PA, et al. Loperamide toxicity: recommendations for patient monitoring and management. *Clin Toxicol*. 2020;58(5):355–359. doi:10.1080/15563650.2019.1681443
5. Food and Drug Administration. Drug safety communication: FDA warns about serious heart problems with high doses of the antidiarrheal medicine loperamide (Imodium), including from abuse and misuse. FDA. 2021. https://www.fda.gov/

drugs/drug-safety-and-availability/fda-drug-safety-communication-fda-warns-about-serious-heart-problems-high-doses-antidiarrheal

6. Killinger JM, Weintraub HS, Fuller BL. Human pharmacokinetics and comparative bioavailability of loperamide hydrochloride. *J Clin Pharmacol.* 1979;19(4):211–218. doi:10.1002/j.1552-4604.1979.tb01654.x

7. Kim KA, Chung J, Jung DH, Park JY. Identification of cytochrome P450 isoforms involved in the metabolism of loperamide in human liver microsomes. *Eur J Clin Pharmacol.* 2004;60(8):575–581. doi:10.1007/s00228-004-0815-3

8. Vandenbossche J, Huisman M, Xu Y, Sanderson-Bongiovanni D, Soons P. Loperamide and P-glycoprotein inhibition: assessment of the clinical relevance. *J Pharm Pharmacol.* 2010;62(4):401–412. doi:10.1211/jpp.62.04.0001

9. Teigeler T, Stahura H, Alimohammad R, et al. Electrocardiographic changes in loperamide toxicity: case report and review of literature. *J Cardiovasc Electrophysiol.* 2019;30(11):2618–2626. Doi:10.1111/jce.14129

10. Food and Drug Administration. Drug development and drug interactions | Table of substrates, inhibitors and inducers. FDA. 2022. Accessed March 24, 2022. https://www.fda.gov/drugs/drug-interactions-labeling/drug-development-and-drug-interactions-table-substrates-inhibitors-and-inducers

11. Litovitz T, Clancy C, Korberly B, Temple AR, Mann KV. Surveillance of loperamide ingestions: an analysis of 216 poison center reports. *J Toxicol Clin Toxicol.* 1997;35(1):11–19. doi:10.3109/15563659709001159

12. Minton NA, Smith PG. Loperamide toxicity in a child after a single dose. *BMJ.* 1987;294(6584):1383–1383. doi:10.1136/bmj.294.6584.1383

13. Sahi N, Nguyen R, Santos C. Loperamide. StatPearls [Internet]. Accessed November 2, 2021. http://www.ncbi.nlm.nih.gov/books/NBK557885/

14. Vaz RJ, Kang J, Luo Y, Rampe D. Molecular determinants of loperamide and N-desmethyl loperamide binding in the hERG cardiac K+ channel. *Bioorg Med Chem Lett.* 2018;28(3):446–451. doi:10.1016/j.bmcl.2017.12.020

15. Bruccoleri RE, Burns MM. A literature review of the use of sodium bicarbonate for the treatment of QRS widening. *J Med Toxicol.* 2016;12(1):121–129. doi:10.1007/s13181-015-0483-y

16. Food and Drug Administration. FDA limits packaging for anti-diarrhea medicine loperamide (Imodium) to encourage safe use. FDA. 2019. Accessed March 24, 2022.https://www.fda.gov/drugs/drug-safety-and-availability/fda-limits-packaging-anti-diarrhea-medicine-loperamide-imodium-encourage-safe-use

17. Swank KA, Wu E, Kortepeter C, McAninch J, Levin RL. Adverse event detection using the FDA post-marketing drug safety surveillance system: cardiotoxicity associated with loperamide abuse and misuse. *J Am Pharm Assoc.* 2017;57(2):S63–S67. doi:10.1016/j.japh.2016.11.011

18. Wu PE, Juurlink DN. Clinical review: loperamide toxicity. *Ann Emerg Med.* 2017;70(2):245–252. doi:10.1016/j.annemergmed.2017.04.008

19. American College of Medical Toxicology. ACMT position statement: interim guidance for the use of lipid resuscitation therapy. *J Med Toxicol*. 2011;7(1):81–82. doi:10.1007/s13181-010-0125-3

20. Riaz IB, Khan MS, Kamal MU, et al. Cardiac dysrhythmias associated with substitutive use of loperamide: a systematic review. *Am J Ther*. 2019;26(1):e170–e182. doi:10.1097/MJT.0000000000000585

13 Save a Life, Initiate Buprenorphine: Emergency Department Buprenorphine Administration

Maxwell Kruse and Joshua da Silva

Case Presentation

You are working a busy shift in the ED and decide to pick up a patient who has the chief complaint of "requesting detox." In the room you find a 25-year-old, anxious-appearing man who is diaphoretic and complaining of nausea. He reports a history of fentanyl use, previous opioid overdose, and states that he feels "dope sick." His vital signs are blood pressure 130/70 mm Hg, heart rate 110 beats/min, respiratory rate 18 breaths/min, temperature of 99.5°F/ 37.5 °C, and an oxygen saturation of 98% on room air. On exam, you note that he has slightly dilated pupils at 5 mm and that he appears restless. The remainder of your exam is benign, and his laboratory workup is without concerning findings. The patient appears to be experiencing opioid withdrawal. There is an addiction clinic just down the road, but they typically can't accommodate same-day appointments. You call the clinic and can schedule him an appointment for next week. When you tell him the good news, he begs you for help. He states he feels like he is going to die. He asks if there is anything you can do to help him because he is afraid he will need to use fentanyl again before his appointment.

What Do You Do Now?

DISCUSSION

Background

Since 1999, nearly 500,000 people have died from an opioid overdose, with the death toll continuing to climb despite national initiatives combating the epidemic. In 2019 alone, there were nearly 50,000 opioid-related deaths, six times the number of overdose deaths than 10 years earlier.[1] ED physicians can combat the opioid epidemic with the effective use of medications for opioid use disorder (MOUD). Studies have shown that MOUD with buprenorphine reduces opioid-related overdose and opioid-related mortality and improves retention in treatment programs.[2] Additionally, MOUD programs have shown a reduction of overall costs to the healthcare and criminal justice systems compared to brief interventions and referrals alone.[3] Over the past few years, patients receiving MOUD have more than doubled, with 1.27 million Americans currently receiving therapy.[4] Despite this progress, there is still a lack of vital patient access to these life-saving treatment programs. By learning how to initiate buprenorphine therapy, ED clinicians have an opportunity to bring about meaningful change and save patient lives.

Toxicology and Pathophysiology

Buprenorphine is a semi-synthetic partial agonist of the mu-opioid receptor with favorable pharmacologic properties that enable it to suppress opioid withdrawal, reduce cravings, limit harmful opioid-associated side effects, and allow for infrequent dosing.

Commonly misused opioids such as heroin and fentanyl are strong agonists of the mu-opioid receptor. They elicit profound euphoria and analgesia, joined by serious adverse effects such as respiratory depression. Buprenorphine, however, is a partial or weak agonist of the mu-opioid receptor which enables it to alleviate withdrawal symptoms without causing significant adverse effects. The risk of overdose with buprenorphine is exceedingly low because a ceiling effect in respiratory depression is reached with higher doses.[5]

Although buprenorphine is only a partial agonist, it binds the mu-receptor with remarkably high affinity that is 6.2 times stronger than fentanyl and 120 times stronger than oxycodone. This explains why buprenorphine can "block" the effects of other opioids. As we will explain later, it is important to administer buprenorphine after the effects of other opioids have worn off and the patient is exhibiting signs of withdrawal. You will otherwise "block" the opioids currently in the patient's system and precipitate a rather unpleasant and profound withdrawal syndrome. Additionally, full-agonist opioids have limited ability to displace buprenorphine from mu-receptors, preventing overdose not only by improving abstinence from full opioid agonists (such as heroin) but also by blocking their effects in the case of relapse.[5]

Buprenorphine has a long duration of action and slow dissociation kinetics, which allow for infrequent dosing of once or twice daily. Doses of 32 mg saturate about 98% of mu-receptors.[6] Its half-life varies based on the route of administration but ranges from 24 to 42 hours; it is metabolized by the liver to norbuprenorphine via CYP450-mediated pathways. Although norbuprenorphine is an active metabolite with mu-agonism, it does not reach high enough concentrations in the CNS to achieve any significant clinical effect.[5]

Buprenorphine has high transmucosal, subcutaneous, and intravenous bioavailability, but incredibly low oral bioavailability due to first-pass metabolism. To prevent misuse, it is often prescribed with naloxone, which has poor oral and transmucosal bioavailability but is effective when insufflated or injected. When buprenorphine-naloxone formulations are taken sublingually, the naloxone is essentially inert. However, if a patient attempts to use their buprenorphine-naloxone product by injecting or insufflating it, the naloxone will block opioid receptors and prevent the sensation of "getting high."[5]

Another favorable property of buprenorphine is its kappa-opioid receptor antagonism. The kappa-opioid receptor has been shown to mediate anti-reward pathways resulting in dysphoric and depressive effects. Most misused opioids are weak kappa-receptor agonists, and their activation of this pathway may contribute to the depression associated with opioid dependence. By blocking this kappa-mediated pathway, buprenorphine has been shown to have antidepressant effects, which may prove useful in the treatment of depression especially in the context of opioid addiction.[7]

Workup and Diagnosis

All patients who meet criteria for opioid use disorder should be offered treatment with MOUD and outpatient addiction treatment resources. Patients should be identified for treatment by history and physical exam or by screening protocols, assessing for moderate to severe opioid use disorder based on the criteria set out in the *Diagnostic and Statistical Manual of Mental Disorders* (DSM-5). The clinician then must determine the time since last opioid use, review the patient's medication list, review other illicit substance use, and determine the severity of opioid withdrawal using the Clinical Opiate Withdrawal Scale (COWS), as well as test for pregnancy.[8]

Patients should be in moderate to severe withdrawal (COWS score ≥8) before buprenorphine administration to prevent precipitated withdrawal. If they are not currently in withdrawal, they may be observed for reevaluation in the ED, transferred to an observation unit, or you may consider prescribing buprenorphine for home induction. If the patient is already in a methadone treatment program, they will not be a candidate for buprenorphine administration in the ED due to the long half-life of methadone. Although the concomitant use of opioids and other sedatives can increase the risk of adverse events, the US Food and Drug Administration (FDA) has stated that buprenorphine should not be withheld from patients taking benzodiazepines or other CNS depressants given the significant harm of untreated opioid use disorder.[9]

Pregnant patients should be offered MOUD as opposed to supervised withdrawal as the benefits of improved prenatal care, decreased rate of relapse, and reduction of high-risk behaviors with buprenorphine outweigh the risks of neonatal abstinence syndrome. Recent data show that combination buprenorphine-naloxone products are likely safe in pregnancy, however the use of a buprenorphine monoproduct in pregnant patients is currently the standard of care. The dosing of buprenorphine is the same. Previously, methadone was preferred in pregnancy, but recent guidelines show that buprenorphine is a safe and more feasible alternative with fewer drug interactions. Strongly consider consulting OB/GYN before administering MOUD as patients will require follow-up and fetal monitoring with induction.[10] There is also some evidence that shows the use of buprenorphine in pregnant patients led to shorter duration of treatment and shorter hospital stays.[11]

Treatment

ED clinicians may apply for a Drug Addiction Treatment Act of 2000 X-Waiver through the Drug Enforcement Administration (DEA) to prescribe buprenorphine for more than 30 patients at one time, however, this applies to patients enrolled in an outpatient setting and does not limit the number of patients for whom an ED physician can initiate treatment*. Traditionally, this required an 8-hour training course, which is still recommended and available, but *no longer required* for obtaining the X-Waiver. Providers still must submit a Notice of Intent (NOI) to the Substance Abuse and Mental Health Services Administration (SAMHSA) to obtain an X-waiver. Additionally, ED clinicians may now prescribe up to 3 days of buprenorphine without an X-Waiver (as long as it is in the form of ED take-home packs) for the purpose of initiating treatment for opioid use disorder.[8,9,12] Regular scripts for buprenorphine will still require an X-Waiver. Legislation regarding buprenorphine prescribing is rapidly evolving, and many changes occurred during the writing of this chapter. Providers should verify current regulations with the DEA, SAMHSA, and/or their hospital pharmacy if they are not already familiar with them.

There are many different approaches to treatment with buprenorphine, but there are some important steps to consider:

1. First, assess the patient to ensure they are in moderate to severe opioid withdrawal (COWS score ≥8).
2. If COWS score ≥8, administer the first dose of buprenorphine. We recommend an initial "tester" dose of 2 mg/0.5 mg SL buprenorphine/naloxone.
3. Reassess in 30–60 minutes. If there is no precipitated withdrawal, administer another dose of 6 mg/1.5 mg. This will bring you to the generally accepted starting dose of 8 mg/2 mg SL buprenorphine/naloxone.
4. Aim to eliminate most symptoms of withdrawal in the ED. If the patient is still experiencing withdrawal symptoms after the initial loading dose, consider redosing with 8 mg/2 mg SL buprenorphine-naloxone (the maximum daily dose of buprenorphine-naloxone is 24 mg/6 mg).

* As of 2023, the X Waiver program has been eliminated. The notice of intent is no longer required.

5. If you do not have an X-Waiver, discharge the patient with at least a 72-hour prescription in the form of ED take-home packs and ensure appropriate follow-up (e.g., buprenorphine-naloxone 8 mg/2 mg SL tablet/film BID. Dispense six refills). X-Waivered providers are able and should prescribe additional days of buprenorphine if an outpatient appointment is not available within 3 days.[7] Additionally, you may load the patient with 16–24 mg and allow a slow titration over the course of a couple days until they are able to be seen in follow-up.

There are several protocols for prescribing buprenorphine from the ED, with the best protocol being the one that best matches your practice environment.[8]

Management of Buprenorphine-Precipitated Withdrawal

The best way to treat precipitated withdrawal is prevention by ensuring the patient is not on a long-acting opioid (such as methadone) and has a COWS score ≥8 before induction. However several case reports and case series indicate withdrawal may still occur in patients chronically using high doses of fentanyl.[13,14] As of mid-2022, this scenario is considered rare and has not resulted in a substantiative change in recommended practice. If the patient experiences symptoms of precipitated withdrawal after induction, treat symptomatically with alpha-2 agonists (such as clonidine), antiemetics, and anxiolytics. Alternatively, you may consider attempting to administer additional buprenorphine at 4–8 mg every 30 minutes until symptoms improve.[11]

Long-Term Concerns

Long-term engagement with opioid use disorder treatment and harm reduction is our goal. All patients who receive buprenorphine induction should be offered a referral for outpatient substance use disorder treatment within 3 days. If possible, a face-to-face handoff or interaction with the outpatient provider should be provided. You should also encourage the patient to return to the ED if they are unable to have their buprenorphine prescription filled for any reason.[8,9,12]

CASE CONCLUSION

You remember your X-waiver training and discuss the possibility of starting buprenorphine to bridge the patient until he can be seen in clinic. He agrees and you start with a tester dose of 2 mh/0.5 mg SL and checked on him after getting some notes done about 30 minutes later. The patient says that he is starting to feel better and there is no signs of acute withdraw. You then give him an additional 6 mg/1.5 mg SL and discharge his with a script that would last him for three days. He is very grateful and you see in his record later that he was able to follow-up and is doing much better.

KEY POINTS TO REMEMBER

- ED clinicians have an opportunity to enhance access to treatment and reduce opioid-associated morbidity and mortality by learning to initiate buprenorphine in the ED.
- Buprenorphine is a partial agonist of the mu-opioid receptor with a higher affinity than other commonly abused full-opioid agonists.
- Buprenorphine treatment is effective at reducing opioid-related overdoses and mortality and reducing illicit drug use, and it improves retention in treatment programs.
- Buprenorphine treatment is overwhelmingly safe when compared to the potential harms that come with opioid use disorder.
- Patients must have a COWS score ≥8 for moderate to severe opioid withdrawal before buprenorphine induction.
- Specific and prompt follow-up with outpatient opioid use disorder treatment is essential.

Further Reading

ACEP. Emergency medicine quality network opioid initiative. Accessed April 1, 2022. https://www.acep.org/administration/quality/equal/emergency-quality-network-e-qual/e-qual-opioid-initiative/

Opioid use and opioid use disorder in pregnancy. Committee Opinion No. 711. American College of Obstetricians and Gynecologists. *Obstet Gynecol.* 2017;130:e81–94.

Hawk K, Hoppe J, Ketcham E, et al. Consensus recommendations on the treatment of opioid use disorder in the emergency department. *Ann Emerg Med.* 2021;78(3):434–442. doi:10.1016/j.annemergmed.2021.04.023

SAMHSA. Behavioral health treatment services locator. Accessed April 1, 2022. https://findtreatment.samhsa.gov/

Strayer RJ, Hawk K, Hayes BD, et al. Management of opioid use disorder in the emergency department: a white paper prepared for the American Academy of Emergency Medicine. *J Emerg Med.* 2020;58(3):522–546. doi:10.1016/j.jemermed.2019.12.034

Substance Abuse and Mental Health Services Administration (SAMHSA). Become a waivered buprenorphine practitioner. Accessed April 1, 2022. Updated June 7, 2023. https://www.samhsa.gov/medication-assisted-treatment/become-buprenorphine-waivered-practitioner

References

1. Centers for Disease Control and Prevention (CDC). Opioid data analysis and resources: CDC's response to the opioid overdose epidemic. Updated June 1, 2022. Accessed April 1, 2022. https://www.cdc.gov/opioids/data/analysis-resources.html

2. Wakeman SE, Larochelle MR, Ameli O, et al. Comparative effectiveness of different treatment pathways for opioid use disorder. *JAMA Network Open.* 2020;3(2):e1920622. doi:10.1001/jamanetworkopen.2019.20622

3. Busch SH, Fiellin DA, Chawarski MC, et al. Cost-effectiveness of emergency department-initiated treatment for opioid dependence. *Addiction.* 2017;112(11):2002–2010. doi:10.1111/add.13900

4. U. S. Department of Health and Human Services. Opioid crisis statistics. Accessed April 1, 2022. https://www.hhs.gov/opioids/about-the-epidemic/opioid-crisis-statistics/index.html

5. Coe MA, Lofwall MR, Walsh SL. Buprenorphine pharmacology review: update on transmucosal and long-acting formulations. *J Addiction Med.* 2019;13(2):93–103. doi:10.1097/ADM.0000000000000457

6. Greenwald M, Chris-Ellyn J, Moody D, et al. Effects of buprenorphine maintenance dose on mu-opioid receptor availability, plasma concentrations, and antagonist blockade in heroin-dependent volunteers. *NPP.* 2003;28(11):2000–2009. doi:10.1038/sj.npp.1300251

7. Peciña M, Karp JF, Mathew S, Todtenkopf MS, Ehrich EW, Zubieta JK. Endogenous opioid system dysregulation in depression: implications for new therapeutic approaches. *Mol Psychiatry.* 2019;24(4):576–587. doi:10.1038/s41380-018-0117-2

8. Herring AA, Perrone J, Nelson LS. Managing opioid withdrawal in the emergency department with buprenorphine. *Ann Emerg Med.* 2019;73(5):481–487. doi:10.1016/j.annemergmed.2018.11.032

9. Hawk K, Hoppe J, Ketcham E, et al. Consensus recommendations on the treatment of opioid use disorder in the emergency department. *Ann Emerg Med.* 2021;78(3):434–442. doi:10.1016/j.annemergmed.2021.04.023

10. Opioid use and opioid use disorder in pregnancy. Committee Opinion No. 711. American College of Obstetricians and Gynecologists. *Obstet Gynecol.* 2017;*130*:e81–94.

11. Jones H, Kaltenbach K, Heil S, et al. Neonatal abstinence syndrome after methadone or buprenorphine exposure. *N Engl J Med.* 2010;363(24): 2320–2331. doi:10.1056/NEJMoa1005359

12. Strayer RJ, Hawk K, Hayes BD, et al. Management of opioid use disorder in the emergency department: a white paper prepared for the American Academy of Emergency Medicine. *J Emerg Med.* 2020;58(3):522–546. doi:10.1016/j.jemermed.2019.12.034

13. Varshneya NB, Thakrar AP, Hobelmann JG, Dunn KE, Huhn AS. (2021). Evidence of buprenorphine-precipitated withdrawal in persons who use fentanyl. *J Addict Med.* 2021;10.

14. Silverstein SM, Daniulaityte R, Martins SS, Miller SC, Carlson RG. (2019). "Everything is not right anymore": buprenorphine experiences in an era of illicit fentanyl. Int J Drug Policy. 2019;74:76–83.

14 Tricyclic Antidepressant Toxicity: Management of the Crashing Patient

Matthew Oram and Joshua da Silva

Case Presentation

A 35-year-old man with a past medical history of depression presents to your ED with reports of altered mental status. Medics were called by the patient's girlfriend. She stated that they got into a fight about 2 hours ago; she left the house for about an hour and returned to find the patient with two empty bottles next to him, slurring his words. She is unsure how much medication was left in the bottle, and she hands you an empty bottle of amitriptyline 75 mg immediate-release tablets and a bottle of over-the-counter diphenhydramine 25 mg. The patient is arousable to stimulation and is protecting his airway but is unable to give history. IV access is established, and he is placed on the monitor. Bilateral antecubital IVs are placed by the nurse; point-of-care (POC) glucose is normal. His initial vital signs are heart rate122 beats/min, blood pressure 104/68 mm Hg, respiratory rate 14 breaths/min, temperature 100.6°F/38.1°C; his oxygen saturation

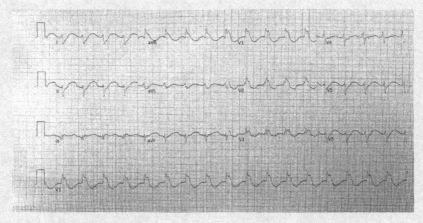

FIGURE 14.1 ECG of patient with tricyclic antidepressant toxicity.

Courtesy of Salman Ahsan, MD

is 92% on room air. Notable physical exam findings
include his somnolence, 5 mm pupils bilaterally
that are poorly reactive, and flushed dry skin. While
you are examining him, he stops responding to
stimulation and has a tonic-clonic seizure lasting for
about 1 minute. You call for 2 mg of IV lorazepam
which promptly aborts the seizure. Repeat vital
signs show heart rate 140 beats/min, blood pressure
70/40 mm Hg, respiratory rate 20 breaths/min,
temperature 101.1°F/38.4°C. After the seizure activity
stops, he remains unresponsive, and the decision
is made to intubate. You call for a 1-L saline bolus
for the hypotension. An ECG obtained shows sinus
tachycardia, R on R′, right axis deviation, and a
widened QRS (Figure 14.1).

What Do You Do Now?

DISCUSSION

Background

Commonly used for treatment of depression in the 1950s, tricyclic antidepressants (TCAs) have become less frequently prescribed with the widespread availability of selective serotonin reuptake inhibitors and serotonin and norepinephrine reuptake inhibitors (SNRIs). The TCA medication class carries with it a narrow therapeutic window and potential for lethal toxicity in overdose, and knowledge of its complications remains vital for any emergency physician because TCAs remain one of the top causes of fatal medication overdose in the United States.[1] Case fatality most commonly occurs from cardiotoxicity mediated primarily via inhibition of fast sodium channels in the His-Purkinje system and myocardium, leading to a variety of conduction abnormalities and potentially fatal arrhythmia. Additional toxic effects of TCAs are mediated by further nonselective inhibition of histamine, muscarinic, gamma-aminobutyric acid (GABA), and alpha-adrenergic receptors in addition to potassium and sodium channel blockade.[1]

Toxicology and Pathophysiology

TCAs are formed by a central three-ring structure, with the presence of one or two methyl side chains which divide TCAs further into secondary and tertiary amines, respectively. While the clinical utility of differentiating secondary versus tertiary amine TCAs is debatable, tertiary TCAs have increased anticholinergic and central histaminergic effects. TCAs' primary therapeutic effect comes via blockade of presynaptic norepinephrine and serotonin reuptake. Absorption of TCAs in the gut occurs rapidly, with peak activity occurring in 2–8 hours. TCAs are highly lipophilic, with a volume of distribution ranging from 10 to 40 L/kg and only a small quantity being found intravascularly in the blood. Tissue levels of TCA may be 10-fold higher than plasma levels, potentially explaining why plasma level may not predict toxicity. In serum, TCAs are largely protein bound. Acidosis decreases binding, potentially exacerbating toxicity in overdose. TCAs undergo first-pass hepatic metabolization; however, in overdose, first-pass metabolism can be overwhelmed, leading to greater than expected oral bioavailability.[1]

TCA overdose can be clinically recognized by toxidromes resulting from its variety of receptor activities. Mental status changes such as sedation, delirium, and hallucinations may occur from the medication's antihistamine and antimuscarinic effects. Typical antimuscarinic findings of pupillary dilation, tachycardia, dry and flushed skin, decreased secretions, and urinary retention are likely; however, diaphoresis can also be found due to inhibition of peripheral norepinephrine uptake. Hypotension may be found in TCA overdose, both mediated by decreased cardiac output from Na^+ channel blockade/arrhythmias and peripheral alpha-1 inhibition causing vasodilation. Seizures can also be seen in TCA overdose, which is likely mediated by GABA inhibition, monoamine reuptake inhibition, and sodium channel blockade.[1]

Workup and Diagnosis

In patients with known TCA overdose, workup is focused on predicting overdose severity and evaluating complicating factors such as co-ingestions and comorbidities that may worsen clinical course. There is little value to obtaining quantitative serum concentrations of TCA because, as stated previously, the pharmacodynamics are varied and there is poor correlation between serum levels and toxicity.[2] Qualitative testing for the TCA using a urine immunoassay may be helpful in completely undifferentiated patients with an atypical presentation, but false positives can occur with various substances including quetiapine, diphenhydramine, carbamazepine, and cyclobenzaprine due to structural similarity.[1]

When evaluating altered patients with limited historical information, understanding of ECG changes is essential to recognize TCA overdose, and QRS length can be used to gauge severity of overdose. Wide complex arrhythmias are a hallmark of TCA toxicity, however more subtle ECG changes can be found prior to potentially lethal arrhythmia. Na^+ channel blockade results in impaired depolarization through the His-Purkinje system and ventricular myocardium leading to multiple conduction abnormalities, most notably widened QRS. In one prospective cohort study of acute TCA overdose, a QRS greater than 100 ms was associated with a 34% incidence of seizures and a 14% incidence of ventricular arrhythmias compared to no seizures or ventricular arrhythmia in those with QRS of less than 100 ms.[3] Other ECG findings of significance include increased R wave amplitude in aVR (RaVR) greater than 3 mm (sensitivity 81%) or R-wave/S-wave ratio in lead aVR (R/SaVR) greater than 0.7 (sensitivity 75%). In one multiple logistic-regression analysis, RaVR greater than 3 mm predicted seizure and arrhythmia in TCA overdose while QRS greater than 100 mm and R/SaVR greater than 0.7 did not.[4] A Brugada ECG pattern can also rarely be seen in TCA overdose, but it may not be associated with increased frequency of arrhythmias and appears to resolve with appropriate treatment.[1]

Treatment

ECG Changes

Sodium bicarbonate should be considered in patients with a QRS of greater than 100 ms in suspected TCA overdose. In patients with old ECGs available demonstrating interventricular conduction delays and stable QRS interval, the QRS interval alone should not determine treatment. An initial bolus sodium bicarbonate will increase extracellular sodium, partially reversing TCA-induced sodium channel blockade through increased electrochemical gradient across cell membranes. In a bolus of sodium bicarbonate, the alkalinization is rapidly buffered but may be maintained with infusion. Alkalinization decreases sodium channel binding and decreases bioavailability of TCA through increased protein binding. Potassium concentrations should be closely monitored during sodium bicarbonate administration as potassium/hydrogen exchange to buffer bicarbonate may lead to hypokalemia through intracellular shift. The initial dose of sodium bicarbonate is widely accepted to be 1–2 mEq/kg, but it should be titrated based on improving QRS interval (on serial ECGs) and hypotension because there are case reports of patients receiving greater than 2,000 mEq of sodium bicarbonate total prior to achieving these goals.[1] In a survey of US poison center medical directors, 71% of respondents reported administering sodium bicarbonate as an initial bolus followed with infusion.[5] A target serum pH of 7.50 to 7.55 is recommended but care must be taken not to overalkalinize due primarily to increased risks of arrhythmia and seizure.[1] If this pH is reached without a narrow QRS interval, hypertonic saline is a reasonable alternative. In pig models, hypertonic saline may be even more effective at increasing blood pressure than sodium bicarbonate alone although sodium dosing in this study (15 mEq/kg) was five-fold that of sodium bicarbonate (3 mEq/kg).[6] It may be reasonable to provide hypertonic saline in equivalent Na+ dosage in substitute for sodium bicarbonate, especially when limited by excess alkalinization, noting that ionic concentration of Na+ in 3% saline is about half that of 8.6% sodium bicarbonate (twice the volume of 3% Na+ to get the same amount of Na+). Sodium acetate is a reasonable alternative to sodium bicarbonate as it provides both sodium and alkalinization because acetate is rapidly converted to bicarbonate through hepatic metabolization.

When sodium bicarbonate is not readily available at a given institution in volumes required for appropriate resuscitation, hypertonic saline and mechanical hyperventilation is a reasonable approach to achieve similar changes in sodium and pH. When comparing hyperventilation alone to hypertonic saline or sodium bicarbonate in pig models with TCA toxicity, there is decreased survival at 1 hour and no survival benefit compared to control.[7] Hyperventilation should only be considered as an adjunct to achieve target pH in patients receiving either sodium bicarbonate or hypertonic saline as primary therapy.

GI Decontamination

TCAs are almost completely absorbed from the GI tract. Early treatment should focus on decreasing GI absorption. Activated charcoal decreases the bioavailability of TCAs up to 4 hours following ingestion[7] and should be given to all neurologically intact patients who are not vomiting. Aspiration of charcoal may cause significant harm through pneumonitis and vomiting, or somnolence may be indications to intubate patients for airway protection to facilitate GI decontamination. Anecdotally, in a reliable story of a large TCA overdose (10–20 mg/kg) it would be reasonable to prophylactically intubate for GI decontamination in asymptomatic patients.

Hypotension

Hypotension in TCA overdose is a combination of cardiogenic and distributive shock. Sodium bicarbonate should be administered to all patients with suspected TCA overdose and hypotension. Sodium bicarbonate is the mainstay of treatment in TCA overdose and is useful in treatment of cardiogenic shock both by reversing cardiac fast Na^+ channel blockade via Na^+ overload and by decreasing intracellular binding of TCA to these channels via serum alkalinization. Sodium bicarbonate dosing and serum alkalinization are discussed in detail above.

Norepinephrine and epinephrine should be administered in patients who remain hypotensive despite appropriate volume expansion, sodium loading, and serum alkalinization. The primary benefit of these medications is likely peripheral alpha-adrenergic agonism, increasing vascular tone, as well as beta-adrenergic agonism to increase cardiac output. They also are direct-acting, which is beneficial as TCA toxicity may deplete intracellular stores of catecholamines by reuptake inhibition. Vasopressin may also be considered for refractory hypotension, given its unique mechanism through V_1 receptors leading to vasoconstriction and increased preload. While there are no trials documenting its efficacy in TCA toxicity, case reports and data from sepsis trials support at least consideration.[8]

Arrhythmias

Similar to hypotension, treatment of ventricular arrhythmias is primarily through sodium bicarbonate infusion at 1–2 mEq/kg to narrow the QRS segment, but be aware that, in TCA overdoses, arrhythmias may be refractory to treatment. For persistent ventricular arrhythmias despite maximal treatment, lidocaine and magnesium should be considered. Amiodarone should be avoided due to risk of QTc prolongation and further precipitation of ventricular arrhythmias. Class 1a and 1c antiarrhythmics should also not be used due to their inhibition of phase 0 depolarization. Although lidocaine has Na^+ channel blocking activity and is considered a class 1b antiarrhythmic, it does not affect phase 0 depolarization like TCAs, class 1a, and class 1c antiarrhythmic medications. Additionally, as it is a class 1b antidysrhythmic, it rapidly unbinds the sodium channel and does not prolong the QRS duration. Lidocaine may be more effective as an antiarrhythmic in amitriptyline and nortriptyline toxicity due to their prolonged duration of Na^+ channel binding.[9] The initial dose of lidocaine is a 1–2 mg/kg bolus over 1–2 minutes with subsequent infusion of 1–2 mg/min. Magnesium should also be considered in cases of persistent ventricular arrhythmia and is given as a 1–2 g initial bolus with repeat dosing of 1g every 6 hours for a QRS greater than 100 ms. While there are case reports of its efficacy in TCA overdose, randomized controlled trial data are poor, with significant heterogeneity in cases/controls.[10] Defibrillation is unlikely to reverse underlying Na+ channel blockade responsible for arrhythmia and is therefore unlikely to be helpful in either ventricular tachycardia or fibrillation.

Seizures

Treatment of seizures in the setting of TCA overdose does not significantly differ from standard protocols in first administering GABA agonists. Metabolic acidosis from seizures is, however, particularly dangerous in TCA toxicity as acidosis will liberate more of the protein-bound TCA molecules, potentially worsening the toxicity. Therefore, rapid control of seizure activity is essential. Benzodiazepines remain first-line for immediate treatment as TCA-induced seizures likely occur from central GABA inhibition. Administer additional benzodiazepines or another GABA-ergic agent such as propofol or a barbiturate for recurrent or prolonged seizures. Despite the antiepileptic and class Ib antiarrhythmic activity of phenytoin, it should be avoided due to conflicting evidence in animal trials, minimal human trial data, and concern for worsening of Na+ channel blockade. Last, the propylene glycol used as insipient with phenytoin may have a negative effect on arrhythmias and hypotension.[1]

Additional Therapy

Experimental therapies may be justified in patients with large overdose who are refractory to previously mentioned treatments. IV lipid emulsion infusion may be beneficial; however, it may not be readily available in many institutions, and supporting data are limited to case reports and animal studies. A possible mechanism of activity is by increasing the volume of distribution of the highly lipid-soluble TCA, resulting in shuttling of the medication away from the myocardium. There are several risks with IV lipid emulsion, particularly with prolonged use, including pancreatitis and acute respiratory distress syndrome, among others. Most studies dose IV lipid emulsion at 1.5 mL/kg bolused over 1–2 minutes as an initial dose.[11] Venoarterial extracorporeal membrane oxygenation

(VA ECMO) may also be considered for cardiopulmonary support in cases refractory to aggressive resuscitation.[1] TCAs are not readily filtered by hemodialysis as they have a large volume of distribution and are highly protein-bound. Therefore, hemodialysis is not a viable option for enhanced elimination.

Expected Course

After initial stabilization, patients with TCA toxicity may require prolonged serum alkalinization in the ICU setting. Despite maximum TCA serum concentrations being achieved in most patients within 24 hours, the half-life of TCA may be greatly extended and variable (half-life 25.3–81.4 hours in one case series) in overdose due to overwhelmed hepatic first-pass metabolization, correlating with prolonged intoxication.[12] TCA toxicity may also be seen in patients without overdose on chronic therapy: limited case reports describe anticholinergic symptoms, confusion, and ECG changes including QRS prolonged in patients with altered TCA metabolism, and TCA dose adjustment is recommended in these settings.[13] It may be difficult to distinguish chronic from acute toxicity in emergent settings if limited historical information is available.

Long-Term Concerns

There are no expected long-term sequelae in patients who recover from a TCA overdose.

CASE CONCLUSION

With the patient's clinical presentation and history, you are very concerned for a significant TCA overdose. You know the ECG changes and vital signs are indications for bicarbonate therapy and you start him at 1 mEq/kg as a bolus. You follow this by mixing 150 mEq of bicarbonate in 1 L of D5W infusing at 250 mL/hr. Due to his lack of response to fluids, you start him on a low-dose peripheral norepinephrine drip while the bicarbonate is infusing. Slowly, the patient's vitals begin to normalize, and his clinical picture improves. You call the ICU and are even able to stop the norepinephrine before the patient leaves the department.

- TCA toxicity can present with a variety of symptoms including antimuscarinic, anticholinergic, sympathomimetic toxidromes. Diagnosis of TCA toxicity requires strong clinical suspicion aided by characteristic ECG changes.
- The mainstay of treatment for TCA toxicity is serum alkalinization and hypernatremia with sodium bicarbonate, which should be administered to patients with suspected TCA overdose and QRS of greater than 100 ms, hypotension, ventricular arrhythmia, and seizure in an initial dose of 1–2 mEq/L.
- Activated charcoal and gut decontamination may have an increased role in TCA overdose due to delayed gastric emptying from anticholinergic effects.
- Lidocaine, despite sodium channel blockade, is the antiarrhythmic of choice in ventricular arrhythmia refractory to sodium bicarbonate.
- Additional therapies, such as extracorporeal membrane oxygenation (ECMO) and IV intralipid, may be indicated but are institution-dependent.

Further Reading

Abeyaratne DD, Liyanapathirana C, Gamage A, Karunarathne P, Botheju M, Indrakumar J. Survival after severe amitriptyline poisoning with prolonged ventricular tachycardia and cardiac arrest. *BMC Res Notes*. 2016;9:167. doi:10.1186/s13104-016-1963-0

Goldfrank's Toxicologic Emergencies. 10th ed., McGraw Hill; 2015: chapter 71.

Gupta V, Gupta R, Wander GS. Role of ECMO in life threatening intoxication. *Egypt J Crit Care Med*. 2018;6(3):103–109.

Odigwe CC, Tariq M, Kotecha T, et al. Tricyclic antidepressant overdose treated with adjunctive lipid rescue and plasmapheresis. *Proc (Bayl Univ Med Cent)*. 2016;29(3):284–287. doi:10.1080/08998280.2016.11929437

References

1. Liebelt EL. Cyclic antidepressants. In: Hoffman RS, Howland M, Lewin NA, Nelson LS, Goldfrank LR. eds. *Goldfrank's Toxicologic Emergencies*. 10th ed. McGraw Hill; 2015. Accessed March 16, 2022. https://accessemergencymedicine.mhmedical.com/content.aspx?bookid=1163&sectionid=65097419

2. Lavoie F M, Gansert G M, Weiss R M. Value of initial ECG findings and plasma drug levels in cyclic antidepressant overdose. *Ann Emerg Med.* 1990;19(6):696–700.

3. Boehnert M, Lovejoy F. Value of the QRS duration versus the serum drug level in predicting seizures and ventricular arrhythmias after an acute overdose of tricyclic antidepressants. *N Engl J Med.* 1985;313:474–479. doi:10.1056/NEJM198508223130804

4. Liebelt EL, Francis PD, Woolf AD. ECG lead aVR versus QRS interval in predicting seizures and arrhythmias in acute tricyclic antidepressant toxicity. *Ann. Emerg. Med.* 1995;26(2):195–201.

5. Seger D, Hantsch C, Zavoral T, Wrenn K. Variability of recommendations for serum alkalization in tricyclic antidepressant overdose: a survey of U.S. poison center medical directors. *J Clin Toxicol.* 2003;41(4):331–338.

6. McCabe JL, Daniel J, Cobaugh J, Menegazzi JJ, Fata J. Experimental tricyclic antidepressant toxicity: a randomized, controlled comparison of hypertonic saline solution, sodium bicarbonate, and hyperventilation. *Ann Emerg Med.* 1998;32(3):329–333.

7. Dawling S, Crome P, Braithwaite R. Effect of delayed administration of activated charcoal on nortriptyline absorption. *Eur J Clin Pharmacol.* 1978;14(6):445–457. doi:10.1007/BF00716388

8. Barry JD, Durkovich DW, Williams SR. Vasopressin treatment for cyclic antidepressant overdose. *J Emerg Med.* 2006;31(1):65–68. doi:10.1016/j.jemermed.2005.08.01

9. Barber MJ, Starmer CF, Grant AO. Blockade of cardiac sodium channels by amitriptyline and diphenylhydantoin. evidence for two use-dependent binding sites. *Circulation Research.* 1991;69(3):677–696. doi:10.1161/01.res.69.3.677

10. Emamhadi M, Mostafazadeh B, Hassanijirdehi M. Tricyclic antidepressant poisoning treated by magnesium sulfate: A randomized, clinical trial. *Drug Chem Toxicol.* 2012;35(3):300–303. doi:10.3109/01480545.2011.61424

11. Chibuzo Clement Odigwe M, Madiha Tariq M, Tulsi Kotecha M, et al. Tricyclic antidepressant overdose treated with adjunctive lipid rescue and plasmapheresis. *Proc (Bayl Univ Med Cent).* 2016;29(3):284–287.

12. Spiker DG, Biggs JT. Tricyclic antidepressants: prolonged plasma levels after overdose. *JAMA.* 1976;236(15):1711–1712. doi:10.1001/jama.1976.03270160033025

13. Giller E, Bialos D, Docherty J, Jatlow P, Harkness L. Chronic amitriptyline toxicity. *Clinical Research.* 1979;136(4):458–459.

15 Don't Lose Your Ear Over Cardiac Glycosides: Cardiac Glycoside Toxicity Management

Marshall Howell, Girgis Fahmy, and Emily Kiernan

Case Presentation

A 62-year-old man with a past medical history of congestive heart failure (CHF) and hypertension presents to the ED with a chief complaint of abdominal pain, diarrhea, and emesis over the past week. The patient is lethargic and unable to provide a history. His wife is at bedside and reports that he was diagnosed with viral gastroenteritis last week. She states that over the past day he has been more fatigued and complained of palpitations. The patient's home medications include aspirin, atorvastatin, lisinopril, digoxin, and torsemide. His vital signs are heart rate 56 beats/min, blood pressure 109/56 mm Hg, respiratory rate 20 breaths/min, temperature 98.7°F/37°C, and O_2 100% on room air. On examination, you see an uncomfortable-appearing male who is actively vomiting. The nurse hands you

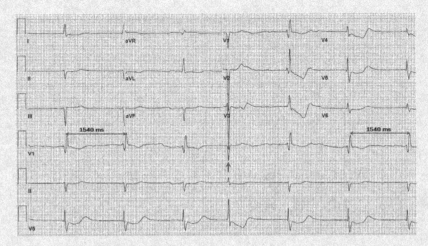

FIGURE 15.1 Triage ECG.

Reprinted from *The American Journal of Medicine*, 131/9, Rami Reddy Manne, J. "Regularized Atrial Fibrillation," 361–363, 2018, with permission from Elsevier.

his triage ECG (Figure 15.1). The patient's labs are notable for potassium 5.4 mEq/L, blood urea nitrogen (BUN) 47 mg/dL, creatinine (Cr) 2.2 mg/dL (previously 1.1 mg/dL), and total digoxin 10.1 ng/mL (normal range is 0.8–2.0 ng/mL).

What Do You Do Now?

DISCUSSION

Background

Digoxin is derived from digitoxin, a cardioactive glycoside found in the fox-glove plant (*Digitalis spp.*). Additional cardiac glycoside-containing plants including pink oleander (*Nerium oleander*), yellow oleander (*Thevetia peruviana*), and lily of the valley (*Convallaria majalis*) have resulted in human toxicity after ingestion. Aside from plants, cardiac glycosides have been isolated from the secretions of the common toad (*Bufonidae* species), which has been used as an aphrodisiac.[1,2] While digoxin is the most commercially available cardiac glycoside in the United States, other preparations, including digitoxin, ouabain, lanatoside C, deslanoside, and gitalin, may be seen internationally.

Despite a roughly 50% decline in digoxin prescriptions from 2013 to 2019,[3] digoxin and other forms of cardiac glycoside toxicity remain prevalent. Digoxin toxicity affects 1% of CHF patients who are treated with digoxin, and 1% of all adverse drug effects in patients older than 40 years are due to digoxin. In the pediatric population, 80% of cardiac glycoside toxicity is due to plant ingestions while the other 20% are due to digoxin.[4]

Toxicology and Pathophysiology

Digoxin inhibits the Na^+-K^+-ATPase in cardiac myocytes. This causes increased intracellular Na^+, which disrupts the typical sodium gradient and leads to an elevated intracellular Na^+, which in turns decreases the activation of the Na^+/Ca^{2+} exchanger, which normally transports three Na^+ ions into the cell in exchange for exporting one Ca^{2+} out of the cell. This in turn leads to an increased intracellular concentration of $Ca2^+$, which causes a Ca^{2+} dependent Ca^{2+} release from the sarcoplasm reticulum. This increased intracellular potassium binds to troponin, which during depolarization causes enhanced inotropy.[1] Within digoxin's narrow therapeutic range, this improves contractility in patients with severe heart failure. In excess, digoxin raises the resting membrane potential, which can lead to myocardial sensitization, dysrhythmia, and risk of sudden cardiac death. In addition, digoxin also increases vagal tone, leading to slowed AV nodal conduction, thus controlling atrial tachydysrhythmias at therapeutic doses.[4]

By this mechanism, digoxin toxicity is associated with a slowed ventricular response in patients with atrial fibrillation.

Digoxin is 70% renally cleared, therefore, compromised kidney function from medication side effects or dehydration can lead to toxicity.[1] Certain medications such as amiodarone, calcium antagonists, and medications that lead to hypokalemia, hypomagnesemia, and hypercalcemia can also potentiate toxicity. Thirty percent of digoxin is protein bound and therefore a reduction in total body protein may increase serum concentrations of unbound, "free" digoxin.[5] Digoxin takes approximately 6 hours after ingestion to fully distribute into body tissues, so levels acquired prior to 6 hours can be deceivingly high,[1] However, the half-life may be up to 40 hours in overdose.[4]

The two mechanisms of activity result in the ECG changes at both toxic and therapeutic digoxin levels. At therapeutic levels, ECGs will show "scooped ST-segments" known as the "Salvador Dali sign," biphasic T-waves, and shortened QT intervals. Digoxin toxicity manifests the same ECG changes seen at therapeutic levels but also may result in nearly any dysrhythmia, except for supraventricular tachycardia due to AV nodal blockade. Box 15.1 demonstrates the wide array of potential dysrhythmias. In acute toxicity, heart block and bradyarrhythmias are more common. However, in chronic toxicity, tachydysrhythmias predominate. Premature ventricular complexes (PVCs) are seen in most cases of digoxin toxicity.[1]

BOX 15.1 Common dysrhythmias in cardiac glycoside toxicity

Atrial flutter or fibrillation with AV block
Bidirectional ventricular tachycardia
Junctional tachycardia
Nonsustained ventricular tachycardia
Premature and sustained ventricular tachycardia
Sinus bradycardia
Ventricular bigeminy
Ventricular fibrillation

From Hack.[1]

Workup and Diagnosis

History and Symptoms

History is one of the most vital components in patients presenting with possible digoxin toxicity. After an acute ingestion, the patient or family member will typically describe an attempt at self-harm, exploratory ingestion by a pediatric patient, or inadvertent overdose. A patient with a chronic ingestion may describe a history of increased fluid loss, decreased oral intake, or some other historical feature that would be concerning for acute renal impairment (as with our patient), initiation or discontinuation of a new medication, or a comorbidity that reduces total body protein.

Clinical symptomatology of digoxin toxicity can be similar in acute and chronic ingestions. The key difference is the onset of symptoms. Most common symptoms seen in both acute and chronic cases include anorexia, nausea, vomiting, and abdominal pain.[4] Patients then typically develop neurological symptoms such as lethargy, confusion, weakness, and visual changes. Visual changes are variable but the most common is xanthopsia or yellow-tinted vision. The neurological symptoms seen in cardiac glycoside toxicity are typically due to distribution of the drug into the CNS, not due to hypoperfusion. However, hypoperfusion can be seen in hemodynamically unstable patients. Patients with acute ingestions are usually asymptomatic, developing symptoms several hours later after full drug distribution. Chronic ingestions have a more indolent onset that can vary from days to months. In addition, symptoms vary from mild GI symptoms to altered mental status (as with our patient), headache, and, rarely, seizures.[6]

Diagnostic Testing

The initial approach to diagnosis and monitoring of the patient with suspected digoxin toxicity centers on total serum digoxin concentration and serum electrolytes, serial ECGs, and continuous telemetry monitoring.

When obtaining serum digoxin concentrations, it is important to understand whether the value provided is total (including protein-bound) or free serum digoxin. Most institutions test for total serum digoxin and have established 0.5–2.0 ng/mL as the therapeutic range. However, this concentration must be interpreted in the context of the absolute serum level, the timing of the last digoxin dose, and the time of the blood draw. Values obtained less than 6 hours from ingestion do not accurately reflect tissue concentration and may be spuriously elevated due to incomplete distribution. Six hours after the last dose, serum total digoxin has been shown to accurately predict cardiac concentrations.[7] The patient's clinical condition should also be considered when interpreting serum concentrations to help guide intervention decisions. While absolute values may vary between facilities, general guidelines indicate aggressive treatment for patients with serum digoxin concentration of 15 ng/mL or greater at any time post-ingestion or 10 ng/mL 6 or more hours after ingestion, regardless of symptoms.[1]

As previously mentioned, acute or chronic renal dysfunction can impair digoxin clearance and may precipitate toxicity. Serum BUN and creatinine for comparison to baseline values may be helpful, if available. Serum electrolyte concentrations in cardiac glycoside overdose are important for prognostication, guiding therapeutic interventions, and preventing worsening toxicity. Serum potassium has been shown to be the most reliable predictor of overdose mortality, greater than ECG changes or serum digoxin concentrations.[8] Hypokalemia, specifically levels of less than 2.5 mEq/L, potentiates digoxin's effects on the Na^+-K^+-ATPase through decreased competitive inhibition at the binding site.[1] Similarly, hypomagnesemia hinders potassium absorption and decreases Na^+-K^+-ATPase function.[1] Both electrolyte deficiencies should be corrected to help with cardiac stabilization in acute or chronic toxicity. Hyperkalemia (>5.0 mEq/L) has been shown to be a predictor of, but not cause for, mortality in both acute and chronic overdose.[8,9] Digoxin blockade of the Na^+-K^+-ATPase prevents transport of potassium into skeletal and cardiac muscle, thus increasing serum concentrations. Renal dysfunction and chronic digoxin toxicity may contribute to hyperkalemia. Severe hyperkalemia (>5–5.5 mEq/L) contributes to AV nodal blockade in a mechanism separate from digoxin, potentiating bradydysrhythmias.

Treatment

Decontamination and Elimination

Activated charcoal (1 g/kg of body weight every 2–4 hours for up to four doses) is recommended in toxic patients to reduce serum concentrations if there is a delay in digoxin-specific antibody fragment (DSFab) administration or when kidney function is decreased.[1] If the patient is encephalopathic or acutely intoxicated, endotracheal intubation may be required prior to administering activated charcoal. Great caution should be used if the patient is experiencing nausea or vomiting due to the concern for charcoal aspiration and pneumonitis. Unfortunately, due to the drug's large volume of distribution and high protein binding, hemodialysis is ineffective. However, dialysis may be used to manage refractory hyperkalemia in end-stage renal disease (ESRD) patients with acute or chronic toxicity.

Digoxin-Specific Antibody Fragments

The definitive therapy for life-threatening digoxin toxicity is DSFab administration. DSFab works to bind intravascular free digoxin and extract free digoxin from the tissues to the intravascular space. The Fab-bound digoxin is inactivated and renally cleared. By removing digoxin from the tissues, the Na^+-K^+-ATPase is freed, leading to influx of potassium into cells and lowered serum potassium concentrations. Each vial contains 40 mg of DSFab, which will bind 0.5 mg of ingested digoxin.[10] Typical DSFab infusions run over 30 minutes but may be bolused for unstable patients. Full effect is seen at 90 minutes, but initial effects begin within 20 minutes.[4] Indications for DSFab administration (Box 15.2) and dosing instructions (Box 15.3) are listed below.

BOX 15.2   **Indications for DSFab administration**

Life-threatening arrhythmias, including wide complex tachycardia, ventricular fibrillation, bradydysrhythmias such as atropine-resistant sinus bradycardia or 3rd-degree AV block)
Potassium >5 mEq/L
Chronic toxicity with dysrhythmias, GI symptoms, or AMS
SDC >15 ng/mL at any time or ≥10 6 hours post-ingestion, regardless of toxidrome
Acute ingestion of ≥10 mg in adults
Acute ingestion of ≥4 mg in a child
Poisoning with a non-dig CAS

Altered mental status (AMS); Cardioactive steroid (CAS); Serum digoxin concentration (SDC).
From Hack.[1]

Number of vials = Serum Drug Concentration (ng/mL) × patient
   weight (kg) ÷ 100
OR
Number of vials = Amount ingested (mg) × 80% bioavailability × 2
   (0.5 mg/vial)
Empiric therapy for acute poisoning: 10–20 vials
Empiric therapy for chronic poisoning: Adults, 3–6 vials; children, 1–2
   vials

From Hack1 and Cummings, Swoboda.4

When assessing for lab value improvement after DSFab administration, it
is important to recognize that, due to its mechanism of action, DSFab dra-
matically *increases* the total serum digoxin concentration. However, much of
that concentration is bound to the antibody fragments and is not contributing to toxicity. Due to this deceivingly elevated value, checking digoxin
levels after DSFab administration is not recommended. Instead, response to
treatment is monitored via resolution of dysrhythmias on ECG or telemetry.[10]

Last, when administering DSFab, it is important to acknowledge potential adverse effects. Particularly in patients taking digoxin for chronic
atrial fibrillation or CHF, DSFab reverses the beneficial effects of digoxin
and may precipitate atrial fibrillation with rapid ventricular response or
acute decompensated heart failure. There are also reports of rebound hypokalemia in pediatric patients since the whole-body potassium stores may
be decreased due to increased renal elimination in response to the increase
extravascular potassium.[11]

Managing Dysrhythmias and Hemodynamic Instability

In the setting of digoxin toxicity with dysrhythmias and hemodynamic instability, the definitive treatment is to administer DSFab. However, before
the advent of DSFab, cardioactive medications, cardioversion/defibrillation,
cardiac pacing, and electrolyte supplementation were used in the treatment
of digoxin toxicity. If DSFab is not readily available, these interventions can
be considered.

Atropine may be used to treat bradydysrhythmias or high-degree AV blocks. Doses of 0.5 mg in adults and 0.02 mg/kg in children have been administered with varying degrees of efficacy, likely attributable to digoxin's AV node depressant action being only partially vagally mediated.[1] Slow infusions of phenytoin (50 mg/min) may increase AV node dromotropy (conduction speed) and suppress supraventricular dysrhythmias with variable success.[1] Lidocaine (1–1.5 mg/kg IV bolus followed by continuous infusion at 1–4 mg/min) may also be used as an antidysrhythmic but has been shown to be less effective than phenytoin.[1,4]

In the setting of digoxin toxicity, synchronized cardioversion is associated with conversion to lethal ventricular arrhythmias and is not recommended.[12] However, unsynchronized defibrillation for pulseless wide complex tachycardia or ventricular fibrillation, in accordance with advanced cardiac life support (ACLS) guidelines, is indicated. Transvenous or transthoracic cardiac pacing are only recommended in the event of delay or failure of DSFab administration.[13]

In patients with dysrhythmia and hypokalemia, DSFab administration should be held until after potassium supplementation as the repletion may treat the dysrhythmia and DSFab may worsen the potassium derangement.[1] However, if the patient is hyperkalemic, medical management of the potassium should be handled judiciously to avoid iatrogenic hypokalemia and potentially worsening toxicity. Hypomagnesemia should also be repleted to help with potassium and calcium homeostasis in the cardiac myocytes.[1]

Typical management of hyperkalemic patients with ECG changes includes calcium gluconate or calcium chloride administration. However, animal and low-level evidence have previously suggested increased mortality in digoxin toxicity after administration of calcium solutions. The hypothesized mechanism, also known as "stone heart" syndrome, involves myocyte hypercontractility and tetany due to calcium supplementation in the setting of increased intracellular calcium due to digoxin.[1] No recent studies have been able to reproduce a similar outcome,[14–16] but calcium continues to be avoided in acute digoxin toxicity due to the availability of DSFab. However, if during the workup and treatment of the patient calcium is ordered in response to hyperkalemia, one should not worry about causing harm as there is no evidence a 1 gm dose of calcium will lead to adverse effects in digoxin toxicity.

CASE CONCLUSION

The patient's history is concerning for acute renal failure in the setting of viral gastroenteritis. This has led to decreased clearance of digoxin and thus has caused toxicity in this patient. This patient's elevated potassium (>5.0 mEq/L) correlated with a higher risk of mortality and will require hemodynamic monitoring in an ICU. DSFab is the primary treatment for digoxin toxicity and was given to this patient. The patient improved overnight in the ICU and was transferred to the floor the following day.

KEY POINTS TO REMEMBER

- While acute toxicity is often accidental or an attempt at self-harm, chronic toxicity is often more insidious, resulting from alterations in serum proteins or renal function.
- Maintaining potassium balance before and after treatment is crucial to the management of digoxin toxicity. Hypokalemia may potentiate digoxin's toxic effects, while hyperkalemia may be a result of toxicity and worsen dysrhythmias.
- DSFab is the definitive treatment for digoxin toxicity. Key indications for DSFab administration include life-threatening dysrhythmias, potassium greater than 5 mEq/L, serum digoxin concentration greater than 15 ng/mL at any time, or more than 10 ng/mL 6 hours post-ingestion.
- After DSFab administration, total serum digoxin levels will be deceptively elevated due to extraction of digoxin from tissues into the intravascular space. Response to treatment is monitored by improvement in dysrhythmias on ECG or telemetry.
- Although toxicity is commonly seen in medication ingestion, toads, plants, and other organisms also can contain cardioactive steroids

---

Further Reading

Cummings ED, Swoboda HD. Digoxin toxicity. StatPearls [Internet]. 2022. Accessed February 28, 2022. http://www.ncbi.nlm.nih.gov/books/NBK470568/

Hack JB. Cardioactive steroids. In: Nelson LS, Howland MA, Lewin NA, Smith SW, Goldfrank LR, Hoffman RS, eds. *Goldfrank's Toxicologic Emergencies*. 11th ed. McGraw-Hill Education; 2019.

Smith SW, Howland MA. Digoxin-specific antibody fragments. In: Nelson LS, Howland MA, Lewin NA, Smith SW, Goldfrank LR, Hoffman RS, eds. *Goldfrank's Toxicologic Emergencies*. 11th ed. McGraw-Hill Education; 2019.

References

1. Hack JB. Cardioactive steroids. In: Nelson LS, Howland MA, Lewin NA, Smith SW, Goldfrank LR, Hoffman RS, eds. *Goldfrank's Toxicologic Emergencies*. 11th ed. McGraw-Hill Education; 2019. Accessed February 28, 2022. accesspharmacy. mhmedical.com/content.aspx?aid=1163013608

2. Brubacher JR, Lachmanen D, Ravikumar PR, Hoffman RS. Efficacy of digoxin specific Fab fragments (Digibind®) in the treatment of toad venom poisoning. *Toxicon*. 1999;37(6):931–942. doi:10.1016/S0041-0101(98)00224-4

3. Digoxin: drug usage statistics, 2013–2019, ClinCalc. Updated Sep 12, 2021. Accessed February 28, 2022. https://clincalc.com/DrugStats/Drugs/Digoxin.

4. Cummings ED, Swoboda HD. Digoxin toxicity. StatPearls [Internet]. 2022. Accessed February 28, 2022. http://www.ncbi.nlm.nih.gov/books/NBK470568/

5. Lip GY, Metcalfe MJ, Dunn FG. Diagnosis and treatment of digoxin toxicity. *Postgrad Med J*. 1993;69(811):337–339.

6. Bhatia SJ. Digitalis toxicity—turning over a new leaf? *West J Med*. 1986;145(1):74–82.

7. Kelly RA, Smith TW. Recognition and management of digitalis toxicity. *Am J Cardiol*. 1992;69(18):108–119. doi:10.1016/0002-9149(92)91259-7.

8. Bismuth C, Gaultier M, Conso F, Efthymiou ML. Hyperkalemia in acute digitalis poisoning: prognostic significance and therapeutic implications. *Clin Toxicol*. 1973;6(2):153–162. doi:10.3109/15563657308990513

9. Manini AF, Nelson LS, Hoffman RS. Prognostic utility of serum potassium in chronic digoxin toxicity. *Am J Cardiovasc Drugs*. 2011;11(3):173–178. doi:10.2165/ 11590340-000000000-00000

10. Smith SW, Howland MA. Digoxin-specific antibody fragments. In: Nelson LS, Howland MA, Lewin NA, Smith SW, Goldfrank LR, Hoffman RS, eds. *Goldfrank's Toxicologic Emergencies*. 11th ed. McGraw-Hill Education; 2019. Accessed February 28, 2022. accesspharmacy.mhmedical.com/content.aspx?aid=1163002783

11. Woolf AD, Wenger T, Smith TW, Lovejoy FH. The use of digoxin-specific fab fragments for severe digitalis intoxication in children. *N Engl J Med*. 1992;326(26):1739–1744. doi:10.1056/NEJM199206253262604.

12. Sarubbi B, Ducceschi V, D'Andrea A, Liccardo B, Santangelo L, Iacono A. Atrial fibrillation: what are the effects of drug therapy on the effectiveness and complications of electrical cardioversion? *Can J Cardiol*. 1998;14(10):1267–1273.

13. Bismuth C, Motte G, Conso F, Chauvin M, Gaultier M. Acute digitoxin intoxication treated by intracardiac pacemaker: experience in sixty-eight patients. *Clin Toxicol.* 1977;10(4):443–456. doi:10.3109/15563657709046282

14. Hack JB, Woody JH, Lewis DE, Brewer K, Meggs WJ. The effect of calcium chloride in treating hyperkalemia due to acute digoxin toxicity in a porcine model. *J Toxicol Clin Toxicol.* 2004;42(4):337–342. doi:10.1081/clt-120039538

15. Fenton F, Smally AJ, Laut J. Hyperkalemia and digoxin toxicity in a patient with kidney failure. *Ann Emerg Med.* 1996;28(4):440–441. doi:10.1016/S0196-0644(96)70012-4

16. Van Deusen SK, Birkhahn RH, Gaeta TJ. Treatment of hyperkalemia in a patient with unrecognized digitalis toxicity. *J Toxicol Clin Toxicol.* 2003;41(4):373–376. doi:10.1081/clt-120022006

16 The (Lack of) Benefit of a Screening Urine Drug Screen

Rebecca Ervin and

Pradeep Padmanabhan

Case Presentation

You are working solo coverage in a small, community ED approximately 50 minutes from a tertiary referral center. Police arrive with a 40-year-old man picked up after a convenience store called for a disruptive customer making violent and suicidal threats. As you are assessing the patient, you are called out of the room.

EMS is rolling in with a seizing 2-year-old girl. She is maintaining her airway with an SpO_2 96% on 15 L facemask. IV access was established en route, and you give 0.05 mg/kg lorazepam intravenously with cessation of seizure activity. She is unresponsive, responding minimally to painful stimuli. There are no external signs of trauma. She has a small laceration to the right side of her tongue. Her cardiopulmonary exam reveals a tachycardic, regular rhythm, and clear breath sounds. Her abdomen is soft with a slightly distended lower abdomen. Her skin is warm and dry.

After appropriately stabilizing both patients, you order a basic laboratory analysis including a urine drug screen (UDS). The lab calls to let you know they are short-staffed, and each UDS will have to be run manually and will take approximately 90 minutes after collection to result.

What Do You Do Now?

DISCUSSION

Background

The National Institute on Drug Abuse (NIDA) was founded in 1974 in response to rising substance use in the 1960s. Its original mission centered around identifying illicit substance use in transportation workers to protect the public from unsafe operators. The NIDA-5 panel screens for marijuana, amphetamines, cocaine, opiates (principally heroin, codeine, and morphine) and phencyclidine. At the time of its development, these were the five most commonly abused substances. In 1975, the Monitoring the Future Survey began monitoring trends in legal and illicit substance use in American teens. In 1992, NIDA became part of National Institutes of Health under the United States Department of Health and Human Research. Much of its work is dedicated to the longitudinal study of the biological, behavioral, and social components of substance use and its impact on society.

Chemistry

The most common UDSs performed in occupational and healthcare settings utilize immunoassays because they are inexpensive, easy to use, and yield rapid presumptive results. Sometimes the antibodies are developed to detect a parent compound, but more frequently they are designed to detect a metabolite of the parent compound. Despite their prevalent use, immunoassay UDSs are neither highly sensitive nor highly specific. Antibodies on the test medium screen for epitopes on an antigen in the urine which identify families of drugs containing similar epitopes. Because the antibody does not bind a single, specific antigen, xenobiotics with similar epitopes can cross-react with the probe, causing a presumptive positive result in the absence of the drug due to a similar chemical structure of the epitope (a false positive)[1]. Similarly, drugs which have been crudely formulated or adulterated may have sufficiently dissimilar chemical structures as not to be bound by the antibody probe and thus missed as a false negative. Immunoassays also depend on a threshold of bound antibody–antigen binding to indicate a positive result. Therefore, delayed testing or dilute specimens are additional reasons for obtaining a false-negative result.

Presumptive positive immunoassays can be confirmed by gas chromatography-mass spectrometry (GC-MS) or liquid chromatography-mass spectrometry (LC-MS). However, these studies are much more expensive, time-consuming, and impractical for routine screening purposes in a hospital setting.

Serum Toxicology Studies

UDSs yield qualitative results. In most circumstances of drugs of abuse, quantity of substance use is rarely, if ever, clinically significant as the clinical severity of presenting symptoms is more important and the actual concentration of the substance may not correlate well with the severity of toxicity depending on the patient's tolerance for the xenobiotic[2]. Substances such as ethanol, salicylates, and acetaminophen have much greater clinical implications at toxic levels. Serum salicylate and acetaminophen studies directly analyze and quantify the parent compounds in the serum reported as mg/dL and guide management in patients with chronic or acute ingestion. Ethanol levels are similarly analyzed and reported in g/dL, commonly referred to as "blood alcohol content."

Limitations

UDSs yield presumptive positive or presumptive negative results. These are determined by a threshold of substance detected, most commonly in ng/mL[3]. Opium is known to be naturally occurring in some commonly consumed foods, such as poppy seeds. When consumed in sufficiently high quantities (greater than what would be found in a single serving of poppy seed cake or a poppy seed bagel), low levels of opiates can be detected by a UDS. However, phencyclidine (PCP) is not known to naturally occur in commonly consumed products. Thus, the threshold for positive PCP result on a UDS is low at 25 ng/mL. To avoid positive results due to incidental ingestion of opiate-containing products, the threshold for a positive screening for opiates is much higher at 2,000 ng/mL. Therefore, interpretation of a negative result must be considered with caution as the xenobiotic may be detectable but below the threshold value for the reporting of a positive result[3].

There is no comprehensive opioid drug screen. Novel non-fentanyl synesthetic opioids are emerging contaminants with varying potency and toxicity. "Nitazenes" such as isotonitazene, metonitazeme, and etonitazene comprise the benzimidazole class. These substances act as mu-receptor agonists in the same way as traditional opiates and opioids but have stronger affinity for the receptor, resulting in increased potency compared to fentanyl[4]. The nitazine metabolite, N-desethylisotonitazene does not cross-react with UDS immunoassays or fentanyl test strips. A patient who used a substance contaminated with a novel non-fentanyl synthetic opioid will demonstrate an opioid toxidrome and can have a negative opioid drug screen.

Timing is a key limitation in urine drug detection. In a patient who used a substance for the first time and immediately comes to the ED, the substance may not have been metabolized and eliminated in the urine in sufficient quantities to be detectable in the urine until 1–2 hours post-exposure[2]. Conversely, because of its high lipid solubility, some heavy users of marijuana may have detectable metabolites for more than 40 days. Most common substances such as cocaine, amphetamines, and benzodiazepines are detectable as early as 1 hour and sufficiently excreted and cleared by hour 48, or 2 days after use[5].

The UDS is most helpful in screening for a specific substance that the UDS is known to be sensitive to. Examples include monitoring intended use of a prescribed, controlled substance such as opiates in patients with chronic pain, or screening for accidental ingestion of a known substance by a child. Although commonly ordered for undifferentiated patients with altered mental status, a negative screen does not adequately rule out substance use contributing to the clinical picture, as discussed below, and a positive screen, even if a true positive, does not necessarily tell you anything about the patient's present condition because the use may have been several days or more ago[5,6].

Specific Tests

Opiate. Opiates are naturally derived from poppy seeds and include morphine and codeine. Heroin is included in this class, since even though it is considered a semisynthetic opioid (diacetyl-morphine), it is metabolized to morphine and will trigger a positive urine opiate UDS. Heroin can be specifically identified by an immunoassay that targets 6-monoacetylmorphine

(6-MAM), a metabolite unique to heroin. Rifampin, the quinolone antibiotic class, dextromethorphan, and consumption of a significant quantity of poppy seeds are all known to cause positive opiate screens[7].

Opioids are synthetic derivatives which are mu-receptor agonists and produce similar effects as opiates. They include drugs such as methadone, hydrocodone, oxycodone, tramadol, and fentanyl, among an ever-growing long list of other synthetic agents. However, there is vast variation in the chemical structures within this class. Thus, it is becoming increasingly common to run separate tests in addition to the UDS to screen specifically for methadone and fentanyl, as discussed below under "other specific tests."

Cannabinoid. 11-nor-Δ^9-tetrahydrocannabinol-9-carboxylic acid (11-nor-Δ^9-THC-9-COOH) is the major urinary metabolite of Δ^9-tetrahydrocannabinol (THC) and is commonly used on standard UDSs[7]. Hemp plants contain very low levels of THC. Some health companies include hemp plant seeds and extracts in powders and energy bars which can cause a positive result for THC on a UDS[7]. Isolation of cannabidiol (CBD) from its THC counterpart for the production and use of homeopathic remedies is an imperfect process, and small amounts of THC can be absorbed and detected. Other common medications such as nonsteroidal anti-inflammatory drugs, efavirenz, and proton pump inhibitors have the potential to cause false positives[5,7]. Dronabinol is a controlled, prescribed synthetic cannabinoid. Patients taking dronabinol as prescribed will have a positive UDS for cannabinoids, making detection of concurrent, illicit cannabinoid use impossible to determine using a traditional immunoassay-based UDS.

In an effort to mimic marijuana's psychoactive effects without detection by drug screen, synthetic cannabinoids such as K2 or "spice" have also risen in popularity. These are commonly made by spraying synthetic cannabinoid compounds onto inert plant or vegetation which is then ground and smoked. Although classified as cannabinoid because of activity at the CB_1 and CB_2 cannabinoid receptor, these chemical structures are dissimilar to that of THC and thus not detected by UDS.

Cocaine. Of all the classes detected by a UDS, cocaine—a methyl ester of benzoyl ecgonine—can be detected with the most accuracy, with few if any instances of false positives or false negatives. Although it is frequently diluted or "cut" with other "white powders," its chemical structure is rarely manipulated or truly adulterated, and the UDS has high sensitivity for benzoylecgonine, its main metabolite[3]. Topical cocaine anesthetic spray is rarely used for medical procedures but can result in a true positive for nonabuse reasons.

Amphetamines. Amphetamines as a class include illicit drugs as well as pharmaceutical agents. Amphetamines and methamphetamines have a relatively simple biochemical structure, which makes development of specific antibody assays for illicit substances challenging. Additionally, both amphetamine and methamphetamine are medications approved by the US Food and Drug Administration (FDA). Many commonly prescribed medications such as labetalol, metformin, promethazine, and trazadone as well as common decongestants such as pseudoephedrine and phenylephrine, can cross-react and cause false-positive UDS amphetamine results[5,7]. The monoamine oxidase B inhibitor selegiline is metabolized to levomethamphetamine and will also result in a positive UDS. Amphetamines have many clinical, therapeutic uses, specifically in treatment of attention deficit disorders and narcolepsy. This class has also been prescribed to military pilots conducting tactical operations during prolonged missions for sustained alertness. Other common illicit substances, such as bath salts (synthetic cathinones) or 3,4-methylenedioxymethamphetamine—more commonly known as MDMA, ecstasy, or molly—can result in false negatives but may also result in a positive analysis depending on the assay used[5].

Phencyclidine. Phencyclidine or "PCP" use has declined in popularity, however, it is occasionally used to adulterate other substances such as marijuana. The classic false-positive example is a patient who has recently taken diphenhydramine. Other substances known to cause false positives include dextromethorphan, tramadol, ketamine, lamotrigine, or venlafaxine[5].

Other Specific Tests: TCA, Fentanyl, Methadone

Tricyclic antidepressants (TCAs) are not commonly thought of as drugs of abuse, but they have a narrow therapeutic index and can be lethal in small doses. Intentional or unintentional ingestion has significant clinical implications, and detection guides management. Thus, specific TCA testing has been developed and is sometimes utilized.

Fentanyl. Fentanyl is a short-acting synthetic opioid used pharmaceutically and found in street drugs. It is well-known and highly potent. Fentanyl is not detected on standard UDSs and thus specific fentanyl immunoassay reagents have been developed[5,8]. In addition to hospital setting drug testing, these tests have also been made available commercially, known as Fentanyl Test Strips (FTS) for community use. However, false positives have occurred with methamphetamine, MDMA, and diphenhydramine[8]. Additionally, the fentanyl class of synthetic opioids is heterogenous and varies in the chemical structure of the class's members. Therefore, while the fentanyl UDS will detect fentanyl with a high degree of accuracy, it should not be expected to detect alfentanil, carfentanil, furanylfentanyl, or many other fentanyl analogs.

Methadone. Methadone is a long-acting synthetic opioid commonly prescribed to treat opioid use disorder but also prescribed to some patients with chronic pain. Unlike buprenorphine, which is a partial agonist, methadone is a full mu-receptor agonist, giving it higher potential for overdose if misused. The primary methadone metabolite is 2-ethylidene-1,5-dimethyl-3,3-diphenylpyrrolidine (EDDP). Methadone maintenance monitoring may utilize the methadone:EDDP ratio to determine compliance[9]. Although less commonly utilized, methadone plasma testing is available and can give a quantified level of active circulating drug to guide management. Generally, concentrations greater than 150 ng/mL are sufficient to counter cravings in patients with a history of opioid use disorder. Concentrations greater than 700 ng/mL can be associated with methadone toxicity.

CASE CONCLUSION

Police inform you they are familiar with the 40-year-old man because he lives with his mother, frequently stops taking his medications for schizophrenia, and is known to use crystal methamphetamine. If medically cleared, you suspect this patient will need psychiatric admission. Although not needed for medical clearance, most accepting psychiatric physicians and facilities require a UDS prior to accepting for transfer.

The 2-year-old child's babysitter arrives to provide more history: the sitter was in the kitchen making dinner and the child was playing in another room when the sitter's dog started barking. The sitter ran into the room to see the child lying on the floor, eyes rolled back, with tonic-clonic jerking movements. She had not heard any sounds or crying to make her believe the child had fallen or hit anything. The sitter's home was built within the last 20 years. The babysitter states she smokes marijuana infrequently and does not keep it in the home. She keeps basic medications such as acetaminophen and ibuprofen on a high shelf in the kitchen, no medications in her purse or bookbag.

Both patients have indications for a UDS. The adult male likely needing psychiatric admission will need to be transferred to another facility, which will likely not accept him until a UDS has been completed. He is hemodynamically stable, but delaying his UDS will take up a bed and significant personnel resources in the form of a sitter.

The undifferentiated, seizing girl is critical. Although obtaining a catheterized urine specimen on her may not be a top priority, doing so may lead to a diagnosis, specific toxicologic treatment, and disposition. Her UDS is positive for TCAs. Upon further questioning, the sitter's dog is given amitriptyline whenever there is thunder or lightning in the area. She keeps it under the sink in the bathroom where the child accessed it; she estimates that 10 20-mg tablets of amitriptyline are missing. With this information, an ECG is obtained demonstrating changes consistent with TCA toxicity. In addition to supportive care, sodium bicarbonate is added to the fluids and the child clinically improves. She is medically stable and transported to the nearest pediatric hospital for further care.

(For further reading on TCA toxicity, refer to Chapter 14 of this text, "Tricyclic Antidepressant Toxicity.")

KEY POINTS TO REMEMBER

- Urine drug screens (UDSs) significantly increase ED costs and length of stay while rarely changing management.
- False positives and false negatives are common and can misdirect management or provide a false sense of reassurance.

- The most effective use of a UDS is identification of an ingested substance which is causing physiologic harm and able to be directly, specifically treated based on the result.
- If a test result does not alter management, the necessity of its use should be heavily scrutinized in consideration of cost and resource utilization.

References

1. Moeller K, Kissack J, Atayee R, Lee K. Clinical interpretation of urine drug tests. *Mayo Clin Proc.* 2017;92(5):774–796. Accessed November 17, 2021. https://doi.org/10.1016/j.mayocp.2016.12.007

2. Riccoboni S, Darracq M. Does the U stand for useless? The urine drug screen and emergency department psychiatric patients. *J Emerg Med.* 2018;54(4):500–506. Accessed November 16, 2021. https://doi.org/10.1016/j.jemermed.2017.12.054

3. Algren D, Christian M. Buyer beware: pitfalls in toxicology laboratory testing. *Mo Med.* 2015;112(3):206–210. Accessed November 20, 2021. https://www.ncbi.nlm.nih.gov/pmc/articles/PMC6170116/

4. World Health Organization Expert Committee on Drug Dependence. *Critical Review Report: Isotonitazene.* World Health Organization; 2020. Accessed November 17, 2021. https://www.who.int/docs/default-source/controlled-substances/43rd-ecdd/isonitazene-43rd-final-complete-a.pdf

5. Stellpflug SJ, Cole JB, Greller HA. Urine drug screens in the emergency department: the best test may be no test at all. *J Emerg Nurs.* 2020 Nov;46(6):923–931. doi:10.1016/j.jen.2020.06.003. Epub 2020 Aug 22. PMID: 32843202

6. Bahji A, Hargreaves T, Finch S. Assessing the utility of drug screening in the emergency department: a short report. *BMJ Open Quality.* 2018;7:e000414. Accessed November 16, 2021. doi:10.1136/bmjoq-2018-0004147. Saitman A, Park HD, Fitzgerald RL. False-positive interferences of common urine drug screen immunoassays: a review. *J Anal Toxicol.* 2014;38:387–396.

8. Lockwood TLE, Vervoordt A, Lieberman M. High concentrations of illicit stimulants and cutting agents cause false positives on fentanyl test strips. *Harm Reduct J.* 2021;18:30. https://doi.org/10.1186/s12954-021-00478-4\

9. Mohamad N, Salehuddin RM, Ghazali B, Bakar et al. Plasma methadone level monitoring in methadone maintenance therapy: a personalised methadone therapy. In: Gowder S, ed. *New Insights into Toxicity and Drug Testing.* IntechOpen; 2013. Accessed November 17, 2021. https://doi.org/10.5772/54850

17 Diphenhydramine: The Cardiac Poison

Chidiebere Victor Ugwu and
T. Christy Hallett

Case Presentation

A 13-year-old girl is brought into the ED by EMS with altered mental status and hallucinations. The parents found the patient in her room that morning, picking at random things in the air and having nonsensical speech. The mother immediately called 911 to transport her to the nearest ED. The patient had a seizure aborted with IM midazolam on her way to the hospital. IV access was difficult to obtain because the patient continually removed leads and would not stay still. Vital signs on arrival were temperature 102.2°F/39°C, respiratory rate 28 breaths/min, heart rate 171 beats/min, SpO_2 99% on room air, and blood pressure 126/72 mm Hg. On examination, her pupils were dilated to 6 mm bilaterally. She had decreased bowel sounds and a tender bulging mass over the suprapubic area. Her skin appeared dry and flushed. A foley was placed, and 700 mL of urine was expelled. The mother went through the patient's phone, where she found a video of her daughter ingesting an entire bottle of diphenhydramine to achieve "a high" on social media.

What Do You Do Now?

DISCUSSION

Background

First synthesized in 1943, diphenhydramine is recognized as one of the most commonly used over-the-counter antihistamines in the United States. Antihistamines treat a myriad of conditions, including anaphylaxis, pruritus, dystonic reaction, antiemetic, gastroesophageal reflux, and other histamine-mediated disorders. Diphenhydramine has anticholinergic, antitussive, antiemetic, and sedative properties, with many different oral formulations available.

In recent years, there have been increasing reports of diphenhydramine overdose in adults and older children due to recreational use, intentional overdose with suicidal intention, or misuse. Teenagers and young adults have popularized diphenhydramine overdoses via social media platforms. Diphenhydramine overdose, particularly in combination with other xenobiotics, has resulted in fatal outcomes. It also has been listed among the top four most frequently used medications for committing suicide in the United States, making this a pressing public health concern.

Toxicology and Pathophysiology

H_1 receptors are proinflammatory mediators causing vasodilation, increased vascular permeability, and bronchoconstriction. H_1 blockers like diphenhydramine are easily absorbed after oral administration due to their highly lipophilic nature, reaching peak plasma levels in 2–3 hours. In cases of massive overdose, absorption from the GI tract could be prolonged due to its antimuscarinic effect, which decreases bowel peristaltic action and gastric emptying. Diphenhydramine can easily cross the blood–brain barrier and cause CNS effects. This property distinguishes diphenhydramine from second- and third-generation antihistamines that are considered non- or less-sedating[1]. Elimination is via hepatic metabolism with a half-life ranging from 1 to 4 hours. Clinical manifestations of diphenhydramine overdose appear to be dose-dependent and will occur at doses that are 3–5 times the recommended dose.

In overdoses, diphenhydramine affects the muscarinic acetylcholine receptors of the parasympathetic system. Symptoms are usually multisystemic affecting the central nervous, cardiovascular, and GI systems and range from mild to severe. Fatal cases have been documented, mostly in

TABLE 17.1 Diphenhydramine toxidrome, its effects and treatment

Diphenhydramine toxidrome	Effects	Treatment

Antimuscarinic	Dilated pupils
	Flushed dry skin
	Decreased ability to sweat
	  Hyperthermia
	Tachycardia
	Urinary retention
		Supportive
		  management
		Benzodiazepines

Antihistamine	Agitation/delirium Sedation/Coma Ataxia Seizure	Supportive management Physostigmine
Cardiac K Channel blockade	QTc Prolongation	Optimizing serum potassium, calcium, and magnesium levels
Cardiac Na Channel blockade	QRS widening	Sodium bicarbonate

children. Since diphenhydramine can easily cross the blood–brain barrier, it causes symptoms including drowsiness, obtundation, agitation, irritability, ataxia, and seizures mostly in higher doses (Table 17.1).[2,3] Mydriasis, blurred vision, and nystagmus are associated ocular manifestations.

Most patients will present with sinus tachycardia due to muscarinic receptor inhibition. Diphenhydramine has been shown to bind to cardiac sodium and potassium channels leading to prolongation of QRS complexes and QTc prolongation, respectively. Wide complex tachycardias, unmasking of a Brugada pattern, or torsade de pointes may also be seen.

Patients can become hyperthermic and develop rhabdomyolysis from dehydration and impaired heat dissipation from an inability to sweat, which could lead to acute kidney injury. The elderly population is at highest risk of developing renal failure from severe dehydration and rhabdomyolysis.

Workup and Diagnosis

Diphenhydramine overdose is a clinical diagnosis based mainly on a history of ingestion and confirmed with the presence of a typical antimuscarinic toxidrome. Other medications like tricyclic antidepressants that share these antimuscarinic effects should also be strongly considered.

Patients with ingestion of doses higher than 7.5 mg/kg are expected to have significant toxicity and are generally triaged by the poison control centers to the ED. Doses as high as 20–40 mg/kg can be fatal, and children are more sensitive to the toxic effects compared to adults[3].

Treatment

Upon arrival to the ED, airway, breathing, and circulation should be assessed, and patients should be immediately placed on cardiac monitor with an ECG obtained. Other labs including electrolytes, acetaminophen and salicylate levels, urine toxicology screen, and creatinine kinase levels can be considered. A comprehensive urine toxicology assay can be obtained and will detect presence of antihistamines as confirmation. However, results can take days to return and have a delayed role in clinical management. It is also notable that diphenhydramine can cause false positives on many immunoassay-based basic urine drug screens for opiates, phencyclidine, and tricyclic antidepressants.

Vital signs with serial exams should be performed to assess for antimuscarinic symptoms or change in mental status. Treatment is primarily supportive, and an asymptomatic patient should be monitored for at least 6–8 hours after ingestion.

Considerations for use of activated charcoal should be individualized based on the time of ingestion and mental status. Further gut decontamination may be beneficial in some cases because of slowed GI motility. Dialysis has not proved to be effective in elimination of antihistamines due to their large volume of distribution.

Benzodiazepines play a significant role in treatment of an antimuscarinic patient. Administration should be liberal for the treatment of agitation, tachycardia, and seizures.

Patients who are somnolent need frequent monitoring and may require intubation for airway protection. Patients with tachycardia or hypotension may need fluid resuscitation. Profound hypotension may further require administration of vasoactive medications. For cases with hypotension refractory to traditional resuscitative measures, a recently published small sample-sized study suggests that lipid emulsion therapy may be beneficial.

ECGs are necessary to evaluate the QTc and QRS interval. Cardiac sodium and potassium channel blockades cause widened QRS and QTc intervals, respectively. IV sodium bicarbonate is used in the treatment of prolonged QRS (>100 ms) and with evidence of sodium channel blockade, such as terminal R-wave in aVR. The initial dose should be given a 1–2 mEq/kg bolus over 1–2 minutes. A sodium bicarbonate infusion or multiple boluses may be necessary. The patient will need close cardiac monitoring and serial ECGs. A recent study associated the presence of acidemia (pH <7.2), QRS prolongation (QRS >120 ms), and an elevated anion gap (AG >20) with severe outcomes. Consider admitting patients with hypotension, QRS widening, or ventricular dysrhythmia to the ICU. Close monitoring of electrolytes, such as potassium, magnesium, and calcium, is necessary for normalizing QTc interval from the potassium channel blockade.

Patients who are agitated and have decreased ability to sweat are prone to developing hyperthermia, and this includes patients with anticholinergic poisoning. The agitation should be treated with benzodiazepines, as previously mentioned. While the hyperthermia associated with diphenhydramine tends to be mild, drug-induced hyperthermia can be a medical emergency and temperatures higher than 104°F/40°C require aggressive management. Patients with uncontrolled severe hyperthermia may develop multiorgan failure and disseminated intravascular coagulopathy even if initial stabilization is successful. Treatment should focus on cooling the patient as soon as possible, ideally within the first hour of developing hyperthermia. Ice packs, evaporative cooling, ice bath immersion, and other active cooling measures should be considered. Rhabdomyolysis can occur due to dehydration and seizures and should be treated with IV fluids and therapy directed toward the causal factor. Also monitor serial electrolytes, creatinine, and creatinine kinase levels.

Physostigmine is a carbamate which can be used as antidotal therapy in anticholinergic toxicity. It can serve as both a diagnostic and a therapeutic agent. Physostigmine reversibly inhibits acetylcholinesterase and prevents the breakdown of synaptic acetylcholine. Indications include the presence of peripheral or central antimuscarinic manifestations. An ECG should always be performed to check for evidence of Na$^+$ channel blockade, such as a widened QRS or a greater than 3 mm R in AVR, prior to giving this medication because this would be a contraindication to use. The dose of physostigmine ranges between 0.5 and 2 mg given slowly intravenously over

5 minutes and can be repeated every 10–15 minutes. Its duration of action is 20–30 minutes and the patient should be reexamined for possible return of antimuscarinic effects. When administered rapidly, or if the patient is not suffering from the toxic effects of an antimuscarinic agent, physostigmine can lead to vomiting, hypersalivation, bradycardia, bronchorrhea with possible respiratory difficulty, and seizures. Atropine reverses the effect of physostigmine when there is excessive cholinergic tone and should always be at the bedside when administering physostigmine. Tricyclic antidepressant ingestion is a relative contraindication to the use of physostigmine though this concern is largely based on outdated literature. Still, this is the reason to avoid physostigmine if the QRS is prolonged.

Long-Term Concerns

Diphenhydramine overdose has a good prognosis as most patients will recover completely without any long-term effects. Very few cases have been reported to be fatal.

The teenager who intentionally overdosed on diphenhydramine was admitted to the ICU for close monitoring of her vital signs and mental status. She received doses of benzodiazepines for agitation. Her mental status gradually improved, and agitation subsided within 24 hours of her admission. The patient was then able to be transferred to the psychiatric unit.

CASE CONCLUSION

For our patient, she was admitted to intensive care unit, where she received supportive management, including fluid resuscitation and a few additional doses of benzodiazepine for agitation and hyperthermia. Her EKG was monitored and remained stable throughout her stay. Over the next 24 hours, she showed improvement with stable vitals, and a result, she was discharged home.

- Diphenhydramine overdose presents early after ingestion with multisystemic antimuscarinic symptoms.
- Physostigmine can be used as a diagnostic and/or therapeutic agent in diphenhydramine overdose.
- Rapid administration of physostigmine can lead to bradycardia, hypersalivation, and seizures; atropine should be at bedside.
- Physostigmine administration is relatively contraindicated in patients with Na^+ channel toxicity as evidence by related ECG changes.

Further Reading

Clemons J, Jandu A, Stein B, Chary M. Efficacy of lipid emulsion therapy in treating cardiotoxicity from diphenhydramine ingestion: a review and analysis of case reports [published online ahead of print, 2022 Feb 16]. *Clin Toxicol (Phila)*. 2022;1–9. doi:10.1080/15563650.2022.2038187

Hughes AR, Lin A, Hendrickson RG. Toxicology Investigator's Consortium (ToxIC). Clinical and patient characteristics associated with severe outcome in diphenhydramine toxicity. *Clin Toxicol (Phila)*. 2021;59(10):918–925. doi:10.1080/15563650.2021.1891244

Nemanich A, Liebelt E, Sabbatini AK. Increased rates of diphenhydramine overdose, abuse, and misuse in the United States, 2005–2016. *Clin Toxicol (Phila)*. 2021;59(11):1002–1008. doi:10.1080/15563650.2021.1892716

References

1. Gosselin S. Antihistamines and decongestants. In: Nelson LS, Howland M, Lewin NA, Smith SW, Goldfrank LR, Hoffman RS, eds. *Goldfrank's Toxicologic Emergencies*. 11th ed. McGraw Hill; 2019. Chapter 49, pg. 6,7.
2. Kearney TE. Diphenhydramine. In: Olson KR, Anderson IB, Benowitz NL, Blanc PD, Clark RF, Kearney TE, Kim-Katz SY, Wu AB, eds. *Poisoning and Drug Overdose*. 7th ed. McGraw Hill; 2018. Chapter 3-25, pg. 1.
3. Manning B. Antihistamines. In: Olson KR, Anderson IB, Benowitz NL, Blanc PD, Clark RF, Kearney TE, Kim-Katz SY, Wu AB, eds. *Poisoning and Drug Overdose*. 7th ed. McGraw Hill; 2018. Chapter 2-15, pg. 1–2.

18 A Long Way from Woodstock: Synthetic Cannabinoids

Daniel Nogee

Case Presentation

A 27-year-old man is brought in by ambulance from a local park for decreased mental status. The patient is unresponsive to painful stimuli; no external signs of trauma are found on exam. Pupils are 3 mm bilaterally and sluggishly reactive. Vital signs are heart rate 119 beats/min, respiratory rate 14 breaths/min, blood pressure 128/74 mm Hg, temperature 98.9°F/37.2°C, and 96% on room air. Fingerstick glucose is 94 mg/dL. He does not respond to 4 mg of naloxone IV and is quickly intubated for airway protection. Urine drug screen is negative for cannabinoids, cocaine, methadone, benzodiazepines, PCP, opiates, and fentanyl. Ninety minutes after intubation, the patient suddenly awakens, pulls out his endotracheal tube, and elopes from the department. Over the course of your shift, several other patients are brought in by EMS from the same park with varying presentations, including agitation, delirium, seizures, and vomiting. Several patients, including your original one, present to the ED multiple times on the same day, with differing symptoms on each visit.

What Do You Do Now?

DISCUSSION

Background

Over the past decade, multiple outbreaks of synthetic cannabinoid (SC) mass overdoses have occurred within the United States, resulting in thousands of ED encounters and several deaths.[1,2] The terms "synthetic cannabinoids" or "synthetic cannabinoid receptor agonists" (SCRAs) encompasses dozens of structurally distinct laboratory-created chemicals with effects on human cannabinoid receptors: a variety of "street names" are listed in Table 18.1. Originally created by academic and pharmaceutical industry research chemists to investigate cannabinoid receptors and develop new medications, SCs are different in both structure and effects from delta-9-tetrohydrocannbainol (THC), the psychoactive chemical found in *Cannabis* (AKA marijuana); "bath salts" (synthetic cathinones) are also structurally and mechanistically different from SCs or THC.[3] SCs were first identified in the US recreational drug supply in the 2000s; because they were not explicitly illegal, SCs were sold in gas stations, head shops, and others similar establishments as a "safe and legal" alternative to THC. SCs are usually sold as metal-foil packages of plant matter sprayed or mixed with SCs, though they have also been identified in liquid form (for use in e-cigarettes or vapes) or as a component of counterfeit prescription narcotics. SCs are generally smoked but can also be ingested.

As they have gradually been recognized as a public health issue, the US Drug Enforcement Agency has worked to regulate/ban individual SC chemicals identified in outbreaks. However, this has led to a wider structural

TABLE 18.1 **Synthetic cannabinoid "street names" and packaging labels**

Spice or Spice 99	Herbal incense
Fake Weed	Synthetic marijuana
Super Strong Incense	Smacked
K2 [various flavors]	AK-47
Scooby Snak	Joker

Not an inclusive list- "brand names" on packaging change frequently!
Included SC(s) may also vary within the same "brand."
From New York State Department of Health.[4]

variety of SCs appearing on the market in an effort to stay one step ahead of law enforcement, often leading to new and unexpected side effects as novel SCs "outbreaks" pop up in unexpected areas.[5] Their chemical structural differences from THC and other illicit substances has also led to SC use among people who may be subject to urine drug testing (such as those in substance use disorder treatment programs, correctional settings, or the military) because they do not cause a positive test result on most commercially available immunoassay-based urine drug screens. Testing for SCs in urine or product samples can be done by specialized labs with liquid/gas-chromatography mass-spectrometry equipment, though this requires knowledge of the specific chemical structure(s) in question and has become more difficult as more varied and novel SC structures appear. Far from a "safe and legal" alternative to THC, the "dirty" nature of SCs has led to a variety of clinical consequences for users.

Toxicology and Pathophysiology

Most currently available SCs have significant structural differences from THC but act as agonists of the same cannabinoid receptors that THC and endocannabinoids bind, CB_1 and CB_2. Compared to THC, SCs have a higher binding affinity for the CB_1 and CB_2 receptors and have active metabolites that can also bind those receptors; the combination of these two factors makes SCs significantly "stronger" CB_1 and CB_2 agonists than THC and leads to greater severity and duration of intoxication and side effects.[3,6] CB_1 receptors are primarily found in the central and peripheral nervous systems and thus are responsible for the "intoxicating" effects of THC and SCs on cognition, memory, and motor function.[7,8] CB_1 receptors have also been identified in the heart, lung, liver, and vascular endothelium, which may explain the non-neurological side effects of SC use. CB_2 receptors are found primarily in the immune system, and in lower levels than CB_1 in the CNS; their role in clinical effects of THC and SCs are less understood.

The wide variety of SC structures, dosages, and interactions with other substances consumed by users, including other SCs, can lead to a wide variety of clinical effects.[6,8,9] Neurological symptoms are the most common, specifically agitation, delirium, confusion, and psychosis; depressed mental status and coma can also occur but appears to be less common.[2] Clinically significant vital signs abnormalities, including tachycardia, bradycardia, hypertension, hypotension, and hyperthermia, may occur. Other symptoms include nausea, vomiting, seizures, and anxiety. Major complications can include acute kidney injury, myocardial infarctions, and strokes. Deaths have occurred, though the exact number and proximate causes are unclear. As with other sedating overdoses, lethal hypothermia can occur in low ambient temperatures. Drug contaminants can also have significant clinical effects independent of the SC, such as the large-scale outbreak of a long-acting anticoagulant rodenticide (LAAR) containing SCs in Illinois in 2018, leading to severe coagulopathy in users.[10] Subsequent outbreaks of LAAR-contaminated SCs have occurred in Israel and Florida and led to multiple deaths, suggesting this problem may continue to grow in frequency and severity.[11]

Workup and Diagnosis

The clinical presentations of SC intoxication overlap significantly with those of other psychoactive substances and can be difficult to distinguish from other drugs of abuse. Demographically, most users of SCs are young (median age 25–26) and male (80–84%).[2,6] As with many other intoxications, clinical history is often the key to diagnosis: suspicion for SC intoxication should be raised if the patient has had similar prior presentations or appears as one of multiple patients in an "outbreak" of similar clinical appearance. Patients may admit to recreational SC use, though usually under the name of a specific brand of substance or other street name. Co-ingestions of other substances are not uncommon (5.7–17.5% of cases), though patients who have a reason to avoid substances that might show up on a urine drug screen (military, athletes, etc.) may have taken SCs specifically because of the lower likelihood of a positive urine drug test.

Most patients should not require significant, if any, diagnostic workup outside of a physical exam, vital signs, and fingerstick glucose. For patients with severe symptoms, such as seizures, hemodynamic instability, or coagulopathy, targeted workup should include CNS imaging (CT head) and labs (including metabolic panel/renal function, creatine phosphokinase [CPK], troponin testing) as appropriate to the presenting symptoms. If there are any signs of coagulopathy that could suggest LAAR contamination, coagulation testing (PT/INR, PTT, thromboelastogram, etc.) should be performed. Workup should focus on identification of SC-induced end organ injury requiring admission and treatment, including acute kidney injury, rhabdomyolysis, and myocardial infarction, and exclusion of non-SC causes of symptoms, such as intracranial hemorrhage, stroke, sepsis, seizure disorders (particularly in the postictal state), hypoglycemia, electrolyte abnormalities, environmental hypo-/hyperthermia, other poisonings (carbon monoxide, etc.), or withdrawal from alcohol, benzodiazepines, or other substances. Commercially available immunoassay-based urine drug screens are not likely to pick up synthetic cannabinoids due to structural differences from THC but may identify other recently ingested substances that could contribute to the patient's presenting symptoms; however, the presence of other positives on a urine drug screen would not exclude SCs as a cause of symptoms. Reference labs may be able to test for a number of different SCs, though not within a clinically useful timeframe. If such a test is performed and is negative, this unfortunately cannot rule out a SC exposure as only substances with a known standard can be identified.

The differential diagnosis of SC intoxication includes many other recreationally ingested illicit substances. For patients with minimal symptoms consider (non-synthetic) THC exposure. Significant agitation and subsequent amnesia in the setting of suspected illicit substance use could indicate PCP or ketamine intoxication. Severe agitation without memory disturbances may indicate an amphetamine, cocaine, or synthetic cathinone intoxication. Severe sedation/coma with preserved respiratory drive and later rapid awakening could be caused by gamma-hydroxybutyrate (GHB) intoxication. Alcohol (ethanol or toxic alcohols), cocaine, and benzodiazepine use, particularly in combination, could also present similarly to SC intoxication. Psychiatric conditions, particularly new-onset schizophrenia and psychoses, may be difficult to distinguish from SC use, outside of waiting hours to days to ensure any SCs in the patient's system have been fully metabolized and excreted.

Treatment

Most patients with SC intoxication will have a benign clinical course and will require little if any treatment. For patients with significant side effects, there is little evidence to support specific treatments outside of symptomatic/supportive care. There is no direct reversal agent for SC intoxication.

Patients with acute agitation can be treated with benzodiazepines or antipsychotics titrated to resolution of agitation. Patients with seizures should receive rapid-acting benzodiazepines; it is unclear if there would be any additional benefit to adding antiepileptic drugs. Mild tachycardia can be treated with IV fluids or benzodiazepines, depending on if it appears secondary to dehydration or acute agitation. If symptoms resolve, the patient has returned to their baseline mental status, and there is no concern for other intoxications or illnesses, then discharge from the ED is appropriate.

For patients presenting with significantly decreased mental status, consider intubation depending on the ability to protect the airway and respiratory drive. A trial of naloxone (starting with 0.4 mg and up to 4 mg) is reasonable if the patient has pinpoint pupils or bradypnea suggesting concurrent opioid intoxication. Flumazenil is not recommended as it could provoke difficult to treat seizures if the patient has underlying physiological dependance on alcohol or benzodiazepines. Obtain labs to rule out rhabdomyolysis and acute kidney injury and admit or observe until mental status returns to baseline.

Patients with cardiac effects, including significant tachycardia, bradycardia, dysrhythmias, chest pain, or hypotension, should rapidly be placed on a monitor, have IV access obtained, have a 12-lead ECG, and have labs drawn, including metabolic panel and troponin testing. Treatment will depend on the specific symptoms experienced, but in general should follow advanced cardiac life support guidelines. If admitted, it should be to a monitored bed, and/or ICU depending on severity of symptoms.

Consider further workup and admission for patients who have mild to moderate symptoms that fail to resolve after several hours of observation. Possible explanations include particularly long-lasting SCs, intoxication with other co-ingestions, or a non-SC cause of symptoms. Consider psychiatric evaluation if patients have agitation, delirium, hallucinations, or other neuropsychiatric symptoms without major lab or vital signs abnormalities and that do not resolve after 24 hours.

Patients with coagulopathy from suspected or confirmed LAAR contamination should be admitted and treated with vitamin K; blood product transfusions and/or prothrombin complex concentrate may be needed to treat cases with severe bleeding. Prolonged admission or establishment of close outpatient follow-up may be necessary to ensure patients are treated until coagulation laboratory parameters return to baseline. Local public health authorities should be notified to assist with identification and referral to appropriate care of other potentially affected SC users.

As with most intoxications, contacting a local poison center and/or on-call toxicologist is beneficial for both the individual patient and the medical system. Reporting SC cases to local poison centers can help improve recognition of SC outbreaks and contributes to the advancement of knowledge about the diagnosis and management of SC intoxication. Poison centers and toxicologists may also be aware of locally significant trends in SC use, such as contamination with dangerous substances requiring further workup. They may also be able to assist with identification of SCs and potential contaminants through referral to specialized reference labs and federal agencies.

Long-Term Concerns

Little is known about the long-term consequences of SC use because these substances have only become commonly available in the past decade. End-organ injury (acute kidney injury or myocardial infarction) caused by acute SC use can be permanent. Chronic use (possibly even one-time use) may result in chronic cognitive impairment or psychiatric illness.[3] Based on comparisons to chronic THC use and animal models of SC use, chronic SC users may also experience physiological and behavioral effects, including gradual development of tolerance and mild to moderate withdrawal symptoms, such as agitation or irritability, from CB_1/CB_2 receptor desensitization and downregulation.[7,8] It is unclear if there are in-utero effects of maternal SC use.

As law enforcement agencies seek to identify and regulate various SC compounds as they appear, SC manufacturers synthesize and distribute new SC chemical structures in an effort to evade identification and regulation. This ongoing game of "cat and mouse" or "whack-a-mole" has led to the proliferation of new SC chemical structures; while there is some animal and human experimental data from the older SC compounds as part of their initial creation for pharmacological investigation purposes, little is known about the pharmacological effects of novel SC compounds. The potential for outbreaks with new and unpredictable symptoms remains high.

CASE CONCLUSION

The cases described above are based on the personal experience of the author in responding to a large-scale SC mass overdose. Given the wide variety of SCs and their varied clinical effects, future mass overdoses may present similarly or with completely different symptoms; contamination with LAARs or other dangerous chemicals may confound the picture further. Clinicians should maintain a high index of suspicion for SCs when "mass overdoses" of multiple patients present in close geographic and temporal proximity with similar symptoms and should involve local poison centers, toxicologists, and public health authorities early and often.

KEY POINTS TO REMEMBER

- Consider SC intoxication in the young male patient (particularly those with a reason to avoid THC and other lab-detectable drugs) presenting with acute agitation, delirium, confusion, or coma.
- Extensive diagnostic workup is not necessary in most mild cases, but in severe cases should focus on identification of end-organ injury and exclusion of other potential causes of symptoms.
- There is little evidence to drive treatment, so focus on treating symptoms and excellent supportive care.
- Call your local poison center (1-800- 222-1222) or toxicologist, particularly if you see multiple cases or new or unusual symptoms; it's a win-win situation as they can give you advice about treatment based on local trends and you can help them identify outbreaks and novel SC structures.

Further Reading

Adams AJ, Banister SD, Irizarry L, Trecki J, Schwartz M, Gerona R. "Zombie" outbreak caused by the synthetic cannabinoid AMB-FUBINACA in New York. *N Engl J Med.* Jan 19 2017;376(3):235–242. doi:10.1056/NEJMoa1610300

Takakuwa KM, Schears RM. The emergency department care of the cannabis and synthetic cannabinoid patient: a narrative review. *Int J Emerg Med.* 2021;14(1):10–10. doi:10.1186/s12245-021-00330-3

Tamama K. Synthetic drugs of abuse. In: Makowski GS, ed. *Advances in Clinical Chemistry*. Elsevier; 2021:191–214.

References

1. Trecki J, Gerona RR, Schwartz MD. Synthetic cannabinoid–related illnesses and deaths. *N Engl J Med*. 2015;373(2):103–107. doi:10.1056/NEJMp1505328
2. Monte AA, Calello DP, Gerona RR, et al. Characteristics and treatment of patients with clinical illness due to synthetic cannabinoid inhalation reported by medical toxicologists: a ToxIC database study. *J Med Toxicol*. Jun 2017;13(2):146–152. doi:10.1007/s13181-017-0605-9
3. Tamama K. Synthetic drugs of abuse. In: Makowski GS, ed. *Advances in Clinical Chemistry*. Elsevier; 2021:191–214.
4. New York State Department of Health. Synthetic marijuana packaging samples. Revised September 2015. Accessed June 30, 2022. https://www.health.ny.gov/professionals/narcotic/synthetic_cannabinoids/sample_images.htm
5. Adams AJ, Banister SD, Irizarry L, Trecki J, Schwartz M, Gerona R. "Zombie" outbreak caused by the synthetic cannabinoid AMB-FUBINACA in New York. *N Engl J Med*. Jan 19 2017;376(3):235–242. doi:10.1056/NEJMoa1610300
6. Takakuwa KM, Schears RM. The emergency department care of the cannabis and synthetic cannabinoid patient: a narrative review. *Int J Emerg Med*. 2021;14(1):10–10. doi:10.1186/s12245-021-00330-3
7. Banister SD, Connor M. The chemistry and pharmacology of synthetic cannabinoid receptor agonists as new psychoactive substances: origins. In: Maurer HH, Brandt SD, eds. *New Psychoactive Substances: Pharmacology, Clinical, Forensic and Analytical Toxicology*. Springer International Publishing; 2018:165–190.
8. Castaneto MS, Gorelick DA, Desrosiers NA, Hartman RL, Pirard S, Huestis MA. Synthetic cannabinoids: epidemiology, pharmacodynamics, and clinical implications. *Drug Alcohol Depend*. 2014;144:12–41. doi:10.1016/j.drugalcdep.2014.08.005
9. Tai S, Fantegrossi WE. Pharmacological and toxicological effects of synthetic cannabinoids and their metabolites. *Curr Top Behav Neurosci*. 2017;32:249–262. doi:10.1007/7854_2016_60
10. Kelkar AH, Smith NA, Martial A, Moole H, Tarantino MD, Roberts JC. An outbreak of synthetic cannabinoid–associated coagulopathy in Illinois. *N Engl J Med*. September 27 2018;379(13):1216–1223. doi:10.1056/NEJMoa1807652
11. Feinstein DL, Hafner J, Breemen R van, Rubinstein I. Inhaled synthetic cannabinoids laced with long-acting anticoagulant rodenticides: a clear and present worldwide danger. *Toxicol Commun*. 2022;6(1):28–29.

19 Beyond Benzos: Alcohol and Sedative-Hypnotic Withdrawal

Kyle Suen

Case Presentation

A 55-year-old man well known to hospital staff presents to the ED after he is found somnolent and with an altered mental status by bystanders. Witnesses who called EMS reported possible seizure-like activity while he was lying on a park bench. EMS reports that this man is homeless and has a history of alcohol use. En route to the hospital, the patient had a generalized tonic-clonic seizure and was given intramuscular midazolam, 5 mg, with cessation of the seizure shortly thereafter. IV access was established, and the patient was given an additional 5 mg diazepam by prehospital providers. Vitals upon arrival to the hospital are heart rate 132 beats/min, blood pressure 150/99 mm Hg, respiratory rate 25 breaths/min, temperature 100.1°F/37.8°C (rectal), and 96% on room air. On exam he appears disheveled and malnourished. He is alert and oriented to person, place, but not time. Exam reveals pupils 7 mm and reactive, tongue fasciculations, bilateral upper extremity tremors. Review of electronic records reveals that the patient is prescribed thiamine, alprazolam, and zolpidem.

What Do You Do Now?

DISCUSSION

Background

The patient presentation described in the clinical vignette should point to the diagnosis of a sedative-hypnotic withdrawal, which may be from alcohol withdrawal syndrome (AWS), benzodiazepine or barbiturate withdrawal, or a combination of these medications. AWS was initially described by Pliny the Elder in the first century BC.[1] He describes alcohol withdrawal in a person whose "drunkenness brings pallor and sagging cheeks, sore eyes, and trembling hands that spill a full cup, of which immediate punishment is a haunted sleep and unrestful nights."

Alcohol use and its related medical problems are commonly encountered by healthcare providers. Studies have shown that up to 8% of admitted patients, 16% of postsurgical patients, 21% of medical ICU patients, and 31% of all trauma patients developed some form of AWS.[2–3] The presence of AWS in postsurgical and trauma patients is associated with nearly a 3-fold increase in mortality.[1]

People who develop mild withdrawal symptoms may often self-treat by "self-medicating" with more alcohol, precluding the need for medical management. However, should access to alcohol become impeded, problems may occur. At the beginning of the COVID-19 global pandemic, many businesses, including liquor stores, were mandated to close. One study found a 12.5% increase in medical toxicology consults for AWS management when comparing pre-closure versus post-closure of liquor stores.[4]

Toxicology and Pathophysiology

The biochemical pathways underlying alcohol use and withdrawal are complex but are also important because they provide insight into the different treatment options for AWS. Chronic heavy alcohol consumption leads to persistent stimulation of the gamma-aminobutyric acid (GABA) A subtype receptor (GABA-Ar), a chloride channel and the chief inhibitory channel class in the CNS. In response, the GABA-Ars in the body undergo conformational changes and receptor downregulation. Conversely, chronic alcohol use also induces conformational changes in the N-methyl-D-aspartate (NMDA) glutamate receptor (one of the primary excitatory receptors in the CNS) and subsequent upregulation of these receptors. It is believed that these receptor changes allow the alcohol user to maintain a normal level of consciousness during periods of elevated alcohol concentrations in the CNS that would otherwise sedate nontolerant individuals.[1,5]

After discontinuation of alcohol use, there is a global decrease in GABA-Ar-mediated inhibitory function and increased NMDA receptor-mediated stimulatory function in the CNS. Loss of inhibitory signals and concomitant increased excitatory signals is believed to cause the clinical effects seen and experienced in AWS.[1,5]

Signs, Symptoms, and Differential Diagnosis

The *Diagnostic and Statistical Manual of Mental Disorders*, 5th edition (DSM-5) defines AWS as the cessation of heavy or prolonged alcohol use resulting, within a period of a few hours to several days, in the development of two or more of the clinical findings listed in Box 19.1. AWS can

---

BOX 19.1 **DSM-5 diagnostic criteria for alcohol withdrawal syndrome (AWS)**

A. Cessation of or reduction in alcohol intake, which has previously been prolonged or heavy

B. Criterion A, Plus any 2 of the following symptoms developing within several hours to a few days

- Anxiety
- Autonomic hyperactivity
- Hallucinations[a]
- Insomnia
- Nausea and vomiting
- Psychomotor agitation
- Seizures (generalized tonic clonic)
- Tremor (worsening)

C. The above symptoms cause clinically significant distress or impairment in social, occupational, or other important areas of functioning.

D. The above symptoms are not attributable to other causes; for example, another mental disorder, intoxication, or withdrawal from another substance.

[a]Specify if hallucinations (usually visual or tactile) occur with intact reality testing, or if auditory, visual, or tactile illusions occur in the absence of a delirium.

---

be characterized based on severity of disease. There are multiple scoring criteria to characterize severity, but currently there is no universally accepted severity score. The three most used scores are the Clinical Institute Withdrawal Assessment of Alcohol Scale, Revised (CIWA-Ar) score, the Glasgow Modified Alcohol Withdrawal Scale (GMAWS), and the Richmond Agitation and Sedation Scale (RASS).[1]

AWS can begin as soon as 6 hours after cessation of drinking and can manifest as any of the clinical findings in Box 19.1. AWS can last for 3–7 days if untreated. In addition to the symptoms listed, patients may experience one or all of the following: alcoholic hallucinosis (AH), delirium tremens (DT), or alcohol withdrawal seizures. AH occurs in 7–9% of patients with AWS and is characterized by transient, vivid, hallucinations that are typically tactile or visual in nature. Patients can experience AH 12–24 hours after cessation of drinking, and the hallucinations are often transient but may infrequently last for weeks.[1] AH may occur with or without the other milder findings of AWS. Patients with AH will have a clear sensorium, whereas those who develop DTs do not.[5]

DTs is a serious manifestation of AWS and is reported to occur in up to 3–5% of patients.[5] It was not until 1955 that it was concluded that withdrawal of alcohol in chronic users can precipitate DTs. DTs typically takes up to 48–96 hours after alcohol cessation to occur, but it has been reported to occur as early as 8 hours from last alcoholic drink.[4] It is characterized by all findings of AWS, but with either (1) a disturbance in consciousness with reduced ability to focus, sustain, or shift attention, delirium, confusion, and frank psychosis; or (2) a change in cognition or the development of a perceptual disturbance that is not better accounted for by a preexisting, established, or evolving dementia. Unlike the previously described clinical findings of AWS, which may last for up to 3–7 days, DTs can last for up to 2 weeks.[1–3,5]

Alcohol withdrawal seizures are another serious complication of AWS and have been described to occur in up to 10% of patients, 40% of whom have an isolated seizure and 3% developing status epilepticus.[1]

There are factors that may help predict how severe a patient's AWS will be. The Prediction of Alcohol Withdrawal Severity Scale (PAWSS) takes into consideration the patient's alcohol use history as well as a select number of clinical and biochemical variables and has demonstrated a 93% sensitivity for predicting complicated alcohol withdrawal among hospitalized patients.[1]

Treatment

Many patients who end up seeking medical attention for AWS may be safely managed as outpatients (Figure 19.1). The successful use of sedative-hypnotics, specifically benzodiazepines, for the treatment of AWS was

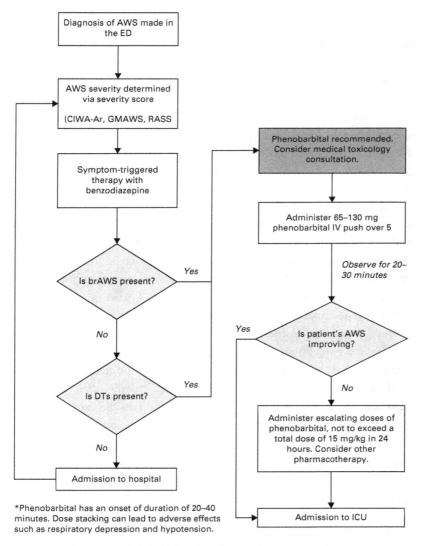

FIGURE 19.1 Approach to alcohol withdrawal syndrome in the emergency department.

demonstrated in a landmark study by Kaim, Klett, and Rothfield in 1969. They performed a double-blind, controlled trial in 537 patients with AWS comparing treatment with either chlordiazepoxide, hydroxyzine, chlorpromazine, thiamine, or placebo over a 2-week period. They concluded that treatment with chlordiazepoxide resulted in a significantly lower incidence of both DTs and alcohol withdrawal seizures.[6]

Benzodiazepines continue to be the first-line medication for treatment of alcohol withdrawal in the ED. Benzodiazepines work via modulation of the GABA-Ar, allowing for increased frequency of GABA-Ar channel opening in the presence of a true GABA-Ar agonist.[1–3,6] In addition to chlordiazepoxide, other benzodiazepines, including diazepam and lorazepam, have been studied for the management of AWS and there is ongoing debate as to which benzodiazepine is the most efficacious.[5] Benzodiazepines are often administered based on the severity of AWS using scales described previously, with frequent provider evaluations to assess need for additional doses; this is referred to as *symptom-triggered therapy*.

While most cases of AWS can be managed with benzodiazepines alone, the development of DTs or benzodiazepine-resistant AWS (brAWS) can occur, and additional pharmacologic intervention may be needed. Benzodiazepines require GABA, or another true GABA-Ar agonist to be present at the receptor for the channel to open. Possible explanations for this resistance include situations where there is low endogenous GABA in the chronic alcohol user, potentially from malnourishment; or that chronic alcohol use has downregulated the GABA-Ar to such an extent that activation is not enough to offset the sympathetic surge induced from the increased excitation of the upregulation of NMDA receptors; or, last, the chronic alcohol use induced conformational changes within the GABA-Ar structure, thereby reducing benzodiazepine affinity to the receptor.[1,3] These possible explanations are not mutually exclusive, and all may be present at the same time.

While brAWS has no clear definition, it has been described in the literature as AWS which requires more than 40 mg diazepam or more than 10 mg or lorazepam within the first hour of treatment, or more than 200 mg diazepam or more than 40 mg lorazepam within the first 3 hours of treatment.[1,5] One study found that 5 out of 6 patients who developed brAWS required intubation. These patients received from 240 mg to 2,160 mg of IV diazepam within 24 hours.[7]

Barbiturates have been reported to be effective medications to use for DTs and brAWS.[5] One double-blind randomized controlled trial compared diazepam and barbital treatment in 107 patients with AWS. The authors concluded that, while there was a trend to favor diazepam in milder cases of AWS, barbital was superior to diazepam in the treatment of DTs.[8]

Phenobarbital is the barbiturate most commonly used for treating AWS, and the addition of a barbiturate to benzodiazepines as a pharmacologic agent for cases of brAWS and DTs makes sense biochemically. Barbiturates have multiple mechanisms of action: at low concentrations they increase the duration that a GABA-Ar channel is open when another true GABA-Ar agonist is present, and, in moderate to high doses, they can open the channel independent of the presence of a GABA-Ar agonist (unlike benzodiazepines). Additionally, and potentially most importantly with respect to brAWS, barbiturates inhibit NMDA receptors, directly reducing the sympathetic surge that occurs with alcohol withdrawal.[1-3,5] Barbiturates may even potentiate benzodiazepine binding at the GABA-Ar, thus augmenting benzodiazepine effect.[3]

The use of barbiturates has also been shown to improve morbidity. A retrospective cohort study from 2000 to 2005 showed that, after implementation of a new guideline that incorporated phenobarbital to escalating doses of diazepam for the treatment of patients with AWS, fewer patients receiving phenobarbital required mechanical ventilation when compared to patients who did not receive phenobarbital according to a predetermined protocol (21.9% vs. 47.3%, respectively). The results also trended toward a shorter length of time in an ICU and decreased rate of nosocomial pneumonia.[2] Another study found that phenobarbital given with lorazepam for AWS was associated with fewer ICU admissions than lorazepam alone (8% vs. 25%).[9]

Adverse effects associated with barbiturates include respiratory depression, somnolence, lethargy, and hypotension, which may lead to provider reluctance in using these medications. However, barbiturates have been shown to be safe for use in the treatment of AWS and are not significantly associated with adverse effects. An ED study found that 92% of patients treated with IV phenobarbital followed by oral phenobarbital for AWS were able to be discharged within 4 hours of treatment. None of these discharged patients returned to the ED within a week, which may suggest that phenobarbital is a safe medication to use, but because this study includes a selection bias, it does not definitively prove safety. Another study found that when treating uncomplicated AWS, phenobarbital was not associated with respiratory depression. In cases of DTs, where intensive care is already needed, one study found 9 cases of phenobarbital-associated respiratory depression out of a total of 73 cases.[9]

Many other medications have been studied for the management of AWS in the inpatient and outpatient settings. Propofol, like phenobarbital, potentiates GABA-Ar activity and inhibits NMDA receptor activity, making it a reasonable option for those in refractory DTs.[5] There are also reports supporting the use of carbamazepine, valproic acid, or gabapentin. Ketamine, an NMDA-receptor antagonist, holds promise as an adjunctive medication in patients who have brAWS.

Dosing regimens for medications used in the management of AWS may vary. An evidence-based approach for treatment focuses on symptom-triggered therapy and is typically managed with varying doses of benzodiazepines, with many institutions creating specific dosing protocols for providers to follow.[1–9] The addition of phenobarbital should be considered when the brAWS is present or imminent, or if DTs are present.[1–5,8,9]

While many advocate for the addition of phenobarbital in addition to benzodiazepines, there is no standardized dosing protocol. One reasonable approach is to give escalating doses of 65 to 260 mg phenobarbital IV every 20–30 minutes until symptoms are improved, using one of the alcohol withdrawal severity scores to guide therapy.[1–2] Clinicians should be cognizant that phenobarbital's duration to clinical effect is 20–40 minutes and therefore avoid inadvertent dose stacking. A total maximum phenobarbital dose should not exceed 15 mg/kg in the first 24 hours.

Phenobarbital dosing considerations should include severity of brAWS, patient age, and risk factors that may exacerbate the adverse effects of phenobarbital. Those with cardiovascular disease, chronic obstructive pulmonary disease, and volume depletion may be at higher risk of the respiratory and cardiovascular adverse effects associated with phenobarbital.[1] We recommend consultation with a medical toxicologist when considering the addition of phenobarbital for treatment of brAWS and DTs.

Benzodiazepine Withdrawal

Benzodiazepines fall under the sedative-hypnotic class of medications, and their chronic use, like chronic alcohol use, can lead to downregulation of the GABA-A receptor. Unlike chronic alcohol use, benzodiazepines do not effect NMDA receptors. Subsequent discontinuation of benzodiazepines can create a withdrawal syndrome that manifests similarly to AWS, including progression to delirium and seizures.[10,11]

The timing and severity of the benzodiazepine withdrawal syndrome (BWS) depends on the specific benzodiazepine and its pharmacodynamics and pharmacokinetics. Withdrawal from short-acting benzodiazepines with no active metabolites, such as triazolam, may occur within hours after use is stopped, whereas withdrawal from longer-acting benzodiazepines with active metabolites, such as diazepam, may take 1–2 days to present.[10,11]

A clinical scale, the Clinical Institute Withdrawal Assessment—Benzodiazepines (CIWA-B), has been proposed as a tool to assess and monitor benzodiazepine withdrawal.[12] Current management strategies for BWS are similar to AWS and are based on scoring on the CIWA-B. Benzodiazepines with a taper are the first-line treatment for BWS.[10,11]

Alprazolam is a high-potency triazolobenzodiazepine and is of special interest because its associated withdrawal syndrome has been reported to be difficult to manage with commonly used benzodiazepines such as diazepam and lorazepam.[13,14] It is possible that the triazole moiety in alprazolam's chemical structure causes unique conformational changes in the GABA-Ar with chronic use. These changes may alter the affinity of common benzodiazepines to their binding site at the GABA-Ar and may be the reason underlying why alprazolam withdrawal is resistant to treatment with diazepam and lorazepam.[13] It has been reported that improvement of the BWS associated with alprazolam is achieved only after readministration of alprazolam and a subsequent taper.[13,14] Clonazepam has also been reported to be an option for alprazolam withdrawal syndrome.[13,15]

Other Sedative-Hypnotic Withdrawals

Chronic use of large doses of non-benzodiazepine sleep aids such as zolpidem can cause a withdrawal syndrome resembling benzodiazepine withdrawal. It has been reported that withdrawal from these medications can cause minor symptoms such as anxiety and tremor, but can also cause serious clinical effects such as seizures. Benzodiazepines have been reported as management options.[15,16]

CASE CONCLUSION

The patient is admitted to the ICU for his severe alcohol withdrawal syndrome with delirium tremens. He is initially started on diazepam and given escalating doses with no improvement in his clinical status. Phenobarbital is added to his regimen and he improves over the next 2-3 days. He is also started on alprazolam given his chronic alprazolam use. While in the ICU, he has a few episodes of respiratory depression but does not require intubation and mechanical ventilation. He is discharged from the hospital on a chlordiazepoxide and alprazolam taper and a referral is made for outpatient management of his substance use disorders.

KEY POINTS TO REMEMBER

- Alcohol withdrawal syndrome (AWS) is a commonly encountered diagnosis in healthcare facilities.
- Chronic use of alcohol leads to downregulation of gamma-aminobutyric acid (GABA) A subtype (GABA-A) receptors and upregulation of glutamate N-methyl-D-aspartate (NMDA) receptors. Subsequent cessation can lead to AWS.
- AWS can vary in severity. There is no standard scale to evaluate severity, but the Clinical Institute Withdrawal Assessment of Alcohol Scale, Revised (CIWA-Ar) score is a commonly used tool to evaluate severity. Delirium tremens (DTs) and alcohol withdrawal seizures are serious manifestations of alcohol withdrawal.
- Benzodiazepines are the first-line pharmacologic option for AWS.
- Benzodiazepine-resistant alcohol withdrawal syndrome (brAWS) and DTs can be managed effectively and safely with phenobarbital. Respiratory depression can occur with when benzodiazepines and barbiturates are used for AWS.

- Benzodiazepine withdrawal presents similarly to alcohol withdrawal, and benzodiazepines are used to manage symptoms.

Further Reading

Ait-Daoud N, Hamby AS, Sharma S, Blevins D. A review of Alprazolam use, misuse, and withdrawal. *J Addict Med*. 2018;12(1):4–10. doi:10.1097/adm.0000000000000350

Long D, Long B, Koyfman A. The emergency medicine management of severe alcohol withdrawal. *Am J Emerg Med*. 2017;35(7):1005–1011. doi:10.1016/j.ajem.2017.02.002

Martin K, Katz A. The role of barbiturates for alcohol withdrawal syndrome. *Psychosomatics*. 2016;57(4):341–347. doi:10.1016/j.psym.2016.02.011

References

1. Goldfrank LR, Hoffman RS, Nelson L, et al. Alcohol withdrawal. In: *Goldfrank's Toxicologic Emergencies*. 11th ed. McGraw Hill:1165–1171.
2. Gold JA, Rimal B, Nolan A, Nelson LS. A strategy of escalating doses of benzodiazepines and phenobarbital administration reduces the need for mechanical ventilation in delirium tremens. *Crit Care Med*. 2007;35(3):724–730. doi:10.1097/01.ccm.0000256841.28351.80
3. Hayner CE, Wuestefeld NL, Bolton PJ. Phenobarbital treatment in a patient with resistant alcohol withdrawal syndrome. *Pharmacotherapy*. 2009;29(7):875–878. doi:10.1592/phco.29.7.875
4. Amaducci AM, Yazdanyar AR, Fikse DJ, et al. Influence of Pennsylvania liquor store closures during the covid-19 pandemic on alcohol withdrawal consultations. *Am J Emerg Med*. 2021;50:156–159. doi:10.1016/j.ajem.2021.07.058
5. Long D, Long B, Koyfman A. The emergency medicine management of severe alcohol withdrawal. *Am J Emerg Med*. 2017;35(7):1005–1011. doi:10.1016/j.ajem.2017.02.002
6. Kaim SC, Klett CJ, Rothfeld B. Treatment of the acute alcohol withdrawal state: a comparison of four drugs. *Am J Psychiatry*. 1969;125(12):1640–1646. doi:10.1176/ajp.125.12.1640
7. Dill C, Shin S. High-dose intravenous benzodiazepine. *Acad Emerg Med*. 2000;7(3):308–310. doi:10.1111/j.1553-2712.2000.tb01087.x
8. Kramp P, Rafaelsen OJ. Delirium tremens. *Acta Psychiatr Scand*. 1978;58(2):174–190. doi:10.1111/j.1600-0447.1978.tb06930.x
9. Martin K, Katz A. The role of barbiturates for alcohol withdrawal syndrome. *Psychosomatics*. 2016;57(4):341–347. doi:10.1016/j.psym.2016.02.011

10. American Psychiatric Association. *Diagnostic and Statistical Manual of Mental Disorders*. 5th ed. American Psychiatric Publishing; 2013.

11. Petursson H. The benzodiazepine withdrawal syndrome. *Addiction*. 1994;89(11):1455–1459. doi:10.1111/j.1360-0443.1994.tb03743.x

12. Busto U, Sykora K, Sellers EM. A clinical scale to assess benzodiazepine withdrawal. *J Clin Psychopharmacol*. 1989;9(6):412–416. doi:10.1097/00004714-198912000-00005

13. Ait-Daoud N, Hamby AS, Sharma S, Blevins D. A review of alprazolam use, misuse, and withdrawal. *J Addict Med*. 2018;12(1):4–10. doi:10.1097/adm.0000000000000350

14. Sachdev G. Failure of lorazepam to treat alprazolam withdrawal in a critically ill patient. *World J Crit Care Med*. 2014;3(1):42. doi:10.5492/wjccm.v3.i1.42

15. Patterson JF. Alprazolam dependency: use of clonazepam for withdrawal. *Southern Med J*. 1988;81(7):830–831. doi:10.1097/00007611-198807000-00006

16. Liappas IA, Malitas PN, Dimopoulos NP, et al. Zolpidem dependence case series: possible neurobiological mechanisms and clinical management. *J Psychopharmacol*. 2003;17(1):131–135. doi:10.1177/0269881103017001723

20 All Amped Up and Nowhere to Go: Caffeine and Methylxanthine Overdose

Nicholas Nuveen and
Melissa H. Gittinger

Case Presentation

A 21-year-old college student is brought in by EMS after bystanders at his university library noticed he was agitated and then began vomiting. The patient denies any medical history or illicit drug use and states that he has been stressed and trying to stay awake as finals are approaching. Today he has been drinking coffee and taking a "concentration enhancing" supplement he found called guarana powder. He took a tablespoon of the powder about 1 hour prior to arrival and has been vomiting profusely for the past 15 minutes. His vitals on presentation are heart rate 134 beats/min, blood pressure 160/95 mm Hg, respiratory rate 22 breaths/min, and temperature 99.5°F/37.5°C; he weighs 70 kg. On exam he is flushed, tremulous, and agitated, and is not able to sit still. His pupils are normal in size and are reactive to light. Shortly after the exam he continues to vomit and endorses headache and palpations.

What do you do now?

DISCUSSION

This patient presenting with tachycardia and agitation after an ingestion of a substance should raise concern for illicit stimulant intoxication. However, the primary stimulant in guarana powder, a product of the guarana berry, is caffeine (alongside other methylxanthines) concentrated in powder form.[1] This patient is currently suffering from caffeine intoxication. While tachycardia, tachypnea, and agitation are common symptoms across a variety of ingestions, caffeine ingestion should remain on the differential for patients with these symptoms given its near-ubiquitous use and easy accessibility. Depending on the dose ingested, caffeine toxicity can vary in severity from mild tachycardia and agitation at low doses to severe toxicity including seizures, tachydysrhythmias, and hypotension at high doses. Concentrated, high-dose caffeine supplements can be easily purchased at many retail stores or online without significant barriers.[1,2] These supplements, as demonstrated by this patient's presentation, can cause significant symptoms, and even death, with small physical amounts of product.

Background

Caffeine is part of a broader group of alkaloids called methylxanthines. Prominent members of this group include caffeine, theobromine, and theophylline. Caffeine and theobromine are naturally occurring and are found in a wide variety of consumer products. Caffeine can be found in energy drinks, energy powders and pills, coffee, and tea. Theobromine is found in the cacao plant. Guarana, a berry of *Paullinea cupana* found in South America, contains high concentrations of caffeine, and "guaranine" is synonymous with caffeine as an additive to supplements.[1,2] The US Food and Drug Administration (FDA) has issued multiple warnings to consumers and manufacturers of caffeine supplements regarding the dangers of concentrated caffeine.[3]

Theophylline and its salt, aminophylline, have been used to treat asthma due to their beta-adrenergic agonism reversing bronchospasm. They have largely been replaced in this role by selective beta-2 agonists such as albuterol.[2] However, caffeine and theophylline still play a role in the treatment of apnea and bradycardia of prematurity.[4] Caffeine is also used as an ingredient in analgesics, alongside ibuprofen and acetaminophen, typically marketed as an over-the-counter treatment for headaches and migraines.

Toxicology and Pathophysiology

At therapeutic doses, methylxanthines are used to reduce bronchospasm through a variety of mechanisms, including adenosine antagonism, catecholamine release, and stimulation of beta-adrenergic receptors. At extremely high concentrations, like those seen in severe toxicity, methylxanthines also inhibit phosphodiesterase, causing increases in cyclic adenosine monophosphate (cAMP). Elevated intracellular cAMP can mimic beta-adrenergic stimulation by relaxing smooth muscle and inhibiting histamine release from mast cells.[2,5]

Caffeine and theophylline have nearly 100% oral availability. They are also not subject to first-pass metabolism, making them available in high concentrations shortly after ingestion. Caffeine peak concentration is noted 30–60 minutes after ingestion, and immediate-release formulations of theophylline peak at 60–90 minutes. Sustained-release forms of either caffeine or theophylline display delayed peak concentrations. While both methylxanthines display linear metabolism kinetics at therapeutic ranges, they shift to logarithmic (Michaelis-Menten) kinetics at higher doses.[1,2,5] The half-life is presumed to be around 4.5 hours in those without significant induction or inhibition of relevant liver enzymes.[2]

Tolerance, interindividual differences in metabolism, preexisting diseases, and other factors cause variation in the doses at which methylxanthines induce toxicity. Concentrations at which morbidity and mortality have been noted can also vary widely. For caffeine, doses between 150 mg/kg and 210 mg/kg are potentially lethal, although the minimum toxic dose is not well defined. Theophylline toxicity is more complex, given that chronic users have symptoms indicating toxicity at noticeably lower serum concentrations than people in acute overdose due to chronically elevated levels of theophylline throughout the body. The goal serum concentration of theophylline is 5–15 mg/L; in patients on chronic theophylline, concentrations greater than 40 mg/L are associated with potentially severe toxicity. However, in patients not chronically taking theophylline who acutely overdose on theophylline, levels greater than 80 mg/L are associated with potentially severe toxicity.

A common clinical scenario is the theophylline user who has recently quit smoking. Regular cigarette use upregulates enzymes used in theophylline metabolism, and smoking cessation causes downregulation of those enzymes, causing a previously appropriate dose to become a toxic one due to decreased metabolism of the theophylline. [2]

Data regarding theobromine in humans are scant. It is a noted poison in animals, particularly dogs, when they consume large quantities of chocolate or cacao products, leading to GI effects, tachycardia, and neurologic effects such as tremors.[2]

Workup and Diagnosis

Signs and symptoms of methylxanthine toxicity are similar between the different compounds. Multiple organ systems are affected, with many effects being dose-dependent (Table 20.1). GI symptoms include nausea with severe, intractable emesis. Chronic methylxanthine use also causes increased gastric acid secretion, which, while not a priority in an acute setting, can cause gastritis and esophagitis in chronic use or abuse.[1]

The cardiovascular effects of methylxanthine toxicity can be severe and life-threatening. Sinus tachycardia is universally noted with methylxanthine use, but in toxicity this can progress to tachydysrhythmias including supraventricular tachycardia (SVT), multifocal atrial tachycardia (MAT), atrial fibrillation, ventricular tachycardia, and ventricular fibrillation. Electrolyte disturbances caused by toxicity can further contribute to dysrhythmia formation. Adrenergic stimulation can also precipitate myocardial infarction secondary to increased oxygen demand.[1,2]

Blood pressure changes are also present and variable with methylxanthine use. Dietary and therapeutic dosing cause hypertension initially, although this effect has been noted to decrease with chronic use.[6] The mechanism of this elevation in blood pressure is likely beta-1 adrenergic stimulation as well as increased catecholamine release. Interestingly, with significantly higher methylxanthine serum concentrations in overdose scenarios, hypotension has been frequently reported.[1,2,5] Mechanisms to explain this include dysrhythmias and tachycardia causing decreased cardiac output due to poor filling, as well as extreme phosphodiesterase inhibition and beta-2 agonism causing peripheral vasodilation. There is also a characteristic widened pulse pressure that develops as toxicity progresses.[2]

CNS effects include anxiety, agitation, tremors, hallucinations, headache, and, eventually, seizures that may be severe and refractory to treatment, requiring rapid escalation of care. Intoxication also stimulates the respiratory centers of the brain, increasing the respiratory rate and leading to respiratory alkalosis as well as respiratory distress and failure in severe cases.

Musculoskeletal signs and symptoms include tremors, myoclonus, and fasciculations secondary to CNS and striated muscle stimulation. This stimulation can lead to rhabdomyolysis and hyperthermia if unchecked.[7]

Metabolic changes associated with methylxanthine toxicity are useful in distinguishing it from other stimulants. The most notable electrolyte abnormality is hypokalemia, believed to be due to beta-2 adrenergic stimulation activating the Na+-K+-ATPase, resulting in the shift of potassium into cells.[5] This can cause clinically significant serum hypokalemia while maintaining normal total body potassium levels. Caution should be taken when repleting potassium, as resolution of the methylxanthine toxicity will result in potassium shifting out of the cell, thus putting the patient at risk of hyperkalemia if their initial hypokalemia were aggressively repleted. Other metabolic changes include hypomagnesemia, hypophosphatemia, and hyperglycemia. Leukocytosis may also be present secondary to catecholamine release.[2]

The diagnostic workup for suspected methylxanthine poisoning should include regular electrolyte monitoring, with special attention to serial potassium levels. Serum caffeine and theophylline levels should also be collected when testing is clinically available, and concentrations should ideally be monitored every 1–2 hours to inform management and better assess chronic versus acute poisoning. An ECG and continuous cardiac monitoring are important to monitor for the development of dysrhythmias from adrenergic stimulation as well as hypokalemia. Additionally, labs to evaluate for co-ingestions such as salicylate and acetaminophen levels should be collected if the methylxanthine was taken in a known or suspected suicide attempt. Finally, a total creatine kinase and a urinalysis should be collected to evaluate for rhabdomyolysis.

Treatment

As with all patients, immediate attention should be paid to airway, breathing, and circulation and support given as needed. With methylxanthine ingestions it is important to confirm whether there were co-ingestions, as well as what the time of ingestion and reason for ingestion were. Calculating the dose and assessing whether the toxicity is from chronic or acute use is also valuable information in the evaluation of suspected methylxanthine toxicity.

Initial treatment for patients depends on symptoms displayed as well as time since ingestion. GI decontamination can be effective in reducing the amount of substance available to cause toxicity but is of limited utility in the setting of emesis. If a patient presents within 60 minutes of an ingestion, activated charcoal is recommended to decrease initial absorption of the methylxanthine. For theophylline, multidose activated charcoal (MDAC) is a mainstay of treatment due to this methylxanthine's high enterohepatic recirculation. Additionally, the activated charcoal is effective not only at binding methylxanthine present in the GI tract, but also by facilitating the movement of methylxanthine through the gut wall in what is termed "gut dialysis." Dosage recommendations vary, but 0.5 g/kg every 2–6 hours is thought to be an acceptable regimen.[1,2,8]

System-specific treatments include antiemetics for the recurrent emesis brought on by toxicity. As electrolyte abnormalities such as hypokalemia and hypomagnesemia may cause QT prolongation, it is wise to obtain an ECG to evaluate QT intervals before administering ondansetron or other QT prolonging medications. Also, avoiding phenothiazine antiemetics such as prochlorperazine and promethazine should be considered because they may lower the seizure threshold in these high-risk patients.[1,2]

Cardiovascular management is particularly important as dysrhythmias are life-threatening and may require a departure from usual management in the case of methylxanthine poisoning. For mild tachycardia and symptomatic palpitations, benzodiazepines are a good initial therapy as they are thought to reduce catecholamine levels.[5,9] If SVT develops, the usual treatments of adenosine or cardioversion may only provide transient efficacy given that the presence of methylxanthine is not going to change appreciably after cardioversion. Additionally, methylxanthines act as an adenosine antagonist and may decrease the efficacy of adenosine treatment of SVT. Treatment of SVT should include beta-adrenergic antagonism such as esmolol, alongside the common treatments (adenosine and/or electrical cardioversion), as beta- agonism is a primary driver of the dysrhythmias.[2,5,9]

Treatment of ventricular dysrhythmias such as ventricular tachycardia and premature ventricular contractions also requires specific considerations. The advanced cardiac life support (ACLS) algorithm with the use of amiodarone, lidocaine, and electrical cardioversion should be followed.[2] However, beta-adrenergic antagonists should again be utilized given the dysrhythmia stems from beta-adrenergic agonism. Esmolol is a suggested agent given its rapid onset and quick duration of action if an adverse effect such as bronchospasm occurs. Again, it is important to note that methylxanthine levels will remain elevated and may require recurrent shocks and continuous infusion of medications to control rhythm.[2,10]

For the hypotension that develops with very high serum concentrations, resuscitation with a 20 mL/kg crystalloid bolus is appropriate. However, if hypotension is persistent, using a vasopressor may be necessary. If pressor use is ineffective or dysrhythmia develops, use of beta-adrenergic antagonists such as esmolol is indicated despite the counterintuitive nature of using a beta-adrenergic antagonist to increase blood pressure. This is postulated to be effective due to reducing beta-1–mediated dysrhythmia to allow for improved cardiac filling as well as combating beta-2–mediated vasodilation.[2,5]

Symptoms of CNS excitation ranging from mild anxiety to severe symptoms such as seizures should be treated with benzodiazepines. Patients at extremes of age (younger than 3 or older than 60 years) are most at risk of seizure development.[2] If patients do not respond to initial treatment, it may be necessary to escalate from benzodiazepines to barbiturates or propofol. Given their mechanism of effect, gamma-aminobutyric acid (GABA)ergic agents are preferred versus sodium channel blocking antiepileptic medications. Additionally, due to the long duration of methylxanthines there may be a need for multiple doses of shorter-acting benzodiazepines.[1]

Treatment of methylxanthine-induced hypokalemia is difficult given the total body potassium level is unchanged, but symptomatic hypokalemia with ECG changes (QT prolongation, dysrhythmias) requires treatment. IV or oral replacement as tolerated is acceptable. Serial monitoring for development of hyperkalemia during resolution of toxicity is important.

Finally, extracorporeal elimination of methylxanthines may be necessary under certain conditions. This can be done via intermittent hemodialysis

TABLE 20.1 Clinical findings in methylxanthine toxicity and suggested therapies

System	Clinical findings	Suggested therapies
Gastrointestinal	Nausea Vomiting Gastritis Esophagitis	Benzodiazepines Antiemetics (as permitted by QT)
Cardiovascular	Tachycardia Hypertension Hypotension (at very high serum concentrations) Tachydysrhythmias (SVT, MAT, atrial fibrillation, ventricular tachycardia and ventricular fibrillation)	Benzodiazepines IV Fluid Vasopressors Beta-adrenergic antagonists (for refractory hypotension as well as dysrhythmias) Amiodarone Adenosine Cardioversion
Neurologic	Anxiety Headache Agitation Tremors Seizures	Benzodiazepines Barbiturates Propofol
Metabolic	Hypokalemia Hypomagnesemia Hypophosphatemia Respiratory Alkalosis Metabolic Acidosis Rhabdomyolysis Leukocytosis	Treat symptomatic electrolyte abnormalities only (as abnormalities are due to electrolyte shifts) IV fluids

MAT, multifocal atrial tachycardia; SVT, supraventricular tachycardia.
Modified from Gresham et al.

or continuous renal replacement therapy (CRRT). Hemoperfusion is an alternative but not the preferred method. Some indications for extracorporeal elimination are refractory seizures, life-threatening dysrhythmias, and continued clinical deterioration despite appropriate management. Serum concentrations of theophylline greater than 100 mg/L in acute overdose and greater than 60 mg/L in chronic overdose are also recommended to receive extracorporeal treatment.[11]

CASE CONCLUSION

Returning to our case of the 21-year-old college student who presented after ingesting guarana powder, his initial EKG showed sinus tachycardia without QT prolongation, and he was given ondansetron for his nausea. Providers were unsure of time since ingestion and were concerned about his vomiting, leading them not to administer activated charcoal. His agitation continued and he eventually had a seizure. He was given midazolam with resolution of the seizure and was admitted for further monitoring. He did not have recurrence of seizures nor did he develop an arrhythmia, and he was discharged within 36 hours of admission.

KEY POINTS TO REMEMBER

- Caffeine and theobromine are methylxanthines found in many foods and supplements. Theophylline (and its salt, aminophylline) are compounds used in the treatment of apnea of prematurity and infrequently in the treatment of reversible bronchospastic disease.
- Methylxanthines act to release endogenous catecholamines, primarily causing beta-1 and beta-2 adrenergic agonism. Additionally, they are antagonists of adenosine, acting to prevent histamine release and inhibit phosphodiesterase.
- Caffeine, theobromine, and theophylline have high levels of oral bioavailability; with caffeine, peak concentrations are found 30–60 minutes after ingestion and with theophylline 60–90 minutes after ingestion.
- Signs of methylxanthine toxicity include tachycardia, tachyarrhythmias, hypotension at extreme concentrations, severe emesis, tachypnea, hypokalemia, and CNS excitation including seizures.
- Clinical evaluation should include serial electrolyte measurements, serial methylxanthine concentrations (if available), ECGs, and creatine kinase or urinalysis to detect rhabdomyolysis.

- Mainstays of treatment include:
    - GI decontamination with multidose activated charcoal.
    - Dysrhythmias should be treated with benzodiazepines and beta-adrenergic antagonists such as esmolol and metoprolol.
    - Hypotension should be treated with IV fluid bolus and vasopressors and/or, counterintuitively, with beta-blockers.
    - Seizures and agitation should be treated with benzodiazepines and care escalated rapidly if not responsive.

Further Reading

Gresham C, Brooks DE. Methylxanthines and nicotine. In: Tintinalli JE, Ma O, Yealy DM, Meckler GD, Stapczynski J, Cline DM, Thomas SH, eds. *Tintinalli's Emergency Medicine: A Comprehensive Study Guide*. 9th ed. McGraw Hill; 2020. Accessed February 27, 2022. https://accessmedicine-mhmedical-com.proxy.libr ary.emory.edu/content.aspx?bookid=2353&sectionid=220745204

Hoffman RJ. Methylxanthines and selective β2-adrenergic agonists. In: Nelson LS, Howland M, Lewin NA, Smith SW, Goldfrank LR, Hoffman RS, eds. *Goldfrank's Toxicologic Emergencies.*, 11th ed. McGraw Hill; 2019. Accessed February 27, 2022. https://accessemergencymedicine-mhmedical-com.proxy.library.emory. edu/content.aspx?bookid=2569&sectionid=210274122

Willson C. The clinical toxicology of caffeine: a review and case study. *Toxicol Rep*. 2018;5:1140–1152. doi:10.1016/j.toxrep.2018.11.002

References

1. Gresham C, Brooks DE. Methylxanthines and nicotine. In: Tintinalli JE, Ma O, Yealy DM, Meckler GD, Stapczynski J, Cline DM, Thomas SH, eds. *Tintinalli's Emergency Medicine: A Comprehensive Study Guide*. 9th ed. McGraw Hill; 2020. Accessed February 27, 2022. https://accessmedicine-mhmedical-com.proxy.libr ary.emory.edu/content.aspx?bookid=2353&sectionid=220745204

2. Hoffman RJ. Methylxanthines and selective β2-adrenergic agonists. In: Nelson LS, Howland M, Lewin NA, Smith SW, Goldfrank LR, Hoffman RS, eds. *Goldfrank's Toxicologic Emergencies.* 11th ed. McGraw Hill; 2019. Accessed February 27, 2022. https://accessemergencymedicine-mhmedical-com.proxy.libr ary.emory.edu/content.aspx?bookid=2569&sectionid=210274122

3. U.S. Food and Drug Administration. FDA takes step to protect consumers against dietary supplements containing dangerously high levels of extremely concentrated or pure caffeine. FDA. April 12, 2018. Accessed March 1, 2022. https://www.fda.gov/news-events/press-announcements/fda-takes-step-protect-consumers-against-dietary-supplements-containing-dangerously-high-levels

4. Rostas SE, McPherson C. caffeine therapy in preterm infants: the dose (and timing) make the medicine. *Neonatal Netw.* 2019;38(6):365–374. doi:10.1891/0730-0832.38.6.365

5. Willson C. The clinical toxicology of caffeine: a review and case study. *Toxicol Rep.* 2018;5:1140–1152. doi:10.1016/j.toxrep.2018.11.002

6. Turnbull D, Rodricks JV, Mariano GF, Chowdhury F. Caffeine and cardiovascular health. *Regul Toxicol Pharmacol.* 2017;89:165–185. doi:10.1016/j.yrtph.2017.07.025

7. Campana C, Griffin PL, Simon EL. Caffeine overdose resulting in severe rhabdomyolysis and acute renal failure. *Am J Emerg Med.* 2014;32(1):111.e3–111. e111004. doi:10.1016/j.ajem.2013.08.042

8. Ilkhanipour K, Yealy DM, Krenzelok EP. The comparative efficacy of various multiple-dose activated charcoal regimens. *Am J Emerg Med.* 1992;10(4):298–300. doi:10.1016/0735-6757(92)90006-j

9. Seneff M, et al. Acute theophylline toxicity and the use of esmolol to reverse cardiovascular instability. *Ann Emerg Med.* 1990;19:671–673. [PubMed: 1971502]

10. Laskowski, Larissa K et al. "Start me up!" Recurrent ventricular tachydysrhythmias following intentional concentrated caffeine ingestion. *Clin Toxicol (Philadelphia, Pa.).* 2015;53(8):830–833.

11. Ghannoum M, Wiegand T, EXTRIP Workgroup. Extracorporeal treatment for theophylline poisoning: systematic review and recommendations from the EXTRIP workgroup. *Clin Toxicol (Phila).* 2015;53:215–229. [PubMed: 25715736]

21 Not So Essential Oils: Essential Oil Ingestions

Ashima Goyal Gurkha and
Dhritiman Gurkha

Case Presentation

A 20-month-old otherwise healthy boy presents to the ED extremely drowsy and confused. His heart rate is 70 beats/min and regular, blood pressure is 75/40. His respirations are shallow and irregular at a rate of 8 breaths/min with supplemental oxygen via nonrebreather mask (pulse ox 90%). His exam is notable for confusion, 1 mm pupils bilaterally, and reduced muscle tone with absent deep tendon reflexes. He is noted to have a tonic-clonic seizure lasting 10 minutes. A dose of lorazepam is given without resolution of seizure activity. A second dose of lorazepam is administered but he continues to seize. Point-of-care glucose upon arrival is 98 mg/dL. The child has no previous history of seizures. His liver function tests and serum calcium are normal. In addition to serum ethanol, acetaminophen, salicylate levels, a urine drug screen is also obtained. He is not on any home medications.

What Do You Do Now?

DISCUSSION

Background

When approaching a patient with seizures that is thought to be from a suspected toxic exposure, the following toxidromes should be considered: organophosphates, anticholinergics, cyclic antidepressants, sympathomimetics, isoniazid (or any hydrazine), and methylxanthine. Toxidromes for specific toxins can be helpful for determining the cause of a seizure. When a patient's clinical picture does not fit a particular toxidrome, essential oil toxicity should be considered. Recognizing essential oil toxicity is challenging because the history of a toxic essential oil ingestion is often given by the patient or parent of a child. History of exposure is important because many patients/caregivers may be unaware of the dangers of essential oils and not mention their use when seeking medical care.

Since ancient times, essential oils have been recognized for their medicinal values. The ancient Egyptians used essential oils in medicine and in preparation of bodies for burial through mummification. In Asia, the Vedas codified the uses of perfumes and aromatics for liturgical and therapeutic purposes.[1] Later, Greeks and Romans used distillation to create aromatic derivatives, including soaps and perfumes. During the Renaissance, the use of essential oils was extended throughout the world.[2] Essential oils continue to be used today and in recent years have become increasingly popular in a variety of consumer products and as alternative "natural" treatments for common ailments. The low cost, ease of availability, and perception of low harm only increases their use.

The International Organization for Standardization defines essential oils as a "product obtained from a natural raw material of plant origin, by steam distillation, by mechanical processes from the epicarp of citrus fruits, or by dry distillation, after separation of the aqueous phase-if-any by physical processes."[3] Individual oils may be obtained from species of plants and/or can be produced commercially. These oils are odorous, colorless, and are considered volatile. They are highly complex mixtures of volatile compounds with the major constituents being hydrocarbons, alcohols, aldehydes, ketones, phenolic esthers, oxides, and esthers.[2] Common essential oils include but are not limited to clove, eucalyptus, fennel, sage, tea tree, wintergreen, and woodworm. Essential oils are commonly used to enhance the flavor of food, drinks, fragrances, teas, and spices. They are also used in household products such as candles, detergents, and aromatherapy. The oils are usually applied to the skin, but also can be administered orally, inhaled, or diffused through the air.

All essential oils are hydrocarbons and share the basic toxidrome for hydrocarbons CNS and respiratory depression. As hydrocarbons, essential oils are hydrophobic in that they mimic fat-soluble drugs and therefore are well absorbed through the skin and mucus membranes and can readily cross the blood–brain barrier. They are metabolized by the liver and, following limited phase I enzyme metabolism by glucuronidation or sulfation, eliminated by the kidney in the form of polar compounds or exhaled via the lungs as carbon dioxide.[2] Hydrocarbons can cause nausea and vomiting, which can lead to aspiration pneumonitis due to the dissolution of surfactant and resulting mechanical injury. Thus, airway protection is paramount in nauseous and vomiting patients to prevent aspiration.[4] Along this same line, gastric lavage is contraindicated for hydrocarbon ingestions given the concern of vomiting while placing a nasogastric or orogastric tube, thus iatrogenically causing a hydrocarbon pneumonitis. Urinary output should be carefully monitored, particularly if hypotension is present or if large volumes of oil have been ingested.[5]

Essential oils can cause severe toxicity when ingested, although the exact risk and end-organ damage depends on the specific essential oil (Table 21.1). Toxicity can occur from the essential oil itself or the additive hydrocarbon emulsifier. The onset of toxicity from essential oils is generally rapid and quantities as little as 5 mL can be fatal. Essential oils concentrations typically range from 1% to 20%, but can be higher. Following ingestion, onset of symptoms is usually within 1 hour. Sigs of aspiration can occur immediately but can be delayed up to 6 hours. Volumes of 5–15 mL are likely to cause toxicity in adults, whereas smaller ingestions of 2–3 mL have been associated with toxicity in children.[5] Children are at higher risk of toxicity from these products causing symptoms such as CNS depression, vomiting, or pneumonitis. Children have a greater body to surface area ratio which can cause rapid dissemination of oils applied to the skin and may lead to toxicity. Due to their inherent curiosity, children can swallow oils in liquid form easily. Additionally, the oil can be nauseating, inducing vomiting, which can then cause aspiration pneumonitis. Nonaccidental poisoning in children should be considered when a child's developmental age is inconsistent with exploratory behavior and accidental poisoning.

A recent Australian study reviewed essential oil exposure calls to the New South Wales Poisons Information Centre between July 2014 and June 2018. Most exposures were noted to be accidental or a result of therapeutic error, typically mistaking essential oils for liquid pharmaceuticals, most commonly cough liquids.[6] In this study, the most frequently involved essential oils were eucalyptus (46.4%), tea tree (17.0%), lavender (6.1%), clove (4.1%), and peppermint oils (3.5%).[6] The increase in essential oils among common household products and risk of toxic exposures reflects need for public awareness and continued education. Despite their frequent use and perceived safety, the use of essential oils does not come without potential harm.

Toxicology and Pathophysiology

Tea tree oil comes from the leaves of an Australian tree called *Melaleuca alternifola*. As a traditional medicine, it has been used for treatment of conditions such as head lice, acne, toothaches, and vaginitis, however there is no evidence supporting medical use of tea tree oil. Tea tree oil is a mixture of cyclic hydrocarbons containing 35–40% terpinen-4-ol, 2 to 15% cineole, and 12 other compounds.[7] When taken orally in high concentrations, tea tree oil can cause symptoms such as confusion, vomiting, ataxia, and decreased consciousness. There have been reported cases of irritation to the skin after repeated exposure of topical tea tree oil dermal application.[8,9] Symptoms of irritation to the skin include redness, itching, or burning. There is no antidote available. Treatment is based on the level of toxicity. Mild illness may require skin decontamination with dish soap bathing and supportive care for oral ingestion. The effectiveness of orally administered charcoal is unknown. Great caution should be taken with hydrocarbon ingestions and charcoal because charcoal may induce vomiting, which can lead to aspiration pneumonia of both the essential oil and charcoal, a complication to be avoided at all cost.

Lavender is an essential oil obtained from distillation of flower spikes of different species of lavender. It is primarily composed of linalyl acetate (51%) and linalool (35%).[9] It has traditionally been used for skin applications for massage therapy and aromatherapy. Symptoms of lavender ingestion include difficulty breathing, vomiting, diarrhea, rash, and/or confusion. Lavender oil has estrogenic and anti-androgenic properties and can cause prepubertal gynecomastia.[10,11] Lavender oil in general is not toxic when inhaled during aromatherapy but can be deadly if swallowed in large amounts.[12] It may cause an allergic skin reaction with repeated dermal exposure. There is no reported treatment for lavender toxicity. Supportive care is recommended.

Clove oil is an essential oil obtained from the dried flower buds of *Eugenia caryophyllata* tree and contains 70–90% eugenol.[13] Clove extracts are found in many topical creams, lotions, and bath oils and in toothpaste for its possible effect in alleviating toothache or painful gums. Ingestion of a small amount of clove oil, especially in children, can be fatal. A prior case report notes a 2-year-old boy developing coma with generalized seizures after drinking between 5 and 10 mL of clove oil.[13] Eugenol used in low doses appears to have few side effects other than local irritation, rare allergic reactions, and contact dermatitis, while exposure to or ingestion of a large amount can result in tissue injury and a syndrome of acute onset of seizures and coma, as well as damage to the liver and kidneys.[14] Additionally, eugenol can lead to neuropathy. In high concentrations, eugenol oil has cytotoxic activity and causes acute hepatic necrosis via metabolism of glucuronide and sulphate conjugates. This clinical presentation is similar in nature to acetaminophen hepatotoxicity. For this reason, acetylcysteine can be considered when treating patients with eugenol or clove oil overdose. Although there are no antidotes, acetylcysteine has been thought to contribute to favorable outcomes. Also important is management of electrolyte balance, prevention of hypoglycemia, and use of antiemetics as needed.

Another popular yet deadly essential oil that is common but lacks appropriate concern is pennyroyal. Pennyroyal is an herbal extract or oil derived from leaves of the plant in the mint genus (*Mentha pulegium*). Given its strong spearmint-like fragrance, it was historically used to flavor tea, wine, etc. Furthermore, it was also used as an abortifacient and insect repellent. In modern times, it has been used for aromatherapy. If ingested, pennyroyal oil is highly toxic and has been associated significant hepatotoxicity and death. The principal toxic component of pennyroyal is pulegone, which is converted to other hepatoxic components (menthofuran) by the cytochrome P450 system. Patients can initially present with GI manifestations including nausea, vomiting, and abdominal pain in addition to neurological symptoms of dizziness, lethargy, and agitation. Although there are no known antidotes, glutathione has been reported to detoxify the toxic metabolites of pulegone. Hence, N-acetylcysteine should be administered.[14,15]

Eucalyptus oil is commonly used as a naturopathic treatment for a variety of ailments. Eucalyptus oil is thought to treat cough and colds, muscle aches, and lice infestations.[16] No studies to date have confirmed eucalyptus oil to be an effective treatment for these ailments. Pure eucalyptus oil can contain 70–80% eucalyptol (1,8 cineole), which is the primary toxic compound.[17] Symptoms consistent with a toxic exposure are generally rapid in onset and can include a burning sensation in the mouth and vomiting. Patients will typically exhibit a decrease in respiratory effort, loss of reflexes, and a depressed level of consciousness, which may be profound owing to toxicity that is shared by all hydrocarbons. In adults, death may occur after ingestion of 30 mL but have been reported for ingestions as low as 4–5 mL as well. There is no specific antidote for eucalyptol, and management is primarily supportive. When eucalyptus poisoning is suspected, removal of dermal contamination can be performed by using soap and lukewarm water. Asymptomatic patients and patients with mild oropharyngeal irritation should be observed for a minimum of 4 hours. The greatest risk for seizures is within the first 2 hours of ingestion. Benzodiazepines should be used as first-line treatment for seizures, with repeat doses as needed. Refractory seizures may require intubation and ventilation. In patients with prolonged altered mental status or focal neurological deficits, neuroimaging should be pursued to rule out alterative diagnoses such as a structural lesion. With prompt diagnosis and appropriate management, patients have been shown to have complete recovery within 24 hours without increased risk of future seizures.[18]

Methyl salicylate, more commonly known as oil of wintergreen, is a source for potentially fatal salicylate toxicity. Oil of wintergreen is a topical ointment used for its analgesic, anti-inflammatory, and antiplatelet properties. It is a potent essential oil because it contains a significant concentration of salicylate, which can have serious clinical implications with the smallest exposure. Acute salicylate toxicity can occur by ingestion or topical absorption. Early symptoms may not be present until 6–12 hours after ingestion and can include nausea, vomiting, tachypnea, and/or tinnitus. The primary effects of toxicity include direct stimulation of the CNS respiratory center leading to respiratory alkalosis. Salicylates also uncouple oxidative phosphorylation, leading to increased oxygen consumption and increase in metabolic rate. The Krebs cycle is inhibited, which alters lipid metabolism and causes production of ketones, resulting in metabolic acidosis. These effects can lead to altered mental status and possible seizures.[19] For details regarding treatment, refer to Chapter 2.

Treatment

Initial risk assessment of essential oil toxicity includes determining the suspected oil ingested, amount, concentration, route taken, and any other potential co-ingestants. Examination needs to focus on respiratory status. Specifically, ensure airway patency and respiratory effort in the setting of aspiration and seizures, if they have not already occurred. In addition, hemodynamics should be supported as needed. Finally, side effects on various body systems should be considered including GI (vomiting, diarrhea, hepatotoxicity) and skin (mucus membrane irritation, contact dermatitis).[14]

Acute management is primarily through aggressive supportive care as there is no true antidotal therapy for most essential oils. Charcoal is generally ineffective in hydrocarbon ingestion and contraindicated in the setting of depressed mental status, which is frequently seen after an essential oil ingestion. Furthermore, vomiting and subsequent aspiration can lead to severe pneumonitis. Generally considered treatments include n-acetylcysteine for clove oil and pennyroyal oil, but this should be ordered in consultation with a medical toxicologist. Routine eye irrigation should be completed for possible ocular exposure/irritation. Irritation to the skin should be treated with soap and water and removal of all clothing. Aspiration is managed with supportive care including oxygen and bronchodilators; intubation may be required if the patient's airway is compromised or for respiratory failure. Chest x-ray and blood gas should be considered in children with suspected aspiration pneumonitis who are symptomatic. In children who are asymptomatic with history of a small ingestion, imaging and laboratory evaluation is not initially indicated. Asymptomatic children with significant exposure (>5 mL) should be observed for a period of 4 hours prior to discharge with normal vital signs.[4] If a patient has abnormal physical findings or vital signs, they should be admitted until resolution of their symptoms. For adolescents in particular, admission should be considered for intentional overdose, as there is greater concern for a large ingestion compared to exploratory ingestion by a younger child. Risk assessment should be completed to assess future risk of self-harm if discharge is considered.

CASE CONCLUSION

The child in the case presented to the ED with respiratory depression. Initial management included optimizing oxygenation and ventilation. The child also had seizures which resolved with lorazepam. At 2 hours post admission, his blood pressure, pulse, and respiratory rate returned to normal, although his mental status remained depressed. Electroencephalogram was noted to be normal. Laboratory evaluation for altered mental status was unremarkable, including blood glucose, serum sodium, and calcium. CT head without contrast was noted to be normal. After 4 more hours, the patient regained consciousness and by 24 hours, he was back at baseline. He was discharged home 48 hours after admission. After the patient was stabilized, questions regarding potential environmental exposures were pursued. It was discovered that a half-full eucalyptus oil aromatherapy bottle was found in the mother's bedroom with some spilled oil on the carpet. The patient was suspected to have ingested eucalyptus oil. Key findings of a poisoning include a history of oral ingestion or topical exposure, and the patient may have a scented smell on the breath, oropharyngeal irritation, GI discomfort, and seizures, which may be the first sign of exposure or significant toxicity.

TABLE 21.1 **Toxic essential oils with significant toxicity**

Essential oils	Botanical name	Primary toxin	Primary clinical manifestation
Bergamot	*Citrus aurantium bergamia*	Bergapten (psoralen)	Muscle cramps, paresthesia, blurred vision
Cinnamon	*Cinnamomum zeylanicum*	Cinnamaldehyde	Dermatitis
Clove	*Syzygium aromaticum*	Eugenol	Hepatotoxicity, neuropathy
Camphor	*Cinnamomum camphora*	Terpene	Hepatotoxicity, seizures, neurotoxicity
Eucalyptus	*Eucalyptus globulus*	1,8 cineole	Seizures
Fennel	*Foeniculum vulgare*	Trans anethole, alpha-pinene	Seizures, neurotoxicity, pulmonary edema
Frankincense	*Boswellia sacra*	Alpha-pinene, limonene, sabinene	Dermatitis, diarrhea
Lavender	*Lavandula* spp.	Linalyl acetate and linalool	Dermatitis, difficulty breathing, prepubertal gynecomastia
Nutmeg	*Myristica fragrans*	Myristicin, eugenol	Hallucinations, flushed skin with tachycardia and pinpoint pupils
Pennyroyal	*Hedeoma pulegioides*	Pulegone	Hepatotoxicity, renal failure
Peppermint	*Mentha* spp.	Menthol, menthone	Ataxia, myalgia
Sage oil	*Salvia officinalis*	Alpha or beta Thujone	Seizures, neurotoxicity
Tea tree	*Melaleuca alternifolia*	Mixture of cyclic hydrocarbons	Dermatitis, difficulty breathing, prepubertal gynecomastia

(*Continued*)

TABLE 21.1 **Continued**

Essential oils	Botanical name	Primary toxin	Primary clinical manifestation
Thyme	*Thymus vulgaris*	Thymol, para-cymene	Difficulty breathing, neurotoxicity
Wintergreen	*Gaultheria procumbens*	Methyl salicylate	Tinnitus, altered mental status, seizures, renal failure
Wormwood	*Artemisia absinthium*	Alpha or beta Thujone	Seizures, dementia, neurotoxicity

Clinical manifestations of note: essential oil toxicity primarily presents itself as nausea, vomiting, headache, and abdominal pain.

KEY POINTS TO REMEMBER

- Symptoms are specific to type of essential oil ingested.
- Children are at higher risk for toxicity.
- Aspiration pneumonia is a risk from essential oil ingestions.

Further Reading

El Hattab, M. Algae essential oils: chemistry, ecology, and biological activities. In: Santana de Oliveira M, Almeida da Costa W, Gomes Silva S, eds. *Essential Oils*. IntechOpen; 2020.

Liaqat I, Riaz N, Saleem Q, Tahir H, Arshad M, Arshad N. Toxicological evaluation of essential oils from some plants of Rutaceae family. *Evid Based Complement Alternat Med.* 2018;2018:1–7.

Mathew T, Kamath V, Kumar R, et al. Eucalyptus oil inhalation-induced seizure: a novel, underrecognized, preventable cause of acute symptomatic seizure. *Epilepsia Open.* 2017;2(3):350–354.

Plant R, Dinh L, Argo S, Shah M. The essentials of essential oils. *Adv Pediatr.* 2019;66:111–122.

References

1. Ríos J. Essential oils: what they are and how the terms are used and defined. In: Preedy V, ed. *Essential Oils in Food Preservation, Flavor and Safety*. Academic Press; 2022: 3–10.

2. Djilani A, Dicko A. The therapeutic benefits of essential oils. In: Bouayed J, Bohn T, eds. *Nutrition, Well-Being and Health*. IntechOpen; 2012.

3. Ward JM, Reeder M, Atwater AR. 2020. Essential oils debunked: separating fact from myth. *Cutis*. Apr 2020;105(4):174–176.

4. De Groot A, Schmidt E. Essential oils, part I. *Dermatitis*. 2016;27(2):39–42.

5. Patel S, Wiggins J. 1980. Eucalyptus oil poisoning. *Arch Dis Childhood*. 1980;55(5):405–406.

6. Anas N. Criteria for hospitalizing children who have ingested products containing hydrocarbons. *JAMA*. 1981;246(8):840.

7. Lee K, Harnett J, Cairns R. Essential oil exposures in Australia: analysis of cases reported to the NSW Poisons Information Centre. *Med J Austral*. 2019;212(3):132–133.

8. Morris M, Donoghue A, Markowitz J, Osterhoudt K. Ingestion of tea tree oil (Melaleuca oil) by a 4-year-old boy. *Pediatr Emerg Care*. 2003;19(3):169–171.

9. Greig J, Carson C, Stuckey M, Riley T. *Skin Sensitivity Testing for Tea Tree Oil* [ebook]. Rural Industries Research and Development Corporation. 1999. Accessed February 27, 2022. https://www.agrifutures.com.au/wp-content/uploads/publicati ons/99-076.pdf

10. Veien N, Rosner K, Skovgaard G. Is tea tree oil an important contact allergen? *Contact Dermatitis*. 2004;50(6):378–379.

11. Prashar A, Locke I, Evans C. Cytotoxicity of lavender oil and its major components to human skin cells. *Cell Prolif*. 2004;37(3):221–229.

12. Henley D, Lipson N, Korach K, Bloch C. Prepubertal gynecomastia linked to lavender and tea tree oils. *N Engl J Med*. 2007;356(24):2541–2544.

13. Landelle C, Francony G, Sam-Laï N, et al. Poisoning by lavandin extract in an 18-month-old boy. *Clin Toxicol*. 2008;46(4):279–281.

14. Hartnoll G, Moore D, Douek D. Near fatal ingestion of oil of cloves. *Arch Dis Childhood*. 1993;69(3):392–393.

15. National Institute of Diabetes and Digestive and Kidney Diseases. *LiverTox: Clinical and Research Information on Drug-Induced Liver Injury*. 2012. Accessed February 27, 2022. https://www.ncbi.nlm.nih.gov/books/NBK551727/

16. Woolf A. Essential oil poisoning. *J Toxicol: Clin Toxicol*. 1999;37(6):721–727.

17. Tibballs J. Clinical effects and management of eucalyptus oil ingestion in infants and young children. *Med J Austral*. 1995;163(4):177–180.

18. Kumar K, Sonnathi S, Anitha C, Santhoshkumar M. Eucalyptus oil poisoning. *Toxicol Int*. 2015;22(1):170.

19. Chin RL, Olson KR, Dempsey D. Salicylate toxicity from ingestion and continued dermal absorption. *Cal J Emerg Med*. 2007;8(1):23–25.

22 ME Think You Should Not Use: Methamphetamines Intoxication

Suad Al-Sulaimani

Case Presentation

A 28-year-old man with no prior psychiatric hospitalizations was sent to the ED after his partner called 911; he was concerned that he had become uncharacteristically agitated and irritable after attending a party last night. The patient had started screaming at his partner and threatened him with a knife. When the patient arrived in the ED, he was given intramuscular lorazepam 2 mg and haloperidol 5 mg due to threatening behavior toward ED staff. His vital signs on arrival were heart rate 125 beats/min, blood pressure 170/90 mm Hg, respiratory rate 20 breaths/min, temperature 101.8°F/38.8°C, and saturation 90% on room air. The initial physical examination shows an uncooperative, combative young man. He is pale and diaphoretic. His pupils are dilated and minimally responsive to light, and he is tachypneic with clear lungs bilaterally. The medical record shows multiple prior ED visits for complications of methamphetamine use, as well as concomitant alcohol and tobacco use. The initial ECG showed sinus tachycardia (122 beats/min) with normal QRS and QTc intervals and without evidence of ST elevations or depressions.

What Do You Do Now?

DISCUSSION

Background

The patient in this clinical vignette presents with severe agitation and is violent. Additionally, he is tachycardic, hyperthermic, and hypertensive after an illicit drug exposure. The differential diagnosis is broad and includes organic diseases, psychiatric conditions, and wide range of psychostimulant xenobiotics. Additionally, it is possible that the history of methamphetamine use may be a red herring, masking other toxicological causes of the sympathomimetic toxidrome. The sympathomimetic toxidrome may carry a broad differential diagnosis. Management of methamphetamine toxicity may be complicated by an uncooperative patient; however, active supportive measures to avoid harm to the patient and staff through aggressive sedation is the cornerstone in treating such patients.

Methamphetamine is a widely available illicit drug due to the ease and low cost of manufacturing. There has been a significant surge in methamphetamine use since 2009 in the United States.[1-3] Patients presenting to the ED for complications of illicit methamphetamine use tend to be adolescent and young males.[2] Pediatric exposure to these drugs is expected to continue as phenylethylamine derivatives are approved by the US Food and Drug Administration (FDA) for treatment of attention deficit disorder with hyperactivity (ADHD), obesity, and narcolepsy.[3-5] The National Office on Drugs and Crime and National Poison Data System (NPDS), a database maintained by the American Association of Poison Control Centers, 2019–2000 data showed increased use of amphetamine-type stimulants, particularly methamphetamine, with increasing numbers since 2017. Data showed an increase in the rate and severity of reported cases especially in those 20 years and older.[6,7]

Clinical effects following methamphetamine exposure can vary widely depending on dose, route, duration, and pattern of use.[3] Acute methamphetamine toxicity is associated with anxiety, agitation, hypertensive crises, stroke, acute myocardial toxicity, and sudden cardiac death. CNS effects of methamphetamine use are characterized by being more agitated, violent, and aggressive compared with other psychostimulants such as cocaine.[4] As a consequence of impaired psychomotor and cognitive skills associated with methamphetamine, patients may present with serious trauma such as motor vehicle accidents and falls.[3] Cardiac toxicity may be serious and may lead to cardiogenic shock and death.

Chronic methamphetamine users may present with heart failure because of underlying cardiomyopathy; subsequently they may progress to cardiac ischemia and arrhythmias.[8] Hype-adrenergic surge may lead to hypertensive crises, and vasospasm may lead to serious complications: methamphetamine-related stroke is associated with poor clinical outcomes. Mechanisms of methamphetamine-associated stroke include hypertension, vasculitis, direct vascular toxicity, and vasospasm.[9] Rhabdomyolysis and acute kidney injury (AKI) occur commonly but resolve with supportive care. The potential complications include but are not limited to renal injury, liver failure, cardiac failure, hypotension, acute respiratory distress syndrome (ARDS), coagulopathy, cerebral edema, and death.[3–5,8–10]

Toxicology and Pathophysiology

Methamphetamine belongs to a broader group of compounds called phenylethylamines.[3] Phenethylamines are chemical structures with a backbone of an aromatic ring with a two-carbon side chain leading to a terminal amine (Figure 22.1). Specific substitutions made to the phenylethylamine backbone have led to a wide variety of xenobiotics with different properties.[1–3] Many illicit drugs derive from phenylethylamines, including methamphetamine ("crank," "speed"), 3,4-methylenedioxymethamphetamine (MDMA; "ecstasy" or "Molly"), paramethoxyamphetamine (PMA), methylenedioxymethamphetamine (MDA; "sassafras" or "Sally"), and many others. Some other medically used drugs including duloxetine (Cymbalta), and the ADHD medication d-amphetamine (Adderall: a combination of amphetamine and d-amphetamine mixed salts), dextroamphetamine (Dexedrine), levomethamphetamine (Desoxyn), and methylphenidate (Ritalin) are also derived from phenylethylamines.[11] Methamphetamine is produced by addition of an extra methyl group to the terminal amine in amphetamine. This extra methyl group leads to the additional properties of methamphetamine, making it more lipid soluble, with potent stimulant and cardiovascular effects.[1–3]

The underlying toxicological and pathophysiologic mechanisms of methamphetamines are complex. The primary mechanism of action is the release of catecholamines from presynaptic nerve terminals. The pharmacologic effect results from stimulation of dopamine and norepinephrine and, to a lesser extent, serotonin receptors leading to a hyperadrenergic state. A wide range of clinical effects are related to the binding selectivity to the neurotransmitter. Several other mechanisms contribute to the pharmacological effects of methamphetamines, including inhibition of neuronal reuptake of catecholamines, thereby increasing their availability at the nerve terminal and promoting prolonged activity. Amphetamines also promote the intracellular expression of tyrosine hydroxylase and inhibit monoamine oxidase activity, leading to increased dopamine synthesis and decreased metabolism, respectively.[1-3]

There are multiple routes of methamphetamine administration: nasal insufflation, pyrolysis and inhalation, ingestion, or IV injection. Smoking crystalline methamphetamine is the most common route of use. Powdered "speed" and a yellow paste "base" are also available as pure forms of methamphetamines.[1-12] Methamphetamine is characterized by a prolonged effect on the CNS because of its lipophilicity and long half-life. Plasma levels usually peak 30 minutes after IV or IM injection and 2–3 hours after oral ingestion. The half-life of methamphetamine is approximately 12 hours, compared with about 90 minutes for cocaine. Methamphetamine metabolism occurs in the liver, mainly involving the cytochrome isoenzyme CYP2D.[8] Methamphetamine is excreted predominantly in the urine. There is almost no xenobiotic more potent at increasing dopamine levels in the brain than amphetamines, which underlies their highly addictive potential and the difficulty in treating amphetamine use disorder.

Workup and Diagnosis

The diagnosis of methamphetamine intoxication is usually made on the basis of clinical effects and the predominance of adrenergic effects, characterized by the sympathomimetic toxidrome. The diagnosis of amphetamine intoxication is further supported by clinical presentation of hallucinations, hyperthermia, and excess sympathetic tone.[3] Methamphetamine users are more aggressive, violent, and dangerous compared to other illicit drug abusers and thus more likely to pose a risk to themselves and others. Several laboratory testing modalities may be helpful in the workup of patients presenting with methamphetamine intoxication and should be guided by the clinical presentation. A basic metabolic panel (BMP) can demonstrate electrolyte abnormalities, particularly hyponatremia associated with MDMD use. Hyponatremia is attributed to both increased sweating with a concomitant increase in free water ingestions as well as serotonin receptor selectivity, which may affect the antidiuretic hormone release leading to a syndrome of inappropriate antidiuretic hormone (SIADH).[1] An elevated creatine kinase (CK) level may indicate rhabdomyolysis, which is a common finding. CK levels and renal function should be monitored closely because renal failure, as well as potentially life-threatening hyperkalemia, may develop. Metabolic acidosis, an elevated lactate level, and coagulopathy can develop secondary to dehydration, inadequate peripheral perfusion, seizures, or hyperthermia.[3] An ECG should be obtained to look for interval changes, especially QT prolongation, dysrhythmias, and evidence of ischemia. A chest X-ray and/or CT can be obtained if there is concern for pulmonary edema or aortic dissection.[8] Abdominal imaging should be considered in cases of body stuffing.

Urine immunoassays are a common, widely available test for the detection of amphetamines and amphetamine derivatives. These techniques are highly vulnerable to false negatives and false positives. Further discussion about the utility of the UDS can be found in Chapter 16. A routine amphetamine urine drug screen is neither a highly sensitive nor specific test. Unfortunately, even a true-positive result has limited value in the management of acutely intoxicated patients because it could indicate the use of amphetamines at any time in the past several days. A wide range of xenobiotics may result in false-positive results; for example, many over-the-counter cold and flu preparations that contain pseudoephedrine, an amphetamine derivative, and levomethamphetamine is FDA-approved as an inhaled nasal decongestant. Additionally, selegiline, an MAOI, is metabolized to levomethamphetamine; and bupropion is a cathinone and resembles amphetamine in structure. Other medications that are known to cause a positive UDS screen for amphetamines are trazodone, amantadine, and certain antihistamines.[1-13] Some amphetamines such as MDMA and cathinones are not recognized on standard urinary drug testing and may lead to false-negative results. Urine immunoassays should not be routinely ordered to guide clinical management. The gold standard for drug testing, gas chromatography–mass spectrometry analysis, is used in special situations and is usually not part of the routine workup.[13]

Treatment

Treatment for methamphetamine toxicity is supportive in nature. Based on these concerns, benzodiazepines are recommended as first-line treatments in the management of acute toxicity from amphetamines. Because agitation and violence are predominant features in patients who are acutely intoxicated, temporary physical restraint may be needed to gain pharmacologic control and prevent harm to themselves or others; however, it is essential that pharmacologic agents are the primary means of restraint, and any physical restraints are discontinued as early as possible. High doses of benzodiazepines may be required to achieve control and adequate sedation. Doses exceeding 100 mg of diazepam, or its equivalent, are sometimes required.[6,7,10–14]

Controversy exists regarding the addition of antipsychotics to benzodiazepines to further control agitation. Adjunctive use of antipsychotics is reasonable and supported by evidence, particularly in children younger than 12 years[5] Antipsychotics such as haloperidol and droperidol can be considered as adjuncts to control amphetamine-related psychosis.[14] However, antipsychotic use may be limited by the occurrence of side effects like acute dystonia, seizures, further increases in core temperature, and cardiac dysrhythmia, which are less likely to occur in the pediatric population.[5–13] Seizures are treated with benzodiazepines as a first line. Further pharmacologic treatments for seizures may be required and should focus on agents acting at the gamma-aminobutyric acid (GABA) receptor (e.g., barbiturates, propofol).

In the majority of cases, adequately dosing benzodiazepines is sufficient to calm the patient and prevent injuries inflicted to staff and patient. However, in the rare case of hyperactive delirium with severe agitation, otherwise known as "agitated delirium," more rapid control may be required for the protection of patients and hospital staff. In these patients, the sympathomimetic substance causes a severely hyperagitated state with increased metabolism and metabolic acidosis.[15] Any attempt to subdue this subset of patients physically, even without compromise to their respiratory function, can lead to worsening metabolic acidosis and death owing to the high minute ventilation requirement to compensate for metabolic acidosis. In this case, rapid control is needed, and up to 5 mg/kg of IM ketamine can rapidly cause sympatholysis and sedate the patient. While ketamine is generally safe and should not cause respiratory depression by itself, providers should be aware that patients may stop breathing or, even more rarely, suffer cardiac arrest, and therefore must be prepared for rapid sequence intubation or to begin advanced cardiac life support (ACLS) as necessary.

Cardiac complications are not uncommon. Beyond benzodiazepines, further control of significant hypertension can be achieved using nitroprusside or labetalol, with the goal being to avoid complications such as intracranial hemorrhage and cardiac ischemia. Generally, pure beta-blockers should be avoided as they theoretically may lead to unopposed alpha-adrenergic receptor stimulation. Serial ECGs should be monitored. Ventricular dysrhythmias should be managed following standard ACLS protocols. Correction of electrolyte abnormalities will minimize the risk of dysrhythmia.[8]

Rapid cooling for significant hyperthermia is a necessary and important component of treatment. Severe hyperthermia may develop as a result of disturbance of thermoregulation or increased skeletal muscle hyperactivity because of agitation or seizures. Benzodiazepines should be used followed by active measures. Several active cooling measures can be employed including water mist and fans, ice packs, and ice water immersion. Refractory hyperthermia could also suggest serotonin toxicity; the risk is higher in those taking other therapeutic or recreational serotonergic drugs.[14,16]

Rhabdomyolysis should be treated with aggressive hydration to enhance urinary elimination and prevent acute renal failure.[14,16]

There is limited evidence on the role of activated charcoal in patients following ingestion as long as the ingestion was not a suicidal attempt nor an attempt at eluding law enforcement through orally "stuffing" drugs. The clinical benefit is doubtful because of the rapid absorption of methamphetamines and the risk of aspiration in altered patients. Decontamination needs to be considered in the case of a body stuffer as well as ingestions with suicidal intent. For the specific management of body stuffers toxicity, see Chapter 11.

There are no FDA-approved medications for stimulant use disorder, but a recent study found the combination of injectable naltrexone and oral bupropion was safe and effective in treating adults with moderate or severe methamphetamine use disorder.[17]

Long-Term Concerns

Chronic use of methamphetamines results in serious health problems. Problems related to psychological and cognitive impairment may occur, including depression, psychosis, and movement disorders. Many chronic methamphetamine abusers may suffer from dry xerostomia that can lead to bruxism, dental caries, tooth erosion, tooth loss, and tooth fractures. This has been termed "meth mouth."[13] Poor nutrition is common in methamphetamine users, leading to dramatic changes in physical appearance over short periods of time. Abrupt cessation of repeated methamphetamine use leads to a withdrawal syndrome consisting of depressed mood, anxiety, and sleep disturbance. Chronic users may suffer from serious cardiac complications including cardiomyopathy and congestive heart failure.[8]

CASE CONCLUSION

In conclusion, the case highlights the urgent need for targeted interventions and ongoing support to address the detrimental impact of methamphetamine use on physical, mental, and behavioral aspects of the patient's life. By addressing the root causes of his substance abuse and providing comprehensive care, there is an opportunity to improve his overall well-being and reduce the risk of future complications related to his drug use.

KEY POINTS TO REMEMBER

- Methamphetamine is a highly addictive substance that has reached epidemic surge since 2017.
- Maintain a suspicion for sympathomimetic drug use in patients presenting to the ED with acute psychosis.
- Diagnostic testing should be guided by the clinical manifestation. Urine immunoassay has a low utility to guide clinical management.
- Benzodiazepines and antipsychotics are first-line treatments for acute methamphetamine toxicity. Hyperthermia and rhabdomyolysis should be treated aggressively to reduce sequelae.

Further Reading

Flomenbaum N, Hoffman RS, Goldfrank LR, et al. *Goldfrank's Toxicologic Emergencies*. McGraw-Hill Education; 2019.

National Institute on Drug Abuse. Methamphetamine research report. Revised October 2019. Accessed September 8, 2022. https://nida.nih.gov/download/37620/methamphetamine-research-report.pdf?v=59d70e192be11090787a4dab7e8cd390

Schep LJ, Slaughter RJ, Beasley DM. The clinical toxicology of methamfetamine. *Clinical Toxicology (Philadelphia, Pa.)*. https://pubmed.ncbi.nlm.nih.gov/20849327/

References

1. Flomenbaum N, Hoffman RS, Goldfrank LR, et al. *Goldfrank's Toxicologic Emergencies*. McGraw-Hill Education; 2019.

2. Turner C, Chandrakumar D, Rowe C, Santos GM, Riley ED, Coffin PO. Cross-sectional cause of death comparisons for stimulant and opioid mortality in San Francisco, 2005–2015. *Drug Alcohol Depend*. https://pubmed.ncbi.nlm.nih.gov/29486419/

3. Schep LJ, Slaughter RJ, Beasley DM. The clinical toxicology of methamfetamine. *Clinical Toxicology (Philadelphia, Pa.)*. https://pubmed.ncbi.nlm.nih.gov/20849327/

4. Dargan PI, Wood DM. Comparison of crystalline methamphetamine ('ice') users and other patients with toxicology-related problems presenting to a hospital emergency department. *Med J Austral*. 18 Aug. 2008; https://www.ncbi.nlm.nih.gov/pubmed/18707575

5. Ruha AM, Yarema MC. Pharmacologic treatment of acute pediatric methamphetamine toxicity. *Pediatr Emerg Care*. https://pubmed.ncbi.nlm.nih.gov/17198209/

6. United Nations Office on Drugs and Crime. *World Drug Report 2010 Shows Shift Towards New Drugs and New Markets*. UNODC. https://www.unodc.org/unodc/en/press/releases/2010/June/unodc-world-drug-report-2010-shows-shift-towards-new-drugs-and-new-markets.html

7. Chen T, Spiller HA, Badeti J, Funk AR, Zhu M, Smith GA. Methamphetamine exposures reported to United States poison control centers, 2000–2019. *Clin Toxicol (Philadelphia, Pa.)*. Accessed September 11, 2022. https://pubmed.ncbi.nlm.nih.gov/33403876/

8. Schwarzbach V, Lenk K, Laufs U. Methamphetamine-related cardiovascular diseases. *ESC Heart Fail*. 2020;7(2):407–414. doi:10.1002/ehf2.12572

9. Lappin JM, Darke S, Farrell M. Stroke and methamphetamine use in young adults: a review. *J Neurol Neurosurg Psychiatr*. https://pubmed.ncbi.nlm.nih.gov/28835475/

10. Isoardi KZ, Ayles SF, Harris K, Finch CJ, Page CB. Methamphetamine presentations to an emergency department: management and complications. *Emerg Med Australasia*. https://pubmed.ncbi.nlm.nih.gov/30592564/

11. Malashock HR, Yeung C, Roberts AR, Snow JW, Gerkin RD, O'Connor AD. Pediatric methamphetamine toxicity: clinical manifestations and therapeutic use of antipsychotics-one institution's experience. *J Med Toxicol.* https://www.ncbi.nlm.nih.gov/pmc/articles/PMC8017059/

12. Limanaqi F, Gambardella S, Biagioni F, Busceti CL, Fornai F. Epigenetic effects induced by methamphetamine and methamphetamine-dependent oxidative stress. *Oxid Med Cell Longev.* July 22, 2018. https://www.ncbi.nlm.nih.gov/pmc/articles/PMC6081569/

13. Brahm NC, Yeager LL, Fox MD, Farmer KC, Palmer TA. Commonly prescribed medications and potential false-positive urine drug screens. *Am J Health Syst Pharm.* https://pubmed.ncbi.nlm.nih.gov/20689123/

14. Zun LS. Evidence-based review of pharmacotherapy for acute agitation. part 2: safety. *J Emerg Med.* https://pubmed.ncbi.nlm.nih.gov/29433934/

15. American College of Emergency Physicians. Task force report on hyperactive delirium with severe agitation in emergency settings. June 23, 2021. Accessed November 14, 2022. American College of Emergency Physicians. Task force report on hyperactive delirium with severe agitation in emergency settings. June 23, 2021. Accessed November 14, 2022. https://www.acep.org/siteassets/new-pdfs/education/acep-task-force-report-on-hyperactive-delirium-final.pdf; https://www.acep.org/globalassets/new-pdfs/education/acep-task-force-report-on-hyperactive-delirium-draft-.pdf

16. Wodarz N, Krampe-Scheidler A, Christ M, et al. Evidence-based guidelines for the pharmacological management of acute methamphetamine-related disorders and toxicity. *Pharmacopsychiatry.* https://pubmed.ncbi.nlm.nih.gov/28297728/

17. Trivedi MH, Walker R, Ling W, et al. Bupropion and naltrexone in methamphetamine use disorder. *N Engl J Med.* https://pubmed.ncbi.nlm.nih.gov/334975

23 The Rummy Rum Rums: Alcohol Intoxication

Destiny Horton and Mohan Punja

Case Presentation

A 22-year-old man presents to the ED after his friends called emergency services due to agitation and a minor head injury. Friends state that they were out drinking after their final exams tonight, their friend had consumed a large amount of alcohol and was found on the bathroom floor of his apartment next to a pile of emesis with blood coming from a head injury. Upon arrival in the ED the patient tries to get off the stretcher to leave and begins to scream with slurred speech at your staff; he also pulls out the peripheral IV catheter that your EMS colleagues had placed. EMS reports they have been unable to assess his vital signs due to his level of agitation.

What Do You Do Now?

DISCUSSION

BackgroundEthanol has been used by humans since prehistory as a mood-modifying substance. Dried residues on 9,000-year-old pottery found in northern mainland China imply the use of alcoholic beverages even among Neolithic peoples. It was first synthesized in 1826 by Henry Hennel and was initially used for a multitude of purposes including to fuel lamps and power early Ford Model T cars.

Toxicology and Pathophysiology

Once ingested, ethanol is rapidly taken up from the GI tract with an estimated 80–90% absorbed within 60 minutes. Multiple factors may modify the rate of absorption including medications, food products in the stomach, or mixture with carbonated drinks. There is no specific absorption rate for individuals as this is largely determined by the amount of alcohol dehydrogenase (ADH) enzyme present within the gastric mucosa. Studies have found that the blood ethanol concentration in adults will decrease by approximately 15–20 mg/dL/h (3.26–4.35 mmol/L/h)[4]. Tolerant drinkers, by recruiting the enzyme CYP2E1, may increase their clearance of ethanol to 30 mg/dL/h (6.52 mmol/L/h) or even higher. This estimation comes in handy along with a thorough physical exam and clinical assessment when trying to determine if a patient may be discharged from the ED because discharge is based on clinical judgment and local protocols.

ADH is responsible for oxidizing a percentage of alcohol within the stomach, thus making it unavailable for absorption into the bloodstream[2]. An estimated 95–98% of ethanol is metabolized in the liver, first to acetaldehyde by ADH and then further to acetic acid by aldehyde dehydrogenase (ALDH). Acetic acid is converted to acetyl-CoA, which will then be used within the Krebs cycle[6].

The limiting factor in this pathway is the prevalence of thiamine, which is used for the entry of acetyl-CoA into the Krebs cycle. When thiamine is low, acetyl-CoA builds up and is then instead transformed into acetoacetate, which is reduced to beta-hydroxybutyrate[4]. This is one of the mechanisms causing metabolic acidosis in alcohol intoxication. Acetyl-CoA can also be used in fatty acid synthesis and formation of triglycerides, which is a contributor to the steatosis that can occur in the setting of long-term heavy alcohol use. The use of thiamine in this pathway is the cause of thiamine deficiency in people with high utilization of alcohol, in addition to a dietary deficiency.

Laboratory assessment of alcohol levels has limited use. A patient who drinks chronically is likely to have developed a combined tolerance as they have upregulated CYP2E1 as well as modified their gamma aminobutyric acid (GABA) receptor subunits. It will not be infrequent for a patient to present to the ED with an ethanol level of greater than 300 mg/dL and seem to only be slightly impaired, while a level of 90 mg/dL in a novice drinker can lead to a comatose state.

The main mechanisms of action of ethanol are found to be enhancing the effects of central GABA-A receptors and blocking glutamine transmission at N-methyl-D-aspartate (NMDA) receptors. The GABA pathway is known for its inhibitory actions on the nervous system. By inhibiting NMDA receptor activity, ethanol increases dopamine release from the nucleus accumbens and ventral tegmental area. This translates into a complex cascade of effects on brain function depending on dose and frequency of use[3]. In the frontal lobe, ethanol affects attention and motivation and can lead to disinhibition; in doing so, it affects behavior and emotion. The ultimate effect on the user is thought to depend on the context in which it is consumed. In the cerebellum, ethanol affects coordination and gait. In the amygdala, it can lead to decreased activation of the "fight or flight" response and a general sense of relaxation. In the hippocampus, at high levels, it can cause acute memory impairment, even leading users to "black out," with no memory of the time period following consumption. The "Mellanby effect" is a term given to the perception in a drinker of increased impairment as the blood alcohol level is rising compared to when falling; in other words, a user may feel more sober at the same alcohol level after they have stopped drinking.

Modification of GABA receptors in chronic alcohol users is purported to be one of the mechanisms leading to alcohol withdrawal syndrome because the mechanism for GABA is to function as an inhibitory molecule that modulates excitation pathways within the brain. In response to chronic use, the body attempts to maintain homeostasis by changing the conformation and density of GABA receptors; as a result, a relative lack of alcohol activating the inhibitory function of the receptor leads to a state of neuroexcitation[6].

Workup and Diagnosis

There are generally two types of patients to consider in the context of alcohol: the acutely intoxicated patient and the patient with chronic alcohol use disorder. The medical issues involved and approach to each is generally quite different.

The Acutely Intoxicated Patient

When a patient presents to the ED for evaluation of suspected alcohol intoxication it is very important not to anchor on a diagnosis or you may miss other clinically relevant findings or information. These patients can be difficult to assess because there may be multiple medical problems occurring simultaneously, and the patient may be too inebriated or confused to give a reliable review of systems or history. However, a careful examination for signs of trauma and assessment of appropriate airway protection and vital signs, in addition to testing for blood glucose level, is the only workup that is absolutely required.

If there is concern for a sequela of acute intoxication, such as aspiration or traumatic injury, these should be worked up as usual. Providers should have a low threshold to obtain imaging for traumatic injuries as typical exam features such as tenderness on palpation or changes in the neurological exam may be difficult to elicit.

The Chronic Alcoholic

A patient with chronic alcohol use disorder is quite different. If they have known or suspected cirrhosis, then they should be considered to (1) be functionally immunocompromised, (2) at high risk for GI bleeding, and (3) at higher risk for traumatic injuries due to their coagulopathy and frequent falls. Workup should include some assessment of liver synthetic function such as platelet count and PT/INR. Infection should be aggressively investigated and treated. Patients with ascites and any suspicion for infection should be evaluated for spontaneous bacterial peritonitis (SBP). Any patient with cirrhosis and suspicion for upper GI bleeding will likely need to be admitted for observation and possibly evaluation for variceal bleeding. Variceal bleeding can occasionally be incredibly profuse and, in those situations (massive hematemesis), will require a large volume of blood products, reversal of coagulopathy, and possibly even placement of esophageal tamponade devices such as a Sengstaken-Blakemore or Minnesota tube for short-term stabilization. Octreotide may also be given to help reduce pressure within the varices. The prophylactic antibiotic of choice against SBP is ceftriaxone, which also carries an evidence-based mortality benefit in the setting of variceal bleeding. Patients may present after prophylactic banding of varices with bleeding as well. Emergent consultation with gastroenterology is very important in these patients, and they may decompensate very quickly.

The chronic alcohol user in whom bloodwork shows an anion gap acidosis (anion gap is defined as sodium concentration minus chloride concentration plus bicarbonate concentration, $Na^+ - (Cl^- + HCO_3^-)$); a normal range for an anion gap is 12–16) presents a dilemma[1]. Alcoholic ketoacidosis results from a physiological state of thiamine depletion and diversion of acetyl-CoA from the Krebs cycle, causing metabolic acidosis and lactic acidosis. This condition can have a range of severity, and patients can present without symptoms or can be quite sick with tachypnea and nausea and vomiting. If checked, the clinician may observe an elevated serum osmolar gap. The dilemma with these patients is that a very small minority may have co-ingested a toxic alcohol.

Treatment

Treatment for ethanol intoxication is generally supportive with fluid hydration as main line therapy because these patients may be very dehydrated, unless other medical conditions are found during medical workup. Of note, IV fluid therapy will not help "eliminate" alcohol or speed up sobriety[5]. If the story fits with a patient who is simply too intoxicated to be safely discharged to the care of his or her friends or family, they can simply be monitored in the department until they are clinically sober, or sober enough in the judgment of the provider given the discharge situation. For example, a patient who will be discharged in an urban area to walk home must be much more alert and able to ambulate independently than a patient who will be discharged home with their parent. Often a patient will present severely intoxicated and nearly obtunded but only a few hours later will ambulate to the bathroom and request to leave. We believe that use of the Glascow Coma Scale for assessment of the need to intubate these patients is not appropriate. Ultimately, these patients must be frequently reassessed for gradual improvement, the so-called "sober and go" or "metabolize to freedom" requires this; if not, a more aggressive evaluation should immediately be undertaken.

For patients with a suspected alcoholic ketoacidosis the treatment is repletion of IV thiamine and supplementation of dextrose, preferably by the oral route or intravenously. We recommend giving 100–300 mg IV thiamine in addition to a bolus of D5½ normal saline and encouraging oral intake. It is generally recommended to give thiamine prior to initiating resuscitation with glucose-containing fluids. In addition, in these situations, the provider must consider the possibility of toxic alcohol ingestion. Laboratory assessment of serum osmolarity and the osmole gap will be helpful, and providers can consider consulting a medical toxicologist or a local poison control center.

Combativeness and violence are also common physical manifestations of intoxication. The first step in management of agitation is verbal de-escalation and reducing environmental stimuli. Also, the provider must rapidly assess for capacity if a patient is trying to leave. Some patients may have the capacity to refuse care, but most likely will not have this capacity. If de-escalation techniques are not working, multiple studies have shown that chemical sedatives including benzodiazepines and other medications such as haloperidol or droperidol can be very useful. The goal is to control the patient and stop them from hurting themselves or others and to allow medical staff to appropriately assess the patient for any concurrent medical conditions. Every patient who receives sedatives to control their symptoms should be monitored more closely as they are at risk for excessive respiratory and CNS depression through synergy. We recommend standard pulse oximetry of the patient if they are on room air and use of end-tidal CO_2 detectors in patients who are on supplemental oxygen.

As discussed, patients with a history of alcohol abuse are often given thiamine due to depletion of stores from alcohol use. Lack of thiamine can lead to long-term consequences and cause conditions such as Wernicke's encephalopathy and Korsakoff syndrome. Wernicke's syndrome should be considered in an alcoholic patient who has gait instability (when not acutely intoxicated), worsening confusion, or any nystagmus or oculomotor palsy. In patients with suspected Wernicke's encephalopathy, parenteral thiamine 200–500 mg three times a day should be given for 3–5 days, followed by oral thiamine 250–1,000 mg/day[1].

Another issue is that of *lack* of alcohol. It is important to note that patients can experience withdrawal symptoms at almost any alcohol level. Refer to Chapter 19, on the alcohol withdrawal syndrome, for more information on treatment.

Finally, some patients may present to the department simply requesting assistance with rehabilitation and detoxification from alcohol. The first step is to assess for withdrawal or any concurrent medical or psychiatric conditions. After that, follow your local hospital protocols to connect patients with resources for further care.

CASE CONCLUSION

Indications that a patient may need admission for continued management or workup include continuous altered mental status, intentional self-harm, acute withdrawal, seizures, and severe metabolic derangements. These patients may be very difficult to deal with. In the case of the patient presented at the beginning of this chapter, he was briefly restrained by security and given 10 mg of intramuscular midazolam. This allowed for a CT scan of the head and cervical spine to be performed, in addition to a thorough head-to-toe examination. His blood glucose was 94 mg/dL. His tetanus vaccine was updated and the abrasion on his head was cleaned and dressed. After being medicated he slept quietly while on a cardiac monitor until the morning, whereupon he was quite apologetic and requested to call a ride home. You make sure to counsel him on his dangerous use of alcohol because his high-risk behavior indicates he may have an alcohol abuse disorder. Ultimately, the patient ambulated appropriately with the staff and, after eating a sandwich, was able to be discharged when his friends arrived.

· There is no routine laboratory testing required except for a glucose level in the assessment of the acutely intoxicated patient.

· Frequent reassessment of the acutely intoxicated patient is helpful in ruling out concurrent medical conditions. Patients who do not gradually improve with time require further workup.

· Patients with established or suspected cirrhosis are at high risk for infection, GI bleeding, or traumatic injuries.

· Ethanol withdrawal can occur even if a patient has an elevated ethanol level.

· Alcoholic ketoacidosis is treated with IV thiamine and glucose supplementation.

Further Reading

Finnell JT. Alcohol-related disease. In: Walls RM, Hockberger RS, Gausche-Hill M, et al., eds. *Rosen's Emergency Medicine: Concepts and Clinical Practice*. 9th ed. Saunders; 2018:1838–1851.

Walls RM, Hockberger RS, Gausche-Hill M, et al., eds. *Rosen's Emergency Medicine: Concepts and Clinical Practice*. 9th ed. Elsevier/Saunders; 2018.

Nelson LS, Howland M, Lewin NA, Smith SW, Goldfrank LR, Hoffman RS, eds. *Goldfrank's Toxicologic Emergencies*. 11th ed. McGraw Hill; 2019. https://accesspharmacy.mhmedical.com/content.aspx?bookid=2569&sectionid=210256528 Tintinalli, JE, Stapczynski J, Ma O, et al., eds. *Tintinalli's Emergency Medicine: A Comprehensive Study Guide*. 8th ed. McGraw-Hill Education; 2016.

References

1. Finnell JT. Alcohol-related disease. In: Walls RM, Hockberger RS, Gausche-Hill M, et al., eds. *Rosen's Emergency Medicine: Concepts and Clinical Practice*. 9th ed. Saunders; 2018:1838–1851.

2. Klaassen CD, ed. *Casarett & Doull's Toxicology: The Basic Science of Poisons*. 9th edition. McGraw Hill; 2019. Accessed March 31, 2022. https://accesspharmacy.mhmedical.com/content.aspx?bookid=2462&sectionid=194917645

3. Marx JA, Rosen P. *Rosen's Emergency Medicine: Concepts and Clinical Practice*. 9th ed. Elsevier/Saunders; 2018.

4. Nelson LS, Howland M, Lewin NA, Smith SW, Goldfrank LR, Hoffman RS, eds.). *Goldfrank's Toxicologic Emergencies*. 11th ed. McGraw Hill; 2019. https://accessp harmacy.mhmedical.com/content.aspx?bookid=2569&sectionid=210256528

5. Perri D, Klimaszyk D, Kołaciński Z, Szajewski J. *Ethyl Alcohol (Ethanol)*. *McMaster Textbook of Internal Medicine*. Medycyna Praktyczna. Accessed January 1, 2022. https://empendium.com/mcmtextbook/chapter/B31.II.20.2.1.

6. Tintinalli JE, et al. *Tintinalli's Emergency Medicine: A Comprehensive Study Guide*. 8th ed. McGraw-Hill Education, 2016.

24 The Mu-Agonist Blues: Opioid Overdose and Withdrawal

Tori Ehrhardt and Alaina Steck

Case Presentation

A 45-year-old woman is found down by her roommate, unconscious and "barely breathing." On arrival, EMS noted that the patient had vomited, and they found a needle and syringe next to her on the floor. The roommate was unable to provide any additional medical history for the patient.

EMS administered 1 dose of naloxone 4 mg intranasally en route, but there was no change in the patient's clinical status. They established 2 peripheral IV's and assisted the patient's ventilations with a bag-valve mask.

Primary assessment reveals a patent airway, bradypnea, and regular heart rate with 2+ radial pulses. Vital signs are heart rate 62 beats/min, respiratory rate 5 breaths/min, oxygen saturation 91% on 15 L/min supplemental oxygen, blood pressure 108/58 mm Hg, and temperature 97.1°F/36.2°C. The remainder of her exam is notable for bibasilar crackles, pinpoint pupils, and no obvious signs of trauma upon removal of clothing and cursory inspection.

What Do You Do Now?

DISCUSSION

The history, findings on scene, and physical exam features of central nervous system (CNS) depression, respiratory depression, and miosis are consistent with an opioid overdose. Opioids come in many formulations and can be ingested, insufflated, inhaled, or injected. Furthermore, opioid potency and duration of action can vary substantially among different compounds and routes of use. Opioid overdose deaths are due to respiratory depression and eventual hypoxic respiratory arrest. In this patient's case, administering a second dose of naloxone upon arrival to the ED would result in improvement of her respiratory drive. The sections below discuss the epidemiology and pathophysiology of opioid use and overdose and the workup and management of patients during both acute overdose and withdrawal from opioids.

Background

The 2020 National Survey on Drug Use and Health reported that 9.5 million people ages 12 and older misused opioids in the past year, with 2.7 million people ages 12 and over meeting criteria for an opioid use disorder (OUD).[1] Data from the Centers for Disease Control and Prevention (CDC) show that an estimated 75,673 individuals died from an opioid overdose between April 2020 and April 2021, a 35% increase compared with the prior 12-month period.[2] The addition of potent synthetic opioids—particularly fentanyl and fentanyl analogs—to the drug market is considered largely responsible for the exponential rise in overdose deaths,[3] and the strain and isolation created by the COVID-19 pandemic further exacerbated the death toll due to opioid-involved overdose deaths.[4]

Knowing this information provides clinicians with a few key insights: opioid overdose should always be considered in the differential of any patient with a decreased respiratory rate so that appropriate treatment can be provided. Other conditions which may cause CNS and respiratory depression include toxicity from sedative-hypnotic agents (e.g., benzodiazepines, barbiturates, gamma-hydroxybutyric acid [GHB]), clonidine overdose, hypothyroidism, head trauma, and stroke. Preparation is key not only in medically managing these patients when they present with acute toxicity, but also in knowing what resources to provide them to prevent future overdoses.

Though complex and not fully understood, substance use disorders exhibit neurobiological changes ranging from molecular adaptations to aberrant signal transmission between multiple brain regions[5] and should be viewed as treatable medical conditions rather than dismissed as character flaws or consequences of moral failing. Harm reduction—including overdose education, naloxone provision, and testing and/or prevention services for infectious complications—is a key component of ED care for OUD patients presenting with acute overdose. Specific examples of these strategies are discussed in later sections.

Toxicology and Pathophysiology

Most commonly used opioids are full agonists at the mu opioid receptors, with varying effects on delta and kappa opioid receptors and the opioid receptor like-1 (ORL-1). Mu opioid receptors, the most predominant and well-characterized opioid receptor subtype, are located both centrally and peripherally and mediate supraspinal and spinal-level analgesia, euphoria, sedation, gastrointestinal motility, and respiratory depression. Binding of an endogenous or exogenous opioid to these receptors causes a decrease in neuronal activity; thus, opioid action in the medullary respiratory center and peripheral chemoreceptors decreases both tidal volume and respiratory rate and is responsible for the fatal respiratory depression that can be seen in opioid overdose.[6]

Other pulmonary effects of opioid toxicity include aspiration pneumonitis (due to CNS depression and the inability of a patient to protect their airway) and pulmonary edema (i.e., acute respiratory distress syndrome [ARDS]). There are several hypothesized mechanisms for ARDS in these patients, including pulmonary capillary leak, neurogenic pulmonary edema, hypoxic alveolar damage, anaphylactoid reactions to the opioid itself, and myocardial stunning due to a massive sympathetic response following overdose reversal with naloxone.[7] Ultimately, no definitive cause has been established.

As previously mentioned, potency can vary significantly between specific opioids. For instance, fentanyl is approximately 50–100 times more potent than morphine and approximately 30–50 times more potent than heroin. Coupled with unregulated manufacturing practices, impurities in final products, and narrow therapeutic index (the ratio between a lethal dose and a dose that provides the desired effects), fentanyl and its analogs are particularly likely to cause inadvertent overdoses in end users, even in those experienced with fentanyl use.[3] In clinical settings, potency is often conceptualized in terms of morphine milligram equivalents (MME) or oral morphine equivalents (OME), a standard which provides approximate equivalent doses for a given opioid medication in comparison to morphine, the prototypical mu opioid receptor agonist. While this schema can assist with equianalgesic dosing and risk stratification in a controlled clinical environment, it is less meaningful in the setting of acute opioid toxicity or when discussing risk mitigation with patients.

Last, different opioid compounds, formulations, and routes of administration can impact the clinical course of toxicity and withdrawal. For example, morphine administered intravenously is expected to reach peak serum concentrations within 10 minutes of administration,[8] whereas morphine administered as sustained-release capsules will not reach peak serum concentrations until more than 8 hours following ingestion.[9] Similarly, variable rates of distribution and elimination from the body will impact the duration of toxicity and the time until onset of withdrawal symptoms: the half-life for IV morphine is approximately 2 hours,[10] whereas the half-life for oral methadone may be more than 50 hours.[11] Concurrent hepatic or renal dysfunction may also have a significant impact on the duration of effect following opioid use.

Workup and Diagnosis

Given its prevalence, opioid toxicity should always be on the differential for a patient who presents with decreased mental status and/or diminished respiratory drive. Additional symptoms such as pinpoint pupils, bradycardia, hypotension, hypothermia, or sequelae of injection drug use (venipuncture scars or "track marks," skin and soft tissue infections) may further support the diagnosis; however, lack of such findings does not exclude opioid toxicity. Additionally, unexpected signs and symptoms may occur if the patient has used multiple substances with differing mechanisms of action simultaneously. For example, anticholinergic medications or stimulants can lead to mydriasis and may mask the expected finding of miosis in a patient with acute opioid overdose. The lack of additional signs on presentation should not discourage administration of an opioid antagonist to reverse life-threatening respiratory depression if an opioid overdose is suspected.

A history should be collected, if possible, with specific attention to the type and amount of opioid used and any additional substances that the patient may have used. This information may provide insight into the expected time course of toxicity and anticipated development of additional symptoms. In the United States, alcohol and benzodiazepines are common co-ingestants and can further contribute to respiratory depression via their own mechanisms[12]; but co-use of stimulants and opioids is also on the rise.[13] Additionally, the time of use and any treatment provided by EMS en route is valuable information.

For uncomplicated opioid toxicity (i.e., a patient with a clear history of opioid use, adequate response to naloxone, and no recurrence of opioid effect during an appropriate observation period) little diagnostic testing is needed as opioid toxicity is primarily a clinical diagnosis. On initial presentation, patients with depressed level of consciousness should receive assessment of their blood glucose, most easily performed with point-of-care testing. For those patients who have used multiple substances or who do not respond as expected to an appropriate dose of naloxone (see section on "Treatment"), additional evaluation is required to explore other possible etiologies. Laboratory testing (complete blood count, comprehensive metabolic panel, blood gas, serum lactate, creatine phosphokinase, serum ethanol), radiography (chest x-ray, CT of the head), and ECG should be considered. A routine urine drug screen is not recommended as many opioids—particularly the fentanyl analogs—are not reliably detected on this test and a false-negative result may mislead the clinician. A thorough physical exam, including skin and musculoskeletal evaluation for signs of infection, thrombosis, or compartment syndrome, is also warranted.

In stark contrast to opioid toxicity, patients may instead present in acute opioid withdrawal or require management of withdrawal symptoms that emerge following overzealous naloxone administration for overdose. Patients may report opioid withdrawal outright, or they may be unaware that the symptoms they are experiencing are due to opioid withdrawal. Symptoms include muscle and joint aches, anxiety, irritability, insomnia, chills or hot flashes, piloerection ("gooseflesh"), nausea, vomiting, diarrhea, and abdominal pain. While not life-threatening, these symptoms cause such significant distress to patients that avoidance of withdrawal symptoms is a primary contributor to ongoing use in patients with OUD.[14]

Treatment

As with any emergent presentation, initial assessment should focus on the patient's airway, breathing, and circulatory status. Airway and breathing will be the main concerns for a patient presenting with opioid toxicity. Initial management focuses on assuring or establishing a patent airway and adequate respiratory function. Naloxone, a competitive antagonist at the mu opioid receptor, should be administered once the provider suspects the presence of opioid toxicity as this antidote may obviate the need for endotracheal intubation and mechanical ventilation.

Naloxone may be administered via several routes, as noted in Table 24.1. Naloxone is a safe medication; its side-effect profile depends on whether it is administered to a patient with tolerance to opioids. In patients without underlying physiologic dependence to opioids, naloxone will reverse opioid-induced respiratory and CNS depression without producing adverse effects.

TABLE 24.1 **Routes and suggested starting doses for naloxone administration in suspected opioid overdose**

Route	Dose	Onset (mins)	Time to peak (mins)	$t_{1/2}$	Duration
IV	0.04[a]–2 mg	2	5	0.5–1.5 hours	30–90 minutes, depending on dose and route of administration
IM		2–5	15		
Subcutaneous		2–5	15		
ETT[b]	2–2.5 × IV dose [e.g., 0.08–1 mg]	2–5	–		
Nebulization[c]	2 mg in 3 mL NS	–	–		–
Intranasal	2 mg or 4 mg	8–13	20–30	~2 hours	

[a] Use 0.04–0.05 mg IV as starting dose for suspected opioid-dependent persons.
[b] Off-label, least preferred route, irregular absorption.
[c] Off-label.

Similarly, in patients who present with CNS and respiratory depression but whose symptoms are not due to opioid toxicity, the administration of naloxone will not change the patient's clinical status nor will it cause harm. Thus, in situations where opioid toxicity is on the differential, naloxone should not be withheld due to concerns about adverse effects.

For those patients who do have baseline opioid tolerance, naloxone administration may result in precipitated withdrawal, with severe nausea, vomiting (with risk of aspiration), tachycardia, hypertension, tremor, diaphoresis, and agitation being the most common effects. Less common but more severe sequelae of precipitated withdrawal include seizures, cardiac dysrhythmias, and noncardiogenic pulmonary edema. Pulmonary edema in particular has been suggested to stem from overly aggressive naloxone administration; however, this hypothesis is not universally supported as pulmonary edema also has been observed in opioid-overdose decedents who never received naloxone.[15] Indeed, though the definitive mechanism behind pulmonary edema in opioid overdose has yet to be identified, it should be emphasized that *the benefit of reversing respiratory depression from acute overdose unequivocally outweighs the potential risks associated with naloxone administration.*

The end goal of naloxone administration is to restore adequate ventilatory function. Patients' ventilatory function should be supported with assisted ventilations with a bag-valve mask while awaiting an increase in respiratory rate and tidal volume during naloxone administration. Ideally, patients should be monitored with continuous capnography (end-tidal CO_2 monitoring) during and after naloxone administration.

There are multiple dosing schemes available for naloxone administration. The total effective dose of naloxone depends on several factors, including the patient's existing opioid tolerance, the amount and type of opioid used, the relative affinity of naloxone versus the opioid to be displaced for the mu opioid receptor, the patient's body mass, and the degree to which the opioid partitions into the CNS. The commonly cited initial dose of naloxone 0.4 mg IV is drawn from old anesthesiology literature,[16] in which naloxone was used to reverse excessive postoperative sedation in opioid-naïve patients. Many toxicologists now recommend a lower starting dose of naloxone 0.04 mg IV (pediatric dose: 0.1 mg/kg IV) to avoid precipitated withdrawal in patients who may be opioid-dependent.[17,18] Subsequent doses of naloxone are then escalated until the desired clinical endpoint (adequate ventilatory function) has been reached.

There is also significant variation in the recommended maximum cumulative dose of naloxone that one should administer, with sources citing a maximum dose ranging from 2 mg IV to greater than 30 mg IV.[17,18] These authors suggest that once a 10 mg IV dose of naloxone has been provided (a cumulative dose of 16.44 mg if following the escalating dosing scheme in Figure 24.1), endotracheal intubation and a search for other etiologies of the patient's presentation should be undertaken. However, this is not a hard-and-fast rule, as we note that there are circumstances in which higher total cumulative doses may be warranted, particularly in cases where there is a convincing history or other evidence to suggest that the patient has been exposed to a high-potency, high-affinity opioid.

If the patient's airway status remains tenuous following naloxone administration, endotracheal intubation is the next appropriate intervention. Profound hypotension is uncommon and should prompt evaluation for other causes; it should be treated with IV fluid resuscitation and may require administration of vasopressors, of which push-dose phenylephrine has been associated with lowest odds of in-hospital mortality.[19] Metabolic disturbances or rhabdomyolysis can also occur, requiring further supportive care or hemodialysis.[20]

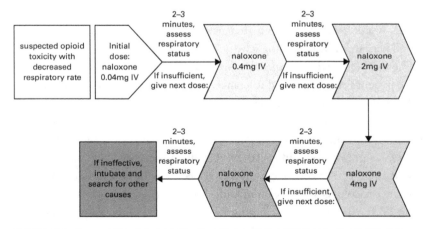

FIGURE 24.1 One possible dosing scheme for naloxone administration in acute opioid toxicity.

Regardless of the complexity of care required, close monitoring of ventilation and oxygenation should be maintained. IV naloxone has a half-life of approximately 1 hour, so longer-acting opioids can outlast the effects of the reversal agent, causing re-emergence of opioid toxicity and respiratory depression as naloxone is cleared from the body. Should a patient require additional naloxone after a period of adequate reversal, a continuous infusion of naloxone may be considered. The infusion is usually started at one-third to one-half of the total effective naloxone dose. Hence, if a patient receives the following sequential naloxone doses—0.04 mg IV, then 0.4 mg IV, then 2 mg IV—in order to achieve an adequate respiratory rate and tidal volume, the total cumulative effective dose is 2.44 mg IV. The continuous infusion can thus be started at a rate of 0.8–1.2 mg/hr (2.44 mg ÷ 3 = 0.8 mg/hr, 2.44 ÷ 2 = 1.2 mg/hr) and titrated to the clinical effect of respiratory depression reversal.

Patients experiencing acute opioid withdrawal should have their symptoms robustly managed as abrupt cessation of opioid medications results in significant patient distress, strong cravings, and recurrent use.[21] The central alpha-2-adrenergic agonist clonidine, though not approved by the US Food and Drug Administration (FDA) for this indication, has been used extensively for the management of opioid withdrawal symptoms. Recommended dosing is orally or transdermally, at doses of 0.1–0.3 mg every 6–8 hours, with a maximum dose of 1.2 mg daily.[22] Additional medications are symptom-targeted and are described in Table 24.2. Acute withdrawal can also be effectively managed with the partial mu receptor agonist buprenorphine; further discussion of the use of this medication is in Chapter 13 of this volume. Beyond the symptomatic treatment of acute withdrawal symptoms, it is important to offer initiation of long-term management of a patient's underlying OUD. The best approach for this is multifaceted and includes both medication and psychosocial support.[22] Medication options shown to decrease both illicit opioid use and mortality include the long-acting full agonist methadone and the partial mu agonist buprenorphine; data for the long-acting antagonist naltrexone show a decrease in illicit use but not mortality.[23] Whether the patient has just experienced an acute opioid overdose or is presenting in acute withdrawal, there is an opportunity to provide harm reduction strategies, offer medications to treat the patient's OUD, or link

TABLE 24.2 Example medications for symptom management in acute opioid withdrawal

Medication	Indication	Dose
Clonidine	Restlessness, anxiety, hypertension, general withdrawal symptoms	0.1–0.3 mg PO every 6–8 hours as needed 0.1–0. 3 mg transdermal patch
Hydroxyzine	Anxiety, irritability, insomnia	25–50 mg PO every 6 hours as needed
Loperamide	Diarrhea	4 mg PO initially, then 2 mg PO every 1 hour while diarrhea persists; maximum 16 mg in 24 hours
Ondansetron	Nausea / vomiting	4 mg SL every 8 hours as needed
Dicyclomine	Abdominal cramps	10–20 mg PO every 6–8 hours as needed
Acetaminophen/ NSAIDs	Myalgias, arthralgias	Per usual analgesic dosing

the patient to other resources that support their recovery. In-depth discussion on buprenorphine, including options for induction from the ED, can be found in Chapter 13.

Long-Term Concerns

Starting medications for the management of a patient's OUD is appropriate and within the scope of the emergency medicine physician. If a system for a "warm handoff" to a long-term OUD treatment provider is not in place, it is important to be aware of local resources with which to connect the patient so that they can continue seeking treatment or harm reduction services. Additionally, ensuring the patient has access to take-home naloxone to carry with them is a simple and effective harm reduction technique that has been demonstrated to minimize mortality from opioid overdose. Provide counseling to these patients and individuals accompanying them in the ED on regional laws which provide criminal liability protections to by-standers who administer naloxone in the case of suspected overdose.

In some areas, syringe service programs operate as a way of providing sterilized syringes to individuals who inject drugs to decrease infectious complications and to provide access to testing and treatment resources. A detailed discussion on potential complications of long-term injection drug use (e.g., abscess, endocarditis, hepatitis C, HIV) is beyond the scope of this chapter but an awareness of these is important to have to maintain an appropriate level of concern for these conditions. Workup of a patient with presenting symptoms or physical exam signs suggestive of possible sequelae of injection drug use should be modified accordingly.

A final long-term consideration is a conversation regarding the patient's substance use, if they are amenable to it, and reinforcement of substance use disorder as a disease, not a character flaw. Though there is a paucity of studies evaluating the effectiveness of counseling tools specifically in patients with opioid use disorder, there are data to suggest that motivational interviewing techniques and referral to peer recovery support services as a component of managing disorders characterized by addictive behaviors lead to improvement in long-term outcomes such as retention on medications for OUD, decreased hospital readmissions, and decreased mortality.[24,25]

CASE CONCLUSION

Our patient received one dose of 0.04 mg IV Naloxone upon arrival to the ED, providing rapid improvement in both respiratory rate from 5 to 13 breaths per minute, and in mental status with the patient awakening and able to answer basic questions such as her name and the year. After a period of observation and monitoring on telemetry and end-tidal CO_2, having remained clinically stable, a discussion was had with the patient regarding her history with substance use. She expressed interest in medications to manage her opioid use, and was admitted to the hospital's observation unit for Buprenorphine induction (see chapter 13 for more information).

- Opioid toxicity should be on the differential diagnosis for patients presenting with CNS and respiratory depression.
- Naloxone is a safe medication. *The benefit of reversing respiratory depression from acute opioid overdose unequivocally outweighs the potential risks associated with naloxone administration.*
- The half-life of the culprit opioid may be longer than that of naloxone; thus, close monitoring for recurrence of respiratory depression is an essential component of care in all patients who have had an overdose reversed with naloxone.
- Opioid withdrawal symptoms should be managed aggressively with medications directed at symptom control or with initiation of buprenorphine.
- All patients with opioid use disorder (OUD) should be offered harm reduction counseling, medications for OUD (methadone, buprenorphine, naltrexone), and provided with overdose education and take-home naloxone (or information on how to obtain naloxone for bystander administration).

Further Reading

Carpenter J, Murray BP, Atti S, Moran TP, Yancey A, Morgan B. Naloxone dosing after opioid overdose in the era of illicitly manufactured fentanyl. *J Med Toxicol.* 2020;16(1):41–48. doi:10.1007/s13181-019-00735-w

Dayer LE, Painter JT, McCain K, King J, Cullen J, Foster HR. A recent history of opioid use in the US: three decades of change. *Subst Use Misuse.* 2019;54(2):331–339. doi:10.1080/10826084.2018.1517175

Degenhardt L, Grebely J, Stone J, et al. Global patterns of opioid use and dependence: harms to populations, interventions, and future action. *Lancet.* 2019;394(10208):1560–1579. doi:10.1016/S0140-6736(19)32229-9

Kosten TR, Baxter LE. Review article: Effective management of opioid withdrawal symptoms: a gateway to opioid dependence treatment. *Am J Addict.* 2019;28(2):55–62. doi:10.1111/ajad.12862

Stoicea N, Costa A, Periel L, Uribe A, Weaver T, Bergese SD. Current perspectives on the opioid crisis in the US healthcare system: a comprehensive literature review. *Medicine (Baltimore).* 2019;98(20):e15425. doi:10.1097/MD.0000000000015425

References

1. Substance Abuse and Mental Health Services Administration. *Key Substance Use and Mental Health Indicators in the United States: Results from the 2020 National Survey on Drug Use and Health* (HHS Publication No. PEP 21-07-01-003, NSDUH Series H-56). Center for Behavioral Health Statistics and Quality, Substance Abuse and Mental Health Services Administration. 2021. Accessed February 28, 2022. https://www.samhsa.gov/data/.

2. Centers for Disease Control and Prevention. Drug overdose deaths in the U.S. top 100,000 annually. National Center for Health Statistics, CDC. November 17, 2021. Accessed February 28, 2022. https://www.cdc.gov/nchs/pressroom/nchs_press_releases/2021/20211117.htm

3. Han Y, Yan W, Zheng Y, Khan MZ, Yuan K, Lu L. The rising crisis of illicit fentanyl use, overdose, and potential therapeutic strategies. *Transl Psychiatry.* 2019;9(1):282. doi:10.1038/s41398-019-0625-0

4. National Center for Drug Abuse Statistics. Fentanyl abuse statistics. 2022. Accessed February 3, 2022. https://drugabusestatistics.org/fentanyl-abuse-statistics/.

5. Uhl GR, Koob GF, Cable J. The neurobiology of addiction. *Ann NY Acad Sci.* 2019;1451(1):5–28. doi:10.1111/nyas.13989

6. White JM, Irvine RJ. Mechanisms of fatal opioid overdose. *Addiction.* 1999;94(7):961–972. PMID: 10707430

7. Mégarbane B, Chevillard L. The large spectrum of pulmonary complications following illicit drug use: features and mechanisms. *Chem Biol Interact.* 2013;206(3):444–451. doi:10.1016/j.cbi.2013.10.011

8. Brunk SF, Delle M. Morphine metabolism in man. *Clin Pharmacol Therapeut.* 1974;16(1):51–57. doi:10.1002/cpt1974161part151

9. Kadian® oral extended-release capsules, morphine sulfate oral extended-release capsules. Package insert. Allergan USA; 2016.

10. Morphine sulfate injection. Mallinckrodt; 2016, https://www.accessdata.fda.gov/drugsatfda_docs/label/2016/020631s001lbl.pdf

11. Dolophine® oral tablets, methadone HCl oral tablets. Roxane Laboratories; 2015, https://www.accessdata.fda.gov/drugsatfda_docs/label/2006/006134s028lbl.pdf

12. Tori ME, Larochelle MR, Naimi TS. Alcohol or benzodiazepine co-involvement with opioid overdose deaths in the United States, 1999–2017. *JAMA Network Open.* 2020;3(4):e202361. doi:10.1001/jamanetworkopen.2020.2361

13. Jones CM, Bekheet F, Park JN, Alexander GC. The evolving overdose epidemic: synthetic opioids and rising stimulant-related harms. *Epidemiol Rev.* 2020;42:154–166. doi:10.1093/epirev/mxaa011

14. Harocopos A, Allen B, Paone D. Circumstances and contexts of heroin initiation following non-medical opioid analgesic use in New York City. *Int J Drug Policy,* 2016;28:106–112.

15. Sterrett C, Brownfield J, Korn CS, Hollinger M, Henderson SO. Patterns of presentation in heroin overdose resulting in pulmonary edema. *Am J Emerg Med.* 2003;21(1):32–34. doi:10.1053/ajem.2003.50006

16. Foldes FF. The human pharmacology and clinical use of narcotic antagonists. *Med Clin N Am.* 1964;48:421–423. doi:10.1016/s0025-7125(16)33474–5

17. Boyer EW. Management of opioid analgesic overdose. *N Engl J Med.* 2012;367(2):146–155. doi:10.1056/NEJMra1202561

18. Connors NJ, Nelson LS. The evolution of recommended naloxone dosing for opioid overdose by medical specialty. *J Med Toxicol.* 2016;12(3):276–281. doi:10.1007/s13181-016-0559-3

19. Clifford C, Sethi M, Cox D, Manini AF. First-line vasopressor and mortality rates in ed patients with acute drug overdose. *J Med Toxicol.* 2021;17(1):1–9. doi:10.1007/s13181-020-00797-1

20. Parthvi R, Agrawal A, Khanijo S, Tsegaye A, Talwar A. Acute opiate overdose: an update on management strategies in emergency department and critical care unit. *Am J Therapeut.* 2019;26(3):e380–e387. doi:10.1097/MJT.0000000000000681

21. Kosten TR, Baxter LE. Review article: Effective management of opioid withdrawal symptoms: a gateway to opioid dependence treatment. *Am J Addict.* 2019;28(2):55–62. doi:10.1111/ajad.12862

22. Kampman K, Jarvis M. American Society of Addiction Medicine (ASAM) national practice guideline for the use of medications in the treatment of addiction involving opioid use. *J Addict Med.* 2015;9(5):358–367. doi:10.1097/ADM.0000000000000166

23. Buresh M, Stern R, Rastegar D. Treatment of opioid use disorder in primary care. *BMJ.* 2021;373:n784. Published 2021 May 19. doi:10.1136/bmj.n784

24. DiClemente CC, Corno CM, Graydon MM, Wiprovnick AE, Knoblach DJ. Motivational interviewing, enhancement, and brief interventions over the last decade: a review of reviews of efficacy and effectiveness. *Psychol Addictive Behaviors.* 2017;31(8):862–887. doi:10.1037/adb0000318

25. Liebling EJ, Perez JJS, Litterer MM, Greene C. Implementing hospital-based peer recovery support services for substance use disorder. *Am J Drug Alcohol Abuse.* 2021;47(2):229–237. doi:10.1080/00952990.2020.1841218

25 GABA-B, the Forgotten Receptor Overlooked No More: Baclofen Overdose and Withdrawal

Nicholas Hoffmann and Jay Bernstein

Case Presentation

A 22-year-old man with a history of cerebral palsy presents via EMS for altered mental status. IV naloxone and D50 were administered in the field with no improvement in mental status. The patient exhibited seizure-like activity en route that was successfully alleviated with 2 mg of lorazepam. Upon arrival to the ED, there was no eye-opening to verbal or painful stimuli. His muscles were flaccid with absent reflexes, and he did not localize to painful stimuli. There was emesis on his shirt. His vital signs were blood pressure 96/60 mm Hg, heart rate 59 beats/min, respiratory rate 8 breaths/min with poor respiratory effort, SpO_2 89% via non-rebreather, and temperature 95.8°F/35.4°C. The physical examination revealed pupils 4 mm bilaterally and minimally reactive. He had no murmurs, he had clear breath sounds bilaterally with obvious bradypnea, his abdomen was soft and nontender, and his skin was cool and pale. When he was suctioned, there was no cough or gag reflex. The oculocephalic and corneal reflexes were negative bilaterally. There were also no obvious external signs of trauma. The exam also revealed the presence of an intrathecal pump. His mother arrived shortly thereafter and stated that the intrathecal pump was recently placed. The patient had a follow-up appointment with his intrathecal baclofen (ITB) pump specialist the day prior. The mother noted that he seemed normal before to going to bed 8 hours prior but was noted to be unresponsive when she tried to awaken him that morning.

What Do You Do Now?

DISCUSSION

Background

Baclofen, beta-chlorophenyl-gamma aminobutyric acid (GABA) (Lioresal, Gablofen, Kemstro, Lyvispah, Ozobax), is the only commonly prescribed GABA-B agonist used to alleviate muscle spasticity and pain caused by cerebral palsy, traumatic or ischemic neurologic injuries, multiple sclerosis, or other neurodegenerative disorders.[1] Less frequently, it has also been used off-label for several other chronic conditions, including nicotine, alcohol, and cocaine use disorders (to decrease cravings) and intractable hiccups.[2] It is commonly administered orally and is quickly absorbed in the GI tract.[2,3] However, it can also be delivered intrathecally via a surgically implanted pump in patients 4 years of age or older for severe cases refractory to oral therapies.[4] Oral baclofen has a bioavailability of 70–85%, with peak blood concentrations occurring 1 to 3.5 hours after ingestion. Thus, signs of toxicity are manifested shortly after ingestion.[5] The half-life is estimated to be 2–6 hours.[2–4,6] Baclofen undergoes first-order elimination and has not been shown to shift to zero-order elimination kinetics even in toxic doses.[3] Baclofen is excreted primarily through renal elimination; thus, elimination may be delayed in those with underlying kidney dysfunction.[4,6] In addition, the lipophilic nature of baclofen results in a much slower elimination from nervous system than from serum. Even after levels are essentially undetectable in the serum, patients may still exhibit signs of toxicity,[3,5] and resolution of symptoms may follow a more protracted course.

GABA-B receptors are widely expressed in the nervous tissue of the brain and spinal cord on both pre- and postsynaptic neurons. Baclofen binds to both presynaptic and postsynaptic receptors. At presynaptic sites, G-protein coupled receptors cause hyperpolarization by closing calcium channels and decreasing neurotransmitter release, resulting in the inhibitory effects. At the postsynaptic sites, potassium and calcium channels are affected and produce an inhibitory effect by increasing the threshold to produce an action potential.[2,5,7] Although inhibitory effects typically prevail, the interaction of baclofen at GABA-B receptors is complex and may occasionally result in excitatory effects (seizures, tachycardia, etc.). Chronic ingestion or infusion may lead to downregulation of receptors, and, upon abrupt discontinuation, a rebound effect with increased postsynaptic excitatory tone causes acute withdrawal symptoms.[8,9]

Toxicology and Pathophysiology

Orally, acute ingestions of 300–970 mg in adults can cause serious toxic effects; ingestions of 1,250–2,500 mg can be fatal.[5] One study found that, with ingestions of 200 mg or greater, patients are more likely to be admitted to intensive care and have longer hospital length of stay.[10] Although reports of suicide attempts are frequently cited in the literature, overdoses have also been seen in accidental pediatric ingestions, as well as recreational use.[11,12] Intrathecally, overdoses can occur with continuous infusions, dose titration, or accidental bolus dosing. Pump malfunctions are less common but have been described.[13]

Baclofen overdoses present with several symptoms that can range from mild to severe and life-threatening depending on several factors that include, but are not limited to, renal insufficiency, age, and chronicity of intoxication.[5,11] Table 25.1 shows the most common presentations. Neurologically,

TABLE 25.1 **Toxic effects of baclofen organized by system and effects**

System	Toxic effects
Neurologic	Headache, dizziness, incoordination, ataxia, myoclonus, fatigue, weakness, areflexia, flaccid extremities, encephalopathy, coma, seizures including status epilepticus, psychosis and confusion, deep coma with brainstem dysfunction
Pulmonary	Respiratory depression and failure
Cardiovascular	Hypertension or hypotension Tachycardia or bradycardia, possibly in alternation Prolonged QTc and first-degree heart block, premature atrial and ventricular contractions, supraventricular tachycardia, atrial flutter, and atrial fibrillation
Gastrointestinal	Nausea and vomiting
Ocular	Blurred vision, horizontal or vertical nystagmus, unreactive pupils, absent corneal reflexes, absent oculocephalic reflex Mydriasis or miosis may be present
Others	Hypothermia and hypersalivation Rarely hyperthermia, as this is more likely withdrawal

From Parker-Pitts et al.[1]

patients with severe intoxication may present with brainstem dysfunction and may even mimic brain death and anoxic encephalopathy.[4,5,13] For this reason, it is imperative that sufficient time be provided for drug elimination prior to even considering a brain death examination in any case of known or suspected baclofen overdose Decorticate posturing, nonreactive pupils, negative oculocephalic reflex, and negative gag reflex may be seen in the ED. It is important to be aware that baclofen overdoses can initially appear identical to a severe brain injury, however this finding is temporary, and a full recovery will typically be seen within 72 hours.[4,5,14] Seizure activity is another possible neurologic complication after overdose, and the pro-epileptic properties of baclofen are not well understood. Given the inhibitory effect on the synaptic junction, antiepileptic properties are typically seen in therapeutic dosing. One possible hypothesis for the seizure activity is that the supratherapeutic levels of the drug causes suppression of inhibitory interneurons that results in cellular hyperpolarization.[15] Hypothermia has also been seen, and rewarming measures are indicated to achieve normothermia.

Workup and Diagnosis

As seen in the presenting case, respiratory depression and respiratory failure can occur requiring mechanical ventilation. Careful and judicious selection of rapid sequence induction (RSI) medications is very important. Patients frequently have underlying neuromuscular disorders and may be at higher risk for concurrent rhabdomyolysis secondary to prolonged immobilization. In some neuromuscular disorders, altered muscle fiber receptors may be hypersensitive to hyperkalemia, which may be induced or worsened by succinylcholine. Therefore, succinylcholine administration can result in cardiac conduction abnormalities or cardiac arrest. While longer acting non-depolarizing paralytics, such as rocuronium, may also have drawbacks, such as masking seizure activity or clinical changes in neurologic status (decline or improvement), they are favored over depolarizing agents like succinylcholine.[5]

Cardiovascular effects in baclofen overdoses may be more varied. Hypotension and hypertension have both been described, as well as tachycardia and bradycardia.[5,10] Supportive care with IV fluids and vasopressors may be warranted. Bradycardia is one of the more commonly described cardiac conduction abnormalities, with several reports supporting use of atropine in 0.5–1 mg slow IV push every 4–6 hours to increase heart rate and blood pressure as needed.[16] Intermittent first-degree heart block with prolonged PR intervals, as well as premature atrial contractions with junctional escape beats have been reported.[17] QTc prolongation, placing patients at risk for fatal arrhythmias such as torsade de pointes, has also been described in the literature.[18] One case report also cited an episode of a serious supraventricular tachyarrhythmia—possibly due to an underlying congenital or structural abnormality or a transient irritable atrial focus secondary to the stressful physiologic effect of the overdose.[19]

Activated charcoal is an appropriate initial consideration in an acute overdose and is typically indicated within 1 hour of ingestion, although in select patients may be given later. The greatest concern with administering activated charcoal is vomiting and aspiration, which may lead to charcoal pneumonitis, particularly in patients who are not fully able to protect their airway.[20,21] Keep in mind that the most common GI effects of baclofen overdose include nausea and vomiting. This places the patient at high risk for aspiration and subsequent charcoal pneumonitis if the patient is obtunded and the airway is not protected early.

One case report supported the use of IV physostigmine with intrathecal overdoses to restore respiratory drive and level of consciousness. The mechanism of how cholinergic potentiation caused this response is not clearly known.[22] More recent case reports and other studies were not able to reproduce this effect and have demonstrated no benefit in the use of physostigmine in baclofen overdose. The potential adverse effects of physostigmine include worsening vomiting, hypersalivation, convulsions, and bradycardia.[23]

As in oral baclofen overdoses, supportive care and management of airway, breathing, and circulation should be strongly considered in the initial presentation of a suspected intrathecal overdose. However, attention should then be directed toward contacting the physician who manages the pump (or other trained professional) to discontinue the pump and provide further consultation and monitoring as an inpatient. The removal of large volumes (15–30 mL) of cerebrospinal fluid (CSF) via lumbar puncture has been performed to limit the effects of large-volume baclofen bolus delivered and may be recommended after the pump is off.[5,13,24] In cases where the cause of the altered mental status is not clear, CSF analysis can also help evaluate for the presence of meningitis, encephalitis, and Guillain-Barré syndrome.

IV lipid infusion has not been studied in human cases of baclofen overdoses. However, there are several successful animal case studies.[25] Flumazenil, a specific benzodiazepine antagonist, has also been cited as a potential adjunct to treatment. In some case reports, it has been successful in counteracting the central inhibitory effects of baclofen, but other case reports cite it is unreliable and ineffective.[14,26,27] Hemodialysis, although un-likely to occur in the ED, is also a useful adjunct—especially in those with abnormal renal function. In baclofen overdose in healthy adults, protein binding is estimated to be 30–35%, and volume of distribution 0.8–2.6 L/kg. In patients with renal dysfunction, the protein binding and volume of distribution is disrupted by fluid shifts and uremia, increasing its ability to be dialyzed.[28] Limited cases have shown efficacy in those with normal renal function, but this is not common practice secondary to the high endogenous clearance and short half-life in those with normal renal function.[29-31] If central venous access is obtained in the ED, placing a catheter capable of allowing temporary hemodialysis may be warranted if the patient has renal dysfunction.

Treatment

Baclofen Withdrawal

Baclofen overdose and withdrawal can present with overlapping signs and symptoms. Baclofen withdrawal classically presents with muscular hypertonicity and hyperthermia rather than muscular flaccidity and hypothermia. Early in baclofen withdrawal, patients may complain of generalized pruritis and progress to disorientation, hyperthermia (up to 43°C or 109.4°F), hemodynamic instability, hallucinations/psychosis, rebound spasticity, myoclonus, seizures, hepatic and kidney dysfunction, rhabdomyolysis, disseminated intravascular coagulation, cardiac arrest, and death.[9] Other important conditions that are in the differential diagnosis, especially if the history and presentation does not clearly point toward baclofen withdrawal, include autonomic dysreflexia, serotonin syndrome, malignant hyperthermia, sympathomimetic toxicity, electron transport chain uncoupler toxicity, and neuroleptic malignant syndrome. The key features and differentiating factors are listed in Table 25.2.

TABLE 25.2 **Key diagnostic and differentiating factors between intrathecal baclofen withdrawal and similar presenting syndromes**

	ITB withdrawal	Autonomic dysreflexia	MH	Serotonin syndrome	NMS
Mechanism	Decreased CNS GABA-B transmission	Disconnection of splanchnic sympathetic outflow from supraspinal control	Ryanodine receptor mutation causing Ca2+ release from sarcoplasmic reticulum	Overload of CNS serotonin transmission	Acute loss of hypothalamic dopaminergic transmission
Key differentiating features	Pruritis, labile blood pressure (may be hypotensive), priapism in men. Medical or pharmacologic history.	Occasional preceding bradycardia, normal consciousness with apprehension, flushing/vasodilation/ sweating above injury; piloerection, pallor, spasticity, and rigidity only below lesion level. T6 or higher SCI.	CK elevation at onset, central acting relaxants ineffective, tetanic muscular contractions. Family or anesthetic history.	Myoclonus. Medical or pharmacologic history— serotonergic medications (SSRI, MDMA, linezolid)	Tremor to generalized rigidity. Medical or pharmacologic history—initiation of dopamine blocking drugs, cessation of dopamine agonist.

ITB, intrathecal baclofen; MH, malignant hyperthermia; NMS, neuroleptic malignant syndrome; SCI, spinal cord injury.
From Coffey et al.[8] and Meythaler et al.[19]

Intrathecal pump malfunctions are true emergencies. Prompt resumption of baclofen therapy is the treatment for withdrawal and can be preventative if timed appropriately. It is important to note that oral doses (sometimes even as high as 120 mg/day in divided doses) are often not effective in preventing or resolving withdrawal. The slow onset of action, low CSF concentration, and poor GI absorption in critically ill patients are all factors in the ineffective nature of oral administration. Bolus and maintenance doses intrathecally are recommended until the ITB pump can be re-started at the patient's baseline dosing.[32] Spasticity and seizures may be treated with benzodiazepines. Antiepileptics should be considered if seizures are refractory to benzodiazepines. Although supportive studies are limited, dexmedetomidine, cyproheptadine, dantrolene, and propofol have also been used.[8,19,33] These adjunctive treatments are also helpful if the patient's presentation and history is not clearly consistent with baclofen withdrawal and other differential diagnoses are being considered. One case report cites dexmedetomidine as a more favorable option in comparison to benzodiazepines or propofol. A better respiratory safety profile, improvement in vital signs, and avoidance of intubation were noted.[33] In support of cyproheptadine, several successful case reports suggest that the abrupt removal of GABA-B inhibition can also cause excessive serotonin release, making cyproheptadine a potentially useful adjunct alongside baclofen and benzodiazepines.[19] Currently however, benzodiazepine use to restore central GABAergic inhibition and continued supportive care are the most supported, logical, and safe treatment options if baclofen withdrawal is the definitive diagnosis.[8,9]

CASE CONCLUSION

In our presentation case, the patient was intubated and mechanically ventilated after his arrival. RSI was used and consisted of weight-appropriate dosing of etomidate and rocuronium. Midazolam was used for sedation and further seizure prevention. CT of the brain did not reveal any acute intracranial bleed, mass, or shift. Two liters of normal saline were administered and blood pressure transiently improved; he eventually required temporary norepinephrine infusion for blood pressure support. His ITB physician came to beside in the ED and stopped the pump. The pump was also interrogated by the manufacturer and was found to be functioning properly. He was transferred to the ICU and was monitored with 24-hour continuous EEG, which revealed increased slow wave activity with periodic epileptic discharges, consistent with baclofen overdose, which resolved by 48 hours.[15]

Large-volume CSF removal via lumbar puncture was performed within the first 24 hours with gradual improvement in neurologic status. CSF studies were negative for viral or bacterial causes, and there was no albuminocytologic dissociation. His ITB physician reinstated his intrathecal baclofen infusion at 48 hours to prevent acute withdrawal. Although his ICU course was complicated by aspiration pneumonia that was treated with antibiotics, he was extubated on day 4 and was discharged home on day 8. The ITB physician opined that the increase in dosing, or perhaps a titration error, may have caused the overdose.

When a patient presents to the ED with a suspected baclofen withdrawal or overdose, emergency physicians must always be cognizant of several key actions. First, early recognition of the need for airway protection and aggressive supportive care. Selecting appropriate RSI medications and avoiding those that will worsen the patient's condition. Watch for concurrent issues such as nonconvulsive status epilepticus, underlying intrathecal pump infections, and the potential for prolonged CNS depression that can mimic brain death. Early lumbar puncture can be therapeutic (for intrathecal overdose) and may help rule-out other possible differential diagnoses. If necessary, placement of a temporary hemodialysis catheter may also promote early dialysis in those with underlying renal dysfunction. Prompt resolution of baclofen therapy once the acute overdose is resolving will help to prevent or lessen the effects of withdrawal. If history is unclear or unavailable, a clinician should have a high index of suspicion for baclofen overdose or withdrawal because routine urine or serum drug screens do not detect baclofen. Other differential diagnoses, including sepsis, hypoglycemia, intracranial pathology, meningitis, intrathecal pump infection, other drug/alcohol withdrawal, co-ingestants, serotonin syndrome, neuroleptic malignant syndrome, and autonomic dysreflexia, should all be considered.[1,9]

- Early recognition of the need for airway protection and aggressive supportive care is essential.
- Select appropriate rapid sequence induction medications and avoid those that will worsen the patient's condition.
- Be aware of nonconvulsive status epilepticus, underlying intrathecal pump infections, and the potential for prolonged CNS depression that can mimic brain death.
- Prompt resolution of baclofen therapy once the acute overdose is resolving will help to prevent or lessen the effects of withdrawal.

Further Reading

Goldfrank LR, Nelson L, Howland MA, et al. *Goldfrank's Toxicologic Emergencies*. 11th ed. McGraw-Hill Education; 2019.

Lioresal® Intrathecal. FDA Access Data. Accessed June 21, 2022. https://www.accessd ata.fda.gov/drugsatfda_docs/label/2019/020075s037lbl.pdf

Ozobax Baclofen oral solution. FDA Access Data. Accessed June 21, 2022. https:// www.accessdata.fda.gov/drugsatfda_docs/label/2019/208193s000lbl.pdf

Roberge RJ, Martin TG, Hodgman M, Benitez JG, Brunswick JE. Supraventricular tachyarrhythmia associated with baclofen overdose. *J Toxicol: Clin Toxicol*. 1994;32(3):291–297. https://doi.org/10.3109/15563659409017961

References

1. Parker-Pitts K, Weymouth W, Frawley T. (Intrathecal baclofen overdose with paradoxical autonomic features mimicking withdrawal. *J Emerg Med*. 2020;58(4):616–619. https://doi.org/10.1016/j.jemermed.2019.12.031

2. Caron E, Morgan R, Wheless JW. An unusual cause of flaccid paralysis and coma. J Child Neurol. 2013;29(4):555–559. https://doi.org/10.1177/0883073813479668

3. Gerkin R, Curry SC, Vance MV, Sankowski PW, Meinhart RD. First-order elimination kinetics following baclofen overdose. *Ann Emerg Med*. 1986;15(7):843–846. https://doi.org/10.1016/s0196-0644(86)80388-2

4. Miller JJ. Baclofen overdose mimicking anoxic encephalopathy: a case report and review of the literature. *Thera Adv Drug Saf*. 2017;8(5):165–167. https://doi.org/10.1177/2042098617693571

5. Stewart E, Tormoehlen LM. Baclofen. In: Brent J, Burkhart K, Dargan P, et al. (eds.), *Critical Care Toxicology*, vol. 2. 2nd ed. Springer International: 1119–1131.

6. Anderson P, Nohér H, Swahn CG. Pharmacokinetics in baclofen overdose. *J Toxicol: Clin Toxicol*. 1984;22(1):11–20. https://doi.org/10.3109/00099308409035078

7. Kohl MM, Paulsen O. The roles of GABAB receptors in cortical network activity. *Adv Pharmacol*. 2010;(58):205–229. https://doi.org/10.1016/s1054-3589(10)58009-8

8. Coffey RJ, Edgar TS, Francisco GE, et al. Abrupt withdrawal from intrathecal baclofen: recognition and management of a potentially life-threatening syndrome. *Arch Phys Med Rehabil*. 2002;83(6):735–741. https://doi.org/10.1053/apmr.2002.32820

9. Kao LW, Amin Y, Kirk MA, Turner MS. Intrathecal baclofen withdrawal mimicking sepsis. *J Emerg Med*. 2003;24(4):423–427. https://doi.org/10.1016/s0736-4679(03)00039-8

10. Leung NY, Whyte IM, Isbister GK. Baclofen overdose: defining the spectrum of toxicity. *Emerg Med Australas*. 2006;18(1):77–82. https://doi.org/10.1111/j.1742-6723.2006.00805.x

11. Drevin G, Briet M, Ghamrawi S, Beloncle F, Abbara C. Baclofen overdose following recreational use in adolescents and young adults: a case report and review of the literature. *Forensic Sci Int*. 2020;316:110541. https://doi.org/10.1016/j.forsciint.2020.110541

12. Weißhaar GF, Hoemberg M, Bender K, et al. Baclofen intoxication: a "fun drug" causing deep coma and nonconvulsive status epilepticus—a case report and review of the literature. *Eur J Pediatr*. 2012;171(10):1541–1547. https://doi.org/10.1007/s00431-012-1780

13. Watve SV, Sivan M, Raza WA, Jamil FF. Management of acute overdose or withdrawal state in intrathecal baclofen therapy. *Spinal Cord*. 2011;50(2):107–111. https://doi.org/10.1038/sc.2011.112

14. Ostermann ME, Young B, Sibbald WJ, Nicolle MW. Coma mimicking brain death following baclofen overdose. *Intens Care Med*. 2000;26(8):1144–1146. https://doi.org/10.1007/s001340051330

15. Sauneuf B, Totouom HK, Savary B, Varin L, Dupeyrat J, Ramakers S, Hanouz JL. Clinical and EEG features of acute intrathecal baclofen overdose. *Clin Neurol Neurosurg*. 2012;114(1):84–86.

16. Cohen MB, Gailey RA, McCoy GC. Atropine in the treatment of baclofen overdose. *Am J Emerg Med*. 1986;4(6):552–553. https://doi.org/10.1016/s0735-6757(86)80018-3

17. Nugent S, Katz MD, Little TE. Baclofen overdose with cardiac conduction abnormalities: case report and review of the literature. *J Toxicol: Clin Toxicol*. 1986;24(4):321–328. https://doi.org/10.3109/15563658608992596

18. Gill D, Mann K, Liu K. QT prolongation by baclofen overdose. *Am J Ther*. 2017;24(5):e625–e627. https://doi.org/10.1097/mjt.0000000000000505

19. Meythaler JM, Roper JF, Brunner RC. Cyproheptadine for intrathecal baclofen withdrawal. *Arch Phys Med Rehabil*. 2003;84(5):638–642. https://doi.org/10.1016/s0003-9993(03)00105-9

20. Juurlink DN. Activated charcoal for acute overdose: a reappraisal. *Br J Clin Pharmacol*. 2015;81(3):482–487. https://doi.org/10.1111/bcp.12793

21. Jung, M. Maryland Poison Control Center. Toxtidbits: baclofen overdose. February 2012. https://mdpoison.com/media/SOP/mdpoisoncom/ToxTidbits/2012/February%202012%20ToxTidbits.pdf

22. Müller-Schwefe G, Penn RD. Physostigmine in the treatment of intrathecal baclofen overdose. *J Neurosurg*. 1989;71(2):273–275. https://doi.org/10.3171/jns.1989.71.2.0273

23. Saltuari L, Kofler M, Baumgartner H. Failure of physostigmine in treatment of acute severe intrathecal baclofen intoxication. N Engl J Med. 1990;322(21):1533–1534. https://doi.org/10.1056/nejm199005243222117

24. Saltuari L, Marosi MJ, Kofler M, Bauer G. Status epilepticus complicating intrathecal baclofen overdose. *Lancet*. 1992;339(8789):373–374. https://doi.org/10.1016/0140-6736(92)91697-7

25. Becker M, Young B. Treatment of severe lipophilic intoxications with intravenous lipid emulsion: a case series (2011–2014). *Vet Medp (Auckl)*. 2017;8:77–85. https://doi.org/10.2147/vmrr.s129576

26. Byrnes SM, Watson GW, Hardy PA. Flumazenil: an unreliable antagonist in baclofen overdose. *Anaesthesia*. 1996;51(5):481–482. https://doi.org/10.1111/j.1365-2044.1996.tb07796.x

27. Saissy JM, Vitris M, Demaziere J, Seck M, Marcoux L, Gaye M. Flumazenil counteracts intrathecal baclofen-induced central nervous system depression in tetanus. *Anesthesiology*. 1992;76(6):1051–1053. https://doi.org/10.1097/00000542-199206000-00027

28. Olyaei AJ, Steffl JL. A quantitative approach to drug dosing in chronic kidney disease. *Blood Purif*. 2011;31(1-3):138–145. doi:10.1159/000321857

29. Chen KS, Bullard MJ, Chien YY, Lee SY. Baclofen toxicity in patients with severely impaired renal function. *Ann Pharmacother*. 1997;31(11):1315–1320. https://doi.org/10.1177/106002809703101108

30. Ghannoum M, Berling I, Lavergne V, et al. Recommendations from the EXTRIP workgroup on extracorporeal treatment for baclofen poisoning. *Kidney Int*. 2021;100(4):720–736. https://doi.org/10.1016/j.kint.2021.07.014

31. Hsieh MJ, Chen SC, Weng TI, Fang CC, Tsai TJ. Treating baclofen overdose by hemodialysis. *Am J Emerg Med*. 2012;30(8):1654.e5–1654.e7. https://doi.org/10.1016/j.ajem.2011.07.013

32. Ross JC, Cook AM, Stewart GL, Fahy BG. Acute intrathecal baclofen withdrawal: a brief review of treatment options. *Neurocrit Care*. 2010;14(1):103–108. doi:10.1007/s12028-010-9422-6

33. Gottula AL, Gorder KL, Peck AR, Renne BC. Dexmedetomidine for acute management of intrathecal baclofen withdrawal. *J Emerg Med*. 2020;58(1):e5–e8. https://doi.org/10.1016/j.jemermed.2019.09.043

26 Is That Chest Pain a Heart Attack, or a Line of Cocaine? Managing Cocaine-Induced Chest Pain

Amir Jamal Mansour, Pradeep Padmanabhan, and Besher Assi

Case Presentation

A 50-year-old man with diabetes and hypertension presented to the ED with the chief complaint of chest pain for the past hour. The chest pain has been ongoing since attending a work party earlier that night. He complains of chest tightness and feels that his heart is racing. He states "I feel like my heart is about to explode." The symptoms started suddenly and have been persistent and severe. When asked about recent drug use, he states he tried some cocaine at the event prior to the onset of his symptoms. He is on metformin and lisinopril. His vitals are heart rate 110 beats/min, blood pressure 172/80 mm Hg, temperature 101.5°F/38.6°C, respiratory rate 23 beats/min, and pulse oximetry 99% on room air. Physical exam is notable for an anxious, obese male in moderate distress with diaphoresis. He has good peripheral pulses with a capillary refill of less than 2 seconds. He has packed his right nostril with a tissue because he had a nosebleed earlier. His lungs were clear, and the remainder of his physical exam is within normal limits.

What Do You Do Now?

DISCUSSION

The recognition, and treatment of cocaine-associated chest pain (CACP) is often challenging. Clinicians who are concerned for acute coronary syndrome (ACS) should treat the patient as such while being cognizant of the other cardiac complications of cocaine ingestion. Patients with CACP may be typically younger and have less risk factors than the traditional myocardial infarction (MI) patient. According to one study, patients with cocaine-associated MI presented with symptoms of substernal chest pain (71.3%) that was pressure-like in nature (46.7%), with shortness of breath (59.3%) and diaphoresis (38.6%).[1] That same study also reported that up to 33% of patients complained of pleuritic chest pain.[2]

Background

Cocaine is a xenobiotic alkaloid derived from the plant *Erthoxylum coca*. The plant is found primarily in South America, specifically in northern parts of the Amazon and in the Andean Highlands. South Americans have chewed dried coca leaves and drank coca tea for thousands of years as part of local religious practices and as a means of enhancing their ability to work long hours through coca's effect of inhibiting thirst and hunger and increasing energy. After coca was brought to Europe, Albert Niemann isolated an active ingredient from coca leaves in 1860 and named it "cocaine." Stories about coca from the Incas as well as preliminary scientific investigations from multiple scientists in the 1800s led to people capitalizing on its medicinal effects. In the 20th century, cocaine was prescribed for headaches, toothaches, GI disorders, neuralgias, and dyspepsia. Anesthetics also began to utilize cocaine, mainly for eye surgery. Not only was cocaine used for medicinal purposes, but it was around this time that coca leaves were used in the production of Coca Cola, and, owing to its widespread availability and addiction forming properties, people began using cocaine recreationally. As early as 1910, there were reports of nasal damage due to nasal insufflation of cocaine. Restrictions and regulation of the use of cocaine has since been ramped up. The Harrison Narcotics act in 1914 regulated the domestic distribution of drugs. The Controlled Substances Act in the 1970s is the foundation of what has now been labeled the "war on drugs" with the creation of the Drug Enforcement Administration (DEA) serving to address drug laws at the federal level.[1]

Today, cocaine is the second most commonly used illicit drug in the United States (just after marijuana) with more than 5.5 million users, or about 2% of the population admitting to cocaine use in the past year. Its use is more common in adults 18–25 years of age, with 5.8% using cocaine in the past year compared to just 1.6% in those older than 26.[3] An estimated 18.2 million people worldwide used cocaine in 2016.[4] In 2018, greater than 1 in 5 drug overdoses in the United States involved cocaine, resulting in 14,666 deaths attributable to cocaine in 2018. This is an alarming triple-fold increase from 2012.[5]

There are two forms commonly used: crack cocaine and cocaine hydrochloride. Crack cocaine is a yellow solid that is smoked, while cocaine hydrochloride is a water-soluble compound, usually a white powder which can be nasally insufflated (snorted) or injected. Slang terms for crack cocaine include black rock, hard rock, snow coke, and candy. Cocaine powder may be referred to as blow, coke, C, snow, rails, and lines.

Toxicology and Pathophysiology

Cocaine's addictive properties are thought to be due to its effects on the mesocorticolimbic dopaminergic system. This system includes dopamine-releasing cells in the ventral tegmental area that project to structures in the forebrain, which includes the nucleus accumbens and prefrontal cortex. The nucleus accumbens plays a critical role in the feeling of reward, while the prefrontal cortex is primarily responsible for the inhibition of behaviors. Cocaine works by blocking monoamine reuptake transporters in presynaptic neurons, effectively increasing synaptic concentrations of dopamine, norepinephrine, and serotonin, which prolongs their effects on the mesocorticolimbic pathway. As a result, there is increased activity, which leads to a heightened feeling of reward as well as a lack of inhibition and impulse control. There are a multitude of symptoms associated with cocaine use many, but not all, of which have been listed in Box 26.1.

Through its ability to block reuptake of monoamines, especially norepinephrine, cocaine stimulates the sympathetic nervous system. Monoamines, like norepinephrine, bind to the adrenergic receptors found on different organs and lead to many of the symptoms seen in Box 26.1. The sodium channel blockade, stimulation of excitatory amino acids, and release of catecholamines also play a role in producing the sympathomimetic effects.[3]

Cocaine is a powerful sympathomimetic agent which increases heart rate and blood pressure while simultaneously reducing left ventricular function and end-systolic wall stress. Through alpha- and beta-adrenergic stimulation, cocaine induces myocardial inotropy and vasoconstriction of cardiac arteries resulting in oxygen demand/supply mismatch.[6] Additional effects of cocaine include activation of platelets, stimulation of platelet aggregation, and potentiation of thromboxane production. All of this ultimately leads to the promotion of thrombus formation, even in low doses, and predisposes individuals to ischemic events.[7]

Workup and Diagnosis
Cocaine use is typically elicited through history. Cocaine use is often under-reported by patients due to concerns about legal issues or stigmatization by healthcare providers. It is metabolized mainly into ecgonine methyl ester and benzoylecgonine by cholinesterase enzymes in the serum and liver. The half-life of cocaine is 45–90 minutes, and it is renally eliminated. The urine drug screen (UDS) for cocaine tests for its benzoylecgonine and ecgonine metabolites. Although there are no known xenobiotics that will cause a false positive for cocaine on the UDS, if the use occurred just prior to testing, there

may not be enough of the benzoylecgonine in the urine to result in a positive test. Cocaine can be detected in urine for 24–48 hours after intranasal use and as long as 22 days after use in chronic users and those with poor kidney function.[8] The ability to result in a positive long after use calls into question the clinical utility of the UDS, and research has shown that emergency drug screens are unlikely to change the management of the patient in the ED.[9]

Patients with suspected CACP should undergo a cardiac workup similar to other patients presenting with chest pain, regardless of whether vasospasm is suspected as the cause. Patients with CACP are also at risk for nonischemic pathology, including cocaine-induced cardiomyopathy, aortic dissection, dysrhythmias, and hemorrhagic alveolitis also known as "crack lung." The hemorrhagic alveolitis is thought to be secondary to forceful inhalation and breath holding when smoking crack from a pipe.[10]

An ECG, chest X-ray, complete blood count (CBC), basic metabolic profile (BMP), serial troponins, and optionally other diagnostic tests further evaluate for other severe effects of cocaine use. A CT scan of the chest should be ordered if there is concern for an aortic dissection owing to the hypertension and injury to vascular walls that results from use.[10] ECGs have been studied in CACP, with up to 89.9% specificity for diagnosing MI; however, the positive predictive value and sensitivity were 17.9% and 35.7%, respectively, making ECG unreliable in the acute setting. So, ECGs, while specific, should not be relied on as a standalone test to assess cardiac effects of cocaine because sensitivity is very low.[10,11]. Cardiac biomarkers, such as troponin, are much better at detecting cardiac injury than are ECGs and, in conjunction, can help with disposition.[12]

Another concern is that ST segment changes may be falsely attributed to benign causes, which can lead to missed diagnosis and poor outcomes. The same is true for troponin, as elevations may not be as significant in patients with cocaine use as compared to those without recent use, but this troponin elevation still needs to be identified and treated accordingly. One study showed that more than 80% of patients with CACP and an elevated troponin had a positive cardiac catheterization, defined as greater than 50% stenosis, with single-vessel disease being the most prevalent, and around 10% having triple-vessel disease. This same study also noted that nearly 20% of these were in the absence of any ECG changes.[13] In summary, it is critical that, in a clinical setting, minimal or even absent ECG changes with marginal elevations in cardiac biomarkers are taken seriously. These findings call for a detailed evaluation, as the study above illustrated that more than 80% of CACP with high troponin levels had positive cardiac catheterization findings. So, although we do obtain the same tests and workup for patients with and without cocaine use, it is important to interpret the tests with the complete clinical picture and associated pathophysiology in mind.

Treatment

In addition to standard therapy, benzodiazepines are a mainstay of treatment for adults presenting to the ED with chest pain and suspected cocaine use. They primarily help control agitation, which is often an accompanying symptom in acutely intoxicated patients.[14] Additionally, they will help reduce psychomotor agitation induced by centrally mediated enhanced sympatric tone and can help reduce hyperthermia caused by this increased muscular tone.[15] By this same mechanism, benzodiazepines can help reduce the increased strain on the heart and vasoconstriction leading to decreased oxygen delivery.[3]

Nitrates can decrease coronary artery vasoconstriction, often easing chest pain and myocardial ischemia, especially when given in conjunction with benzodiazepines.[3] As noted above, regular cocaine use can lead to accelerated atherosclerosis, therefore patients with ECG findings concerning for acute ischemia, particularly ST-elevation, should be discussed with a cardiac catheterization team for possible emergent reperfusion therapy. In the event of ventricular arrhythmias or evidence of sodium channel blockade on ECG, consider sodium bicarbonate. Lidocaine may be considered for ventricular arrhythmias refractory to sodium bicarbonate therapy.

Beta-blocker use in CACP was a controversial topic and was even contraindicated, however this was based on of poor-quality studies and inconclusive research. The debate stemmed from the thought that beta-blockers led to unopposed alpha stimulation, increased coronary vasospasm, seizures, and all-cause mortality; however, this has largely been debunked.[16] In multiple studies there was no statistically significant difference in MI or mortality in patients with CACP regardless of beta-blocker use.[8,17] Therefore, it appears the harms associated with beta-blocker use may have been overstated, although the question of why a beta-blocker would be used over other medications is very apropos. Another medication class to avoid especially in patients with abnormal vital signs is antipsychotics such as haloperidol as these can lower the seizure threshold, worsen hyperthermia, and potentiate dysrhythmias.[8]

Calcium channel blockers (CCB), specifically the nondihydropyridine calcium channel blockers (verapamil or diltiazem) improve coronary vasoconstriction and hemodynamics with no significant adverse outcomes. They work through coronary vasodilation, decreasing cardiac contractility and slowing the AV and sinus nodes. These are best used in conjunction with nitroglycerin and can help relieve many of the symptoms of CACP by decreasing myocardial oxygen demand and improving coronary blood flow.[18] They are contraindicated in patients with left ventricular dysfunction or heart failure.

Other drugs that can be used in addition to standard of care for refractory CACP include phentolamine and dexmedetomidine. Phentolamine can be beneficial in addition to standard therapy due to vasodilatory effects and alpha-antagonism which can help relieve chest pain.[19] Dexmedetomidine is a centrally acting alpha-2 agonist that in some studies has been used to treat CACP, hypertension, and tachycardia; it works through reversing increases in sympathetic nerve activity.[20] One prospective study showed improvement in vasoconstriction when given as in intracoronary infusion as compared to placebo, however this was a small trial of only 22 patients.[21].

Recent literature has suggested the use of an observation unit for patients with CACP and a moderate level of concern for ACS. Monitoring in this setting will include cardiac telemetry, serial ECGs, and serial troponin levels, as well as assurance of sustained symptom resolution. If the patient remains symptomatic, or there is concern based on ECG or troponin changes, further cardiac evaluation with either stress testing or angiography is indicated; however, this decision will likely be made by the cardiologist or per individual hospital protocol. The use of observation units has been shown to be both safe and also cost effective, one study showing no 30-day mortality for patients who were discharged home without evidence of ischemia or cardiovascular complication over the 9- to 12-hour period.[22]

Long-Term Concerns

Overall, research regarding outcomes due to chronic cocaine use has been indeterminate. In a study conducted by Kozor et al., researchers demonstrated that left ventricular (LV) mass was greater in regular cocaine users when compared to cocaine nonusers. Similarly, Maceira et al. found that people who abused cocaine had increased LV end-diastolic volume and right ventricular (RV) end-diastolic volume in addition to increased LV mass. It was noted that frequent cocaine use was associated with decreased LV ejection fraction and RV ejection fraction. These two studies demonstrate an overall negative effect on cardiac function.

For CACP, cessation of cocaine is the primary therapeutic goal, and patients who discontinue cocaine have a commensurate decrease in chest pain and overall mortality.[3] Cardiovascular complications have been routinely demonstrated with continued use, and studies have shown more serious complications with continued use.[22] If available, consider involving social work and/or a peer recovery coach in discharge planning to facilitate counseling, resources, and other services that can aid in recovery.

The Thrombolysis in Myocardial Infarction (TIMI) score is a risk stratification tool that estimate mortality in patients with MI. One study attempted to analyze the clinical utility of this scoring system in patient with CACP. The authors ultimately concluded that the TIMI risk score has no clinical predictive value in this patient population.[23] The HEART score is a similar risk-stratifying tool that looks to identify major adverse cardiac events (MACE) within 30 days. A separate study found that, in CACP, the HEART score was not recommended due to its limited clinical utility in stratifying risk: 14% of patients with CACP who were categorized as low risk experienced MACE within 30 days as compared to only 4% in the general chest pain population.[24]

Last, there have been a few studies that looked at the impact of cocaine use on the development of coronary artery disease (CAD). While some of these studies report an increased likelihood of developing CAD in cocaine users, other studies failed to find that same correlation between cocaine users and CAD.

CASE CONCLUSION

Coming back to our case, the patient had lab work and imaging obtained along with an ECG and symptomatic management included aspirin, sublingual nitro, and Ativan. The patient's initial troponin was not elevated, and ECG was not significant for signs of ischemia and only showed some sinus tachycardia. The repeat troponin did increase slightly though, and so the patient was brought into the observation unit. While in the unit he received serial troponins, which were stable; the patient was agreeable to meeting with the behavioral health team and received resources for drug abstinence and rehabilitation. After about 12 hours the patient had a complete resolution of his symptoms and was discharged and encouraged to follow-up with his primary care physician as well as a cardiologist for further workup and assessment.

KEY POINTS TO REMEMBER

- Normal ECG does not rule out acute myocardial infarction (MI) in patients with cocaine intoxication.
- Troponins have more than 90% sensitivity for acute MI in patients with cocaine-associated chest pain.
- Benzodiazepines improve pain, anxiety, and coronary artery vasospasm.
- If there is concern for MI, prompt cardiology consultation is recommended.

Further Reading

Wightman RS, Perrone J. Cocaine and Amphetamines. In: Tintinalli JE, Ma O, Yealy DM, Meckler GD, Stapczynski J, Cline DM, Thomas SH. eds. *Tintinalli's Emergency Medicine: A Comprehensive Study Guide, 9e*. McGraw Hill; 2020. Accessed August 06, 2023. https://accessemergencymedicine.mhmedical.com/content.aspx?bookid=2353&sectionid=220744818

Heard K, Palmer R, Zahniser NR. Mechanisms of acute cocaine toxicity. *Open Pharmacol J*. 2008;2(9):70–78. doi:10.2174/1874143600802010070. PMID: 19568322; PMCID: PMC2703432.

O'Leary ME, Hancox JC. Role of voltage-gated sodium, potassium and calcium channels in the development of cocaine-associated cardiac arrhythmias. *Br J Clin Pharmacol*. 2010 May;69(5):427–442. doi:10.1111/j.1365-2125.2010.03629.x. PMID: 20573078; PMCID: PMC2856043.

References

1. Drake LR, Scott PJH. DARK classics in chemical neuroscience: cocaine. *ACS Chem Neurosci*. 2018;9(10):2358–2372. doi:10.1021/acschemneuro.8b00117

2. Hollander JE, Hoffman RS, Gennis P, et al. Prospective multicenter evaluation of cocaine-associated chest pain. Cocaine Associated Chest Pain (COCHPA) study group. *Acad Emerg Med*. Jul–Aug1994;1(4):330–339. doi:10.1111/j.1553-2712. 1994.tb02639.x. PMID: 7614278

3. Schwartz BG, Rezkalla S, Kloner RA. Cardiovascular effects of cocaine. *Circulation*. Dec 14, 2010;122(24):2558–2569. doi:10.1161/CIRCULATIONAHA.110.940569. PMID: 21156654

4. Kim ST, Park T. Acute and chronic effects of cocaine on cardiovascular health. *Int J Mol Sci*. 2019;20(3):584. doi:10.3390/ijms20030584

5. Cano M, Oh S, Salas-Wright CP, Vaughn MG. Cocaine use and overdose mortality in the United States: evidence from two national data sources, 2002–2018. *Drug Alcohol Depend*. 2020;214:108148. doi:10.1016/j.drugalcdep.2020.108148

6. Muscholl E. Effect of cocaine and related drugs on the uptake of noradrenaline by heart and spleen. *Br J Pharmacol Chemother*. 1961;16:352–359.

7. Heesch CM, Wilhelm CR, Ristich J, Adnane J, Bontempo FA, Wagner WR. Cocaine activates platelets and increases the formation of circulating platelet containing microaggregates in humans. *Heart*. Jun 2000;83(6):688–695. doi:10.1136/heart.83.6.688. PMID: 10814631; PMCID: PMC1760877

8. McCord J, Jneid H, Hollander JE, et al; American Heart Association Acute Cardiac Care Committee of the Council on Clinical Cardiology. Management of cocaine-associated chest pain and myocardial infarction: a scientific statement from the American Heart Association Acute Cardiac Care Committee of the Council on Clinical Cardiology. *Circulation*. Apr 8, 2008;117(14):1897–1907. doi:10.1161/CIRCULATIONAHA.107.188950. Epub 2008 Mar 17. PMID: 18347214

9. Tenenbein M. Do you really need that emergency drug screen? *Clin Toxicol (Phila)*. Apr 2009;47(4):286–291. PMID:19514875

10. Hollander JE, Hoffman RS, Gennis P, et al. Prospective multicenter evaluation of cocaine associated chest pain. *Acad Emerg Med* 1994;1:330–339.

11. Amin M, Gabelman G, Karpel J, Buttrick P. Acute myocardial infarction and chest pain syndromes after cocaine use. *Am J Cardiol*. 1990;66(20):1434–1437.

12. Hollander JE, Levitt MA, Young GP, et al. Effect of recent cocaine use on the specificity of cardiac markers for diagnosis of acute myocardial infarction. *Am Heart J* 1998;135:245–252.

13. Mohamad T, Niraj A, Farah J, et al. Spectrum of electrocardiographic and angiographic coronary artery disease findings in patients with cocaine-associated myocardial infarction. *Coron Artery Dis*. Aug 2009;20(5):332–336. doi:10.1097/MCA.0b013e32832b906c. PMID: 19543086

14. Richards JR, Garber D, Laurin EG, et al. Treatment of cocaine cardiovascular toxicity: a systematic review. *Clin Toxicol (Phila)*. Jun 2016;54(5):345–364. doi:10.3109/15563650.2016.1142090. Epub 2016 Feb 26. PMID: 26919414

15. Goldfrank LR, Hoffman RS. The cardiovascular effects of cocaine. *Ann Emerg Med*. Feb 1991;20(2):165–175. doi:10.1016/s0196-0644(05)81217-x. PMID: 1996800

16. Pham D, et al. Outcomes of beta blocker use in cocaine-associated chest pain: a meta-analysis. *Emerg Med J.* 2018;35(9):559–563.
17. Richards JR, et al. β-blockers, cocaine, and the unopposed α-stimulation phenomenon. *J Cardiovasc Pharmacol Ther.* 2017;22(3):239–249.
18. Wright RS, Anderson JL, Adams CD, et al; American College of Cardiology Foundation/American Heart Association Task Force on Practice Guidelines. 2011 ACCF/AHA focused update incorporated into the ACC/AHA 2007 Guidelines for the Management of Patients with Unstable Angina/Non-ST-Elevation Myocardial Infarction: a report of the American College of Cardiology Foundation/American Heart Association Task Force on Practice Guidelines developed in collaboration with the American Academy of Family Physicians, Society for Cardiovascular Angiography and Interventions, and the Society of Thoracic Surgeons. *J Am Coll Cardiol.* May 10, 2011;57(19):e215–367. doi:10.1016/j.jacc.2011.02.011. PMID: 21545940
19. Chan, GM, et al. Phentolamine therapy for cocaine-association acute coronary syndrome (CAACS). *J Med Toxicol.*2006;2(3):108–111. doi:10.1007/BF03161019
20. Finkel JB, Marhefka GD. Rethinking cocaine-associated chest pain and acute coronary syndromes. *Mayo Clin Proc.* 2011;86(12):1198–1207. doi:10.4065/mcp.2011.0338
21. Menon DV, Wang Z, Fadel PJ, et al. Central sympatholysis as a novel countermeasure for cocaine-induced sympathetic activation and vasoconstriction in humans. *J Am Coll Cardiol.* 2007;50(7):626–633.
22. Weber JE, Shofer FS, Larkin GL, Kalaria AS, Hollander JE. Validation of a brief observation period for patients with cocaine-associated chest pain. *N Engl J Med.* Feb 6, 2003;348(6):510–517. doi:10.1056/NEJMoa022206. PMID: 12571258
23. Chase M, Brown AM, Robey JL, et al. Application of the TIMI risk score in ED patients with cocaine-associated chest pain. *Am J Emerg Med.* 2007 Nov;25(9):1015–1018. doi:10.1016/j.ajem.2007.03.004. PMID: 18022495
24. Faramand Z, Martin-Gill C, Frisch SO, et al. The prognostic value of HEART score in patients with cocaine associated chest pain: an age-and-sex matched cohort study. *Am J Emerg Med.* 2021;45:303–308. ISSN 0735-6757, https://doi.org/10.1016/j.ajem.2020.08.074.

27 Don't Poke the Snake: The Do's and Don'ts of Snake Bite Management

Katie Lippert and Joshua da Silva

Case Presentation

You are working at your local ED when someone runs to the front desk frantically calling for help. She reports that her husband is in the car and has been bitten by a snake. They were out for a hike on one of the popular trails in the area, and her husband stepped off the path to take a photo of the view. The grass was long; he heard a rattle and then felt a sharp pain on his ankle. He looked down to see a snake slithering away. His wife mentions that the trail was closed due to rattlesnakes, but they decided to hike the area anyway. They regretfully inform you that they were unable to capture the snake for identification, which you inform them is not necessary and not recommended as it often results in more injuries.

You immediately bring the husband back to the resuscitation room for evaluation. The nurse reports his vitals as a heart rate of 110 beats/min, blood pressure is 90/50 mm Hg, respiratory rate is 16 breaths/min, temperature is 98.6°F/37°C; his oxygen saturation is 99% on room air. His left leg is noted to have two puncture wounds with surrounding erythema. While you are evaluating him, he begins to complain of significant nausea as well as worsening pain in his left leg.

What Do You Do Now?

DISCUSSION

Background

Snakes strike fear into the hearts of many, as evidenced by the iconic scene in *Indiana Jones: Raiders of the Lost Ark*, where Jones says, "Snakes! Why did it have to be snakes?" Venomous snakes are so common worldwide (with the exception of the Arctic and some high-altitude locations) that humans have developed evolutionary mechanisms to detect them faster than other stimuli that are less harmful.[1] In the United States, every state has a venomous snake with the exception of Maine, Alaska, and Hawaii.[2] There are two primary families of venomous snakes native to North America: the Elapidae and Crotalidae. The Elapidae family includes coral snakes. The Crotalidae family includes the pit vipers, which are by far the most common cause of snake envenomations in America.[2] Common pit vipers are rattlesnakes, copperheads, and water moccasins. Rattlesnakes, including eastern and western diamondbacks, timber rattlesnakes, pigmy rattlesnakes, and many other species, exist in various parts of the United States. The "pit" in pit viper refers to an organ found under their nose that contains special cells that allows them to detect the heat of their prey.[2] They can also be identified by their retractable front fangs, elliptical pupils, and triangularly shaped heads.[2] Most bites in the United States occur between April and October, with copperheads being responsible for a majority of the bites due to their close proximity to human living spaces. While copperheads may be the most common source of bites, rattlesnakes are responsible for the majority of fatalities. Do not count on a rattle, as, contrary to popular belief, rattlesnakes to not always emit a rattle before striking.[2] Additionally, thanks to events such as Rattlesnake Roundups, rattlesnakes without a rattle are being selected through human intervention. One cannot even count on a snake being decapitated, as the head can bite for up to an hour after removal due to residual reflexes, and this agonal bite can deliver the entire venom load.[2] Snakes do not have more toxic venom during the summer, but they do have increased aggression and venom yield during the hottest months. Venom delivered is controlled by pit vipers, with an offensive bite often delivering more venom than a defensive bite, which are frequently nonenvenomating; hence, "Don't poke the snake."[2]

Many ideas have been proposed for the care of a patient who has been bitten by a snake in the wild. Techniques such as electroshocks, herb concoctions, and cryotherapy have been proposed as methods to inactivate the venom. There are also techniques aimed at trying to remove the venom, which includes suction, incision of the bite wound itself, and irrigation. Last, people have also proposed ways to stop the venom from spreading, such as tourniquets and pressure immobilization.[1] This leads to the question: What is the best way to handle a snakebite, both in the field and in the ED? As more research is published, guidelines have changed and will likely continue to change as the complexity of snake venom is studied further.

Toxicology and Pathophysiology

Snake venom is a complex mixture of chemicals and may contain more than 100 proteins and peptides, both toxic and nontoxic.[3] The protein and non-protein components of the venom cause the toxic effect, having evolved to target specific tissue in the prey, with the aim to immobilize and digest.[3,4] The four main categories of components include enzymes, polypeptides, glycoproteins, and low-molecular-weight compounds.

The enzymes present within the venom "package" are an example of this synergy, with the most common being phospholipase A2, hyaluronidase, collagenase, and metalloproteinase. The most widely studied enzyme is phospholipase A2, as this seems to be present in every family of venomous snake.[4] This enzyme causes damage to red blood cells, peripheral nerve endings, skeletal muscle, and platelets, and it releases histamine, serotonin, and acetylcholine to name a few.[2,4] Hyaluronidase assists with the spread of the venom in tissue by cleaving internal glycoside bonds and mucopolysaccharides and decreasing connective tissue viscosity.[2] Collagenase has a similar breakdown mechanism, with the main result being deeper penetrance and wider spread of the venom.[2] Collagenase and protease present in spitting venom leads to the release of histamine and acetylcholine. Contact with the eye leads to corneal edema, conjunctival inflammation, and uveitis. Thankfully, there has been no evidence of venom spit into the eye passing into systemic circulation.[5] Finally, metalloproteinases cause local tissue destruction and hemorrhage, thought to result from cleaving of the peptide bonds of basement membranes in capillary beds, causing gaps to form which allows extravasation.[5] This action has also been linked to retinal hemorrhages.[5] Secondary to bleeding and reduced perfusion, metalloproteinases also cause myonecrosis and local inflammatory responses.

Crotalidae bites are primarily vasculotoxic, but it is important to note that some species have been found to have neurotoxic venom.[2,4] Specifically, the Mojave, Southern Pacific, and timber rattlesnakes all have been found to cause neurotoxicity. Copperheads cause edema and tissue damage, while cottonmouths cause local tissue necrosis and can cause coagulopathy.[7] Rattlesnakes can also cause local tissue necrosis, angioedema, and anaphylaxis. Hemostatic defects that can occur from envenomation include consumption coagulopathy, vascular damage, disseminate intravascular coagulation-like syndrome, localized clotting, hyperfibrinolysis, thrombocytopenia, and blood vessel injury.[2] Renal failure is the most common presentation prior to death.[4]

Alpha- and beta-neurotoxins are the primary molecules studied in snake neurotoxin. Alpha-neurotoxins act at the motor end plate and bind to acetylcholine receptors, causing flaccid paralysis. Beta-neurotoxins work in conjunction to cause release of acetylcholine at nerve endings and then damage the ending, which blocks any further release of the transmitter.[4] Most neurotoxins bind with high affinity, making reversal of potential paralysis difficult. This toxicity presents as descending paralysis, beginning with ptosis and leading to bulbar and respiratory paralysis.[3] Acetylcholinesterases have been used to sometimes reverse the effects of postsynaptic neurotoxicity. The complexity of snake venom leads to an envenomation syndrome that is a response to metabolizing the individual components of the venom. Those individual components have also been shown to act synergistically.[2] Envenomation from North American Elapidae (coral snakes) will result in minimal local changes, with initial symptoms being nausea, vomiting, abdominal pain, and general malaise. Ptosis will be the initial sign of paralysis, followed closely by descending paralysis leading to respiratory failure and death if not supported and treated.[4]

While the adage "red on black, venom does lack; red on yellow, kills a fellow" can help identify North American coral snakes from nonvenomous snakes that look similar, Elapidae snakes from around the world come in all arrangements of color; therefore, this saying does not help outside of North America. Last, typically Elapidae snakes are associated with neurotoxic venom, however, not all Elapidae snakes in other parts of the world possess neurotoxic properties. Coral snake envenomations are quite rare, and expert consultation should be sought in known or suspected cases. The discussion below focuses primarily on the management of Crotalidae bites.

Workup and Diagnosis

It is important to note that not all snake bites result in envenomation. In fact, 20% of all pit viper bites are dry (non-envenomating).[2] Some people may develop signs of envenomation even with a dry bite due to the high level of anxiety a snakebite provokes.[4] Presentation of a snakebite varies greatly depending on age and size of the patient, the type of snake, and the number of bites, as well as the quantity and toxicity of the venom.[4] Snakes can vary the amount of venom delivered in a strike from none to all venom delivered. This makes care of a patient difficult as there is no way to know ahead of time what type of bite has occurred. Children receive more venom per body size, owing to their small size, and patients with more comorbid conditions will have a higher risk of morbidity and mortality. The size and age of the snake does not factor into the outcome of a patient.[4]

Upon arrival to the ED, airway, breathing, and circulation should be evaluated and treated as needed. Once stabilized from a primary assessment standpoint, patients must be evaluated for local, hematologic, neurologic, and systemic toxicity.[7] Likely the type of snake will not be known, and one must be careful to evaluate for all forms of toxicity. Labs should be obtained to include a complete blood cell count, basic metabolic profile, prothrombin time (PT), activated partial thromboplastin time, fibrinogen, fibrin degradation products, creatine kinase, arterial blood gas (if systemic symptoms), and urinalysis.[4,7] Type and cross-match the patient's blood on arrival, as the effects of both venom and antivenom can affect this later.[4] An ECG should also be obtained. If available, obtain a thromboelastogram (TEG).

Obtain a careful history that includes an attempt to determine that an actual snakebite occurred. Patients should be discouraged from bringing snakes into the ED as Crotalines can cause envenomation even after death. Time elapsed since the bite should be elicited. Obtain a brief medical history, including tetanus status as well as allergies.[4] Physical exam should focus on the bite site for signs of envenomation which include edema, petechiae, bullae, and oozing from the wound. Mark the bite site and measure the circumference of the bitten limb, rechecking every 15 minutes until the swelling has stabilized.[4] A common recommendation is to mark 5 centimeters above and below a major joint and do measurements at the same location each time. Serial negative inspiratory force should be obtained on anyone with concern for possible neurotoxicity. Capnography can also be helpful for early identification of respiratory compromise.[7] Imaging typically is not needed.[7]

To determine appropriate treatment, look for signs of envenomation. If there is rapid extension of swelling in the affected limb or enlargement of local lymph nodes, severe envenomation should be considered. Early systemic symptoms, spontaneous bleeding, and dark urine should also raise concern for severe envenomation.[4] A snakebite severity score is available, but this was intended to be used as a research tool and has not been validated to use clinically. When it has been used clinically it has been shown to result in undertreatment.[7]

Treatment
Antivenom should be administered if there is significant local tissue damage or damage that progresses, if there is hematologic toxicity or systemic toxicity, or if the local edema extends past a major joint. Calling your local poison center (1-800-222-1222) can help determine if the patient you are caring for would benefit from antivenom or not in equivocal cases. If treatment is delayed longer than 6 hours, outcomes are not as good.[7] Currently there are two available antivenoms for pit viper envenomations in the United States: CroFab (FabAV) and ANAVIP (Fab2AV). FabAV is derived from the venom of four snake species (western diamondback, eastern diamondback, Mojave rattlesnake, and cottonmouth) that is immunized into sheep. The immunoglobin is then extracted, purified, and cleaved into the terminal Fab fragment, which allows for better tissue penetration because it is a smaller molecule and carries less antigenicity. The antivenom is cleared renally and may require repeat dosing. It is approved for all envenomations in North America.[6] Initial dosing of FabAV is 4–6 vials, mixed into 250 mL normal saline and given over 1 hour. It is important to note that the dose does not change for children as the treatment is aimed at the venom load and not the patient size. Initially the rate should be 10 mL/hr to observe for adverse reactions. If there are none, then the rate is slowly increased until the entire

dose has been given in 1 hour. If there is progression of symptoms, repeat the 4–6 vial dosing.[6] If control is not obtained after two doses, then consultation with a medical toxicologist or snakebite expert is necessary.[7] After control has been achieved, maintenance dosing consists of 2 vials every 6 hours for 18 hours if the snake was identified as a rattlesnake or the patient had coagulopathy or severe envenomation.[6] If during maintenance dosing there appears to be recurrent swelling, then 4–6 vials should be administered again. After the initial three doses, further maintenance doses may be necessary, but consultation with your local poison center is advisable.

FabAV2 is approved for treatment of rattlesnake bites in North America, but not copperhead and cottonmouth envenomations. FabAV2 is derived from two snake species (*Bothris asper* and *Crotalus duressis*) and immunized in horses; the immunoglobin is then extracted, purified, and cleaved into a fragment that has two binding sites for the venom. (Interestingly, neither snake species used to create this antivenom is native to America. *Bothris asper* is found in Mexico as well as Central and South America and *Crotalus duressis* is found in Brazil.) FabAV2 lasts longer in serum, thus does not require maintenance dosing.[6] The starting dose is 10 vials mixed in 250 mL of normal saline given over 1 hour, followed by 10 more vials if control is not achieved.[6,7]

Very rarely will a snakebite progress to requiring surgical intervention. If there is evidence of increased compartment pressures, the first action is to give more antivenom. If pressures remain consistently elevated, thought can be given to performing a fasciotomy at that time if sufficient antivenom treatment has been given. It is worth noting, however, that prophylactic fasciotomies are never recommended as they will cause more harm than potential benefit. It has been found that the elevated compartment syndrome is caused by the venom, therefore the treatment is to neutralize the venom.[7]

Pre-hospital care has varied throughout the years as far as recommendations from various organizations. First aid in the field has consisted of attempting to suction venom out of the bite site, using tourniquets around the affected limb, and application of ice packs. None of these has any medical benefit and, in fact, can cause harm and should be actively discouraged.[4] Use of a tourniquet can result in venom bolus upon release of the tourniquet. If applied, one must consider releasing it gradually after the initiation of antivenom.[8] Also, due to trapping of tissue-toxic chemicals in the affected limb, necrosis may occur. Electroshocks were once proposed as a viable option for treatment; there is no evidence, either biophysical or biochemical, that stun gun treatment for a snakebite will have any effect on envenomation.[9] This is not a recommended treatment option. There are case reports of people shocking themselves with high-voltage batteries to self-treat their own snake bites. This does nothing for the snake bite but does complicate the care of a now electrocuted individual with burns, trauma, and possible cardiac injury.[9,10] Likewise, cutting the bite site will only lead to further injury, and the snake venom is not amendable to removal by suction. If it is attempted to be sucked out by the victim's or a bystander's mouth, this will only add a bacterial burden, potentially transfer a small amount of venom into the oropharynx, and has not been shown to have any beneficial impact on the snake bite outcome.

Current guidelines recommend reassuring and calming the victim, immobilizing the limb (no tight compression, no tourniquet), and immediate transfer to a hospital.[4] Pressure immobilization has been recommended, which consists of wrapping the affected limb as if it were a sprained ankle. However, studies have shown that this is seldom applied correctly, with no benefit if the limb has been immobilized for more than 10 minutes.[4]

Long-Term Concerns

There is a lack of data following-up snake bite victims long term as most patients are not followed-up after the resolution of their acute symptoms. There have been reports of reduced range of motion in those who do not undergo some form of physical therapy, especially following viperid bites, as well as complex regional pain syndrome and median nerve entrapment syndrome. Chronic local pain and swelling has also been documented, with 6 out of 13 patients after rattlesnake envenomation in California reporting continued pain, numbness, skin peeling, and weakness for up to 12 years after the bite.[11] Rattlesnakes have also been implicated in causing chronic kidney disease.[9] Ultimately, further long-term studies are needed to identify long-term sequelae following envenomation and treatment with antivenom.

CASE CONCLUSION

You quickly identified that the patient brought in after stepping off the trail and feeling a sharp pain was in fact an envenomation by a Crotalidae, likely a rattlesnake given the local area. Recognizing these signs, you quickly ordered FabAV2 because that is what is stocked in your local ED. The patient was monitored closely and his symptoms resolved with one dose. He was able to be discharged from the ED with close follow-up by his family physician.

KEY POINTS TO REMEMBER

- Current first aid for pre-hospital snake bite care involves reassurance of the victim, immobilizing the affected limb (not tight arterial compression), and immediate transfer to a hospital.[4]
- Once envenomation is suspected or confirmed, initiate treatment with antivenom. If no response with two doses, then immediately consult a medical toxicologist or a snakebite expert.[7]
- If a pre-hospital tourniquet was placed, consider the possibility of a venom bolus upon release of the tourniquet, and consider gradually releasing tourniquet after initiation of antivenom.[8]

Further Reading

Bawaskar HS, Bawaska PH, Bawaskar PH. The global burden of snake bite envenoming. *J R Coll Physicians Edinb.* 2021;51(1):7–8. doi:10.4997/JRCPE.2021.102

Benjamin J, Brandehoff N, Wilson B, et al. Joint trauma system clinical practice guideline: global snake envenomation management. *J Spec Oper Med.* 2020;20:43–74.

Langley R, Haskell MG, Hareza D, King K. Fatal and nonfatal snakebite injuries reported in the United States. *South Med J.* 2020;113(10):514–519. doi:10.14423/SMJ.0000000000001156

Lavonas EJ, Burnham RI, Schwarz J, et al. (2020). Recovery from copperhead snake envenomation: role of age, sex, bite location, severity, and treatment. *J Med Toxicol.* 2020;16(1):17–23. https://doi.org/10.1007/s13181-019-00733-y

References
1. Avau B, Borra V, Vandekerckhove P, De Buck E. The treatment of snake bites in a first aid setting: a systematic review. *PLoS Negl Trop Dis.* 2016;10(10):e0005079. doi:10.1371/journal.pntd.0005079

2. Peterson ME. Snake bite: pit vipers. *Clin Tech Small Anim Pract.* 2006;21(4):174–182. doi:10.1053/j.ctsap.2006.10.008

3. Warrell DA. Snake bite [published correction appears in Lancet. 2010 Feb 20;375(9715):640]. *Lancet.* 2010;375(9708):77–88. doi:10.1016/S0140-6736(09)61754-2

4. Ahmed SM, Ahmed M, Nadeem A, Mahajan J, Choudhary A, Pal J. Emergency treatment of a snake bite: pearls from literature. *J Emerg Trauma Shock.* 2008;1(2):97–105. doi:10.4103/0974-2700.43190

5. Chang K-C, Huang Y-K, Chen Y-W, Chen M-H, Tu AT, Chen Y-C. Venom ophthalmia and ocular complications caused by snake venom. *Toxins.* 2020;12(9):576. https://doi.org/10.3390/toxins12090576

6. Patel V, Kong E, Hamilton R. Rattle snake toxicity. StatPearls. 2022. Accessed August 9, 2022. https://www.ncbi.nlm.nih.gov/books/NBK431065/

7. Greene S, Cheng D, Vilke GM, Winkler G. How should native crotalid envenomation be managed in the emergency department? *J Emerg Med.* 2021;61(1):41–48. doi:10.1016/j.jemermed.2021.01.020

8. Bush SP, Kinlaw SB. Management of a pediatric snake envenomation after presentation with a tight tourniquet. *Wilderness Environ Med.* 2015;26(3):355–358. doi:10.1016/j.wem.2015.01.005

9. Davis D, Branch K, Egen NB, Russell FE, Gerrish K, Auerbach PS. The effect of an electrical current on snake venom toxicity. *J Wilderness Med.* Feb 1, 1992;3(1):48–53.

10. Welch EB, Gales BJ. Use of stun guns for venomous bites and stings: a review. *Wilderness Environ Med.* Jun 1, 2001;12(2):111–117.

11. Waiddyanatha S, Silva A, Siribaddana S, Isbister GK. Long-term effects of snake envenoming. *Toxins (Basel).* Mar 31, 2019;11(4):193. doi:10.3390/toxins11040193. PMID: 30935096; PMCID: PMC6521273.

28 You Are Barking Up the Wrong Scorpion: Bark Scorpion Envenomations

Karl Holt and Jonathan de Olano

Case Presentation

A 4-year-old girl near Tucson, Arizona, is brought to the ED complaining of sudden-onset pain to her wrist that began 2 hours ago. Her parents report she has been inconsolable at times, and although she moves her hand, she does not allow them to touch it. She had one episode of emesis at home, and her parents worry she is drooling too much. Both the parents and patient deny recent trauma, prior illness, or known allergies. On exam, there is an area of nonspecific erythema at the left lateral wrist. Copious oral secretions are obvious, and the patient is in a tripod position, but no edema, intraoral lesions, or dyspnea are seen. You observe several isolated instances of muscle twitching, but otherwise her neurologic, pulmonary, and musculoskeletal exams are normal. Vitals are notable for tachycardia at 155 beats/min and systolic blood pressure of 130 mm Hg. After pain medications and labs are ordered, the nurse calls to report the child has increased agitation and salivation, worsening muscle fasciculations, and rapid eye movements.

What Do You Do Now?

DISCUSSION

Background

Epidemiology

Although scorpion stings are the second most common cause of global animal-associated mortality, North American scorpion stings are rarely fatal with appropriate supportive medical care.[1] Southwestern states bear the brunt of scorpion exposures, but eight other states have greater than 100 cases per year that are severe enough to be reported. In the 11 years between 2005 and 2015, 82.7% of the 185,000 cases reported were found in Arizona, Texas, and Nevada, but exposures are routinely reported across the Southern states from Florida to California, predominately in warmer months from May through September.[2] In the United States, the most clinically relevant scorpion is *Centruroides sculpturatus*, otherwise known as the bark scorpion due to its propensity to live close to wooded areas under loose bark and sand rather than burrowing into soil.[3] Nearly 98% of bark scorpion stings occur at or near the victim's residence. With a tan or yellow-colored body, the bark scorpion is further differentiated from other species by curling its tail next to the body rather than straight up. Although relatively small at a maximum length of 5 centimeters, its venom is dispersed from a thin tail with a characteristic subaculear tooth at the end.[1] Children are more likely to have severe complications from envenomations due to a larger venom-to-body-mass ratio. Children younger than 10 represent nearly two-thirds of life-threatening cases, such as respiratory compromise and even respiratory and cardiac arrest, and are the most likely to require hospitalization.[2]

Toxicology and Pharmacology

Venom across all scorpion species is similar in components but differs in clinical manifestations. Many factors can influence the clinical applications victims encounter such as the amount of venom injected, the scorpion's age, its nutritional state, and even the time of year. At the local site of injection, vasodilation occurs allowing further distribution of venom.[4] Like other species, the most dangerous components of bark scorpion venom are neurotoxins.[5] These toxins, comprised of 60–70 amino acids, are highly selective ligands for voltage-gated sodium, potassium, chloride, and calcium ion channels.[6] Not only does this venom act on the sodium channels of excitable cells, but a component known as *a*-toxin acts to inhibit the sodium channel's ability to inhibit its own activity, leading to prolonged sodium current activation.[7] As sodium and calcium flood into excitable cells, they remain in a prolonged excitable state, leading to common clinical manifestations. Repetitive depolarization in the parasympathetic and sympathetic nervous systems results in the exaggerated release of catecholamines and acetylcholine leading to widespread skeletal and smooth muscle contraction. The release of these catecholamines that raise blood pressure, increase oxygen consumption, and elevate heart rate further facilitates venom distribution.

Acetylcholine floods neuromuscular junctions, which produces the characteristic fasciculations seen in bark scorpion sting victims. Indeed, the most severe cases reported in the Southwestern United States involve fasciculations, nystagmus, hypertension, and excessive secretions that can lead to respiratory arrest.[2] The venom itself is toxic to myofibrils, and, because both cholinergic and adrenergic activity increases, a type of "chemical myocarditis" ensues.[7] In some instances, this can lead to acute pulmonary edema and cardiogenic shock.[8] While such extremes are less likely with bark scorpion exposure, they do occur and the clinician should have a low threshold for suspicion and to initiate prompt therapy. The combined effect of an autonomic nervous system in an exaggerated state of hyperactivity and the subsequent arousal of the systemic inflammatory response system (SIRS) conspires to produce the morbidity and mortality observed in those with scorpion exposures.[9]

Workup and Diagnosis

Back to the case: The patient can answer simple questions but is acutely agitated. Obvious rotary nystagmus and involuntary, uncoordinated muscle fasciculations are noted. Along with her work of breathing, both her tachycardia and hypertension are worsening.

What about her presentation should raise suspicion for scorpion envenomation? She complains of focal pain; lives in a region with common scorpion exposures; is becoming more agitated with prominent fasciculations, nystagmus, and hypersalivation; and both her heart rate and blood pressure continue to rise. Which components are most worrisome for a severe case requiring invasive interventions? In multiple studies, the most severe cases routinely involved fasciculations, excessive salivation, hypertension, and rotary nystagmus. In fact, fasciculations and nystagmus are two clinical features unique to bark scorpions compared to other scorpion species prevalent in southern states.[10] But the most acute component of this case is the report of drooling. Bark scorpion envenomations are known to cause involuntary movements of eyes and limbs, but the inability to control oral secretions denotes respiratory distress and impending respiratory failure, specifically in children younger than 10 years, and may be accompanied by acute pulmonary edema.[10]

Airway, breathing, and circulation should be addressed first, but outside of symptom management, the clinician must appreciate the correct insulting agent for adequate resolution. Although scorpionism is the most likely diagnosis, a young patient like this presenting in respiratory distress with hypersalivation and fasciculations should be approached with a broad differential. This includes anaphylaxis, seizures, head trauma, meningitis, tetanus, epiglottitis, and other toxic exposures such as snake or black widow envenomation, organophosphates, serotonin toxicity, and sympathomimetics.

History is a key element when scorpion exposure is suspected. Simply asking if scorpions have been previously seen in the home can influence suspicion as most cases occur in a residence.[11] One study showed 97.8% of cases transpire in a home.[2] Out of those with known exposure, nearly 82% of them had previously seen a scorpion in their home.[10] Such a history coupled with a chief complaint of focal pain elevates suspicion. Pain at the site of potential envenomation is perhaps the most common complaint in nearly 89% of all cases in a recent analysis of more than 185,000 cases during an 11-year period.[2]

The pediatric patient in respiratory distress may have a differential diagnosis including asthma and foreign body ingestion, but when involuntary eye and limb movements are also present, a high degree of suspicion must be placed on scorpion venom, specifically the bark scorpion. Such a patient may require intubation and mechanical ventilation, but, even in the acute phase, it is imperative the provider recognizes this pattern as scorpionism so appropriate treatment may be initiated.

Because hypersalivation has been reported in many cases, organophosphates should also be considered. However, several differentiating hallmarks of organophosphate poisoning should aid providers in ruling in or out this concern. First is the diffuse release of bodily fluids seen with organophosphates including diarrhea, urination, bronchorrhea, and lacrimation, which are not associated with scorpionism. Second, bradycardia is more typical of organophosphate poisoning, whereas scorpion venom causes repetitive axonal firing from activated sodium channels leading to widespread catecholamine release and tachycardia.

An increased cholinergic surge can cause jerking and flailing, but, unlike seizure activity, there is no loss of consciousness or amnesia associated with the abnormal movements involved in scorpion envenomation. Furthermore, the fasciculations seen in scorpionism are completely random and uncoordinated, and patients are conscious of the abnormality.

The hyperactive state observed in scorpionism can also be seen in sympathomimetic intoxication, with tachycardia, tachypnea, and hypertension the most obvious abnormal vital signs observed. However, the sympathomimetic toxidrome is associated with dilated pupils, whereas scorpion venom causes roving and rotary nystagmus and not dilation. However, the similarities between these etiologies have led to several instances of misdiagnosis and even antivenom being inappropriately administered.[12]

Serotonin syndrome should also be considered in any patient who is altered with elevated heart rate and blood pressure, but the widespread involuntary muscular fasciculations in scorpionism is distinguished from the myoclonus observed in the serotonin toxidrome.

Black widow spider bites are an important consideration as they can also present with evidence of adrenergic excess, but the abnormal eye movements and fasciculations seen in scorpion stings are not consistent with widow spider bites. Additionally, there are generally little or no cutaneous signs of a scorpion sting except for complaints of pain, whereas black widow spider bites will produce a characteristic halo lesion at the site.[1]

Important laboratory tests should cover the most likely and most dangerous diagnoses. Electrolytes, blood urea nitrogen, creatinine, creatinine kinase, and liver function tests should be obtained because the constant motor activity can result in rhabdomyolysis, hyperthermia, and end-organ dysfunction. Lipase may be considered if a patient has been stung by *Tityus* or *Leiurus* scorpions because they have been associated with pancreatitis.[13] Imaging may be required if trauma is also a concern.

Treatment

Initial management should focus on maintaining airway, breathing, and circulation. Afterward, secondary measures should focus on pain, agitation, and wound care. Bark scorpion sting victims generally complain of pain, so analgesia should be a top priority. This may be accomplished with oral medications or IV opioids in more severe cases. Fentanyl is ideal because it is not associated with histamine release, is easily titrated, and has a short half-life.[14] Tetanus prophylaxis must be ensured with all patients exposed. Hypersalivation can be treated with atropine, but it is not routinely recommended because it can potentiate cardiopulmonary toxicity. The excessive restlessness and fasciculations should be treated with a rapidly titratable IV benzodiazepine, such as midazolam, and may require high doses.[15] While historically hydralazine and nifedipine have been used,[5] the treatment of severe symptomatic hypertension can be managed with rapidly titratable parenteral options such as nicardipine.

For severe envenomations, specific antivenom is the mainstay of treatment. Research has shown antivenom to be effective and safe. Even in the absence of ICU-level care, antivenom has been proved to reduce the need for transfer.[16] In fact, equine-derived Centruroides-specific F(ab')2 antivenom has shown up to 100% resolution of symptoms within 4 hours of administration without the need for pediatric ICU admission and zero hypersensitivity reactions.[17] The risk of hypersensitivity reactions may be somewhat mitigated by increasing the duration of administration.[18] At the first signs of anaphylaxis, the infusion should be stopped and prompt symptomatic management should include epinephrine, corticosteroids, and diphenhydramine. As with other equine-derived medications, serum sickness may also occur, and patients should be appropriately counseled regarding potential signs and symptoms. Because cholinergic surge is a hallmark feature of scorpionism, antivenom is effective because it neutralizes the venom so it cannot bind to cholinergic receptors.[19] However, the cost of antivenom remains a significant factor. As of August 2022, the cost for one vial was $5,271.[20] The dose is generally 1–3 vials, with the official US Food and Drug Administration (FDA) recommendation being 3 vials. However, recent retrospective studies have evaluated the difference between 1 vial versus the standard 3 vials and concluded there was no clinical difference in outcomes.[21] Out of 141 children who received antivenom, regardless of 1 vial or 3 vials, 100% were asymptomatic within 4 hours and were able to be discharged. This is especially notable in a rural setting where multiple vials may not be available. Cases involving adults receiving antivenom were given 3 vials with complete resolution of symptoms within 1 hour of administration.[22] In less severe cases that do not warrant the cost of antivenom, supportive care and observation is sufficient. Symptoms generally manifest within 4–5 hours, and a period of observation in that timeframe is sufficient.[14]

Long-Term Concerns

There are no long-term complications expected from bark scorpion envenomations.

CASE CONCLUSION

Upon further questioning, the family admits that although an older sibling sustained a scorpion sting in the home several months ago, he had minimal complaints so they had not considered a scorpion could cause such dramatic symptoms. After quickly considering and ruling out other possibilities, her presentation is most consistent with a severe bark scorpion envenomation. You instruct the team to keep her in a position of comfort, to give midazolam due to agitation and fasciculations, and to start nicardipine titrating to her target blood pressure. Meanwhile you place a call to pharmacy to prepare three vials of antivenom for immediate administration. Within 50 minutes, all symptoms appear to be resolved, and she is resting comfortably. After a period of observation, she is finally discharged without further complaint.

Arizona bark scorpion Centruroides sculpturatus. Note the curled tail along with the characteristic subaculear tooth at the end. https://www.inat uralist.org/observations/113420903

Signs and symptoms of acute bark scorpion envenomation.

- Pediatric patients are at high risk for severe toxicity from scorpion stings.
- Bark scorpion venom is a neurotoxin leading to neuroexcitation.
- After emergent stabilization, treatment is largely supportive including tetanus, pain medication, and high doses of titratable benzodiazepines.
- Centruroides-specific antivenom can be administered for severe envenomations.

Further Reading

Boyer LV, Theodorou AA, Berg RA, et al. Antivenom for critically ill children with neurotoxicity from scorpion stings. *N Engl J Med*. 2009;360(20):2090–2098.

Gueron M, Yaron R. Cardiovascular manifestations of severe scorpion sting. clinicopathologic correlations. *Chest*. Feb 1970;57(2):156–162. doi:10.1378/chest.57.2.156. PMID: 5411717

Kang AM, Brooks DE. Geographic distribution of scorpion exposures in the United States, 2010–2015. *Am J Public Health*. 2017;107(12):1958–1963. doi:10.2105/AJPH.2017.304094

References

1. Auerbach PS, Cushing TA, Harris NS. (2017). *Auerbach's Wilderness Medicine*. 7th ed. Elsevier; 2017: 1017–1030.
2. Kang AM, Brooks DE. Nationwide scorpion exposures reported to US Poison Control Centers from 2005 to 2015. *J Med Toxicol*. 2017;13(2):158–165. doi:10.1007/s13181-016-0594-0l'm
3. Klotz SA, Yates S, Smith SL, Dudley S Jr, Schmidt JO, Shirazi FM. Scorpion stings and antivenom use in Arizona. *Am J Med*. 2021;134(8):1034–1038. doi:10.1016/j.amjmed.2021.01.025
4. Weisel-Eichler A, Libersat F. Venom effects on monoaminergic systems. *J Comp Physiol A Neuroethol Sens Neural Behav Physiol*. Sep 2004;190(9):683–690. doi:10.1007/s00359-004-0526-3. Epub May 25, 2004. PMID: 15160282
5. Sofer S, Gueron M. Vasodilators and hypertensive encephalopathy following scorpion envenomation in children. *Chest*. 1990;97(1):118–120. doi:10.1378/chest.97.1.118
6. Tobassum S, Tahir HM, Arshad M, Zahid MT, Ali S, Ahsan MM. Nature and applications of scorpion venom: an overview. *Toxin Reviews*. 2018;39:214–225.

7. Gordon D, Savarin P, Gurevitz M, Zinn-Justin S. Functional anatomy of scorpion toxins affecting sodium channels. *J Toxicol Toxin Rev.* 1998;17(2):131–159. https://doi.org/10.3109/15569549809009247

8. Abroug F, Ouanes-Besbes L, Tilouche N, Elatrous S. Scorpion envenomation: state of the art. *Intensive Care Med.* 2020;46(3):401–410. doi:10.1007/s00134-020-05924-8

9. Reis M, Zoccal K, Gardinassi L, Faccioli L. Scorpion envenomation and inflammation: beyond neurotoxic effects. *Toxicon* 2019;167:174–179. doi.org/10.1016/j.toxicon.2019.06.219

10. Bennett BK, Boesen KJ, Welch SA, Kang AM. Study of factors contributing to scorpion envenomation in Arizona. *J Med Toxicol.* 2019;15(1):30–35. doi:10.1007/s13181-018-0690-4

11. Forrester MB, Stanley SK. Epidemiology of scorpion envenomations in Texas. *Vet Hum Toxicol.* 2004;46(4):219–221.

12. Strommen J, Shirazi F. Methamphetamine ingestion misdiagnosed as Centruroides sculpturatus envenomation. *Case Rep Emerg Med.* 2015;2015:320574. doi:10.1155/2015/320574

13. Albuquerque PLMM, Magalhaes KDN, Sales TC, Paiva JHHGL, Daher EF, da Silva Junior GB. Acute kidney injury and pancreatitis due to scorpion sting: case report and literature review. *Rev Inst Med Trop Sao Paulo.* 2018;60:e30. doi:10.1590/s1678-9946201860030. Epub June 28, 2018. PMID: 29972468; PMCID: PMC6029862

14. Skolnik AB, Ewald MB. Pediatric scorpion envenomation in the United States: morbidity, mortality, and therapeutic innovations. *Pediatr Emerg Care.* 2013;29(1):98–105. doi:10.1097/PEC.0b013e31827b5733

15. Cydulka R, Fitch M, Joing S, Wang V, Cline D, Ma O. *Tintinalli's Emergency Medicine Manual.* 8th ed. McGraw-Hill Education; 2017.

16. Boyer LV, Theodorou AA, Chase PB, et al. Effectiveness of centruroides scorpion antivenom compared to historical controls. *Toxicon.* 2013;76:377–385. doi:10.1016/j.toxicon.2013.07.014

17. Boyer LV, Theodorou AA, Berg RA, et al. Antivenom for critically ill children with neurotoxicity from scorpion stings. *N Engl J Med.* 2009;360(20):2090–2098. doi:10.1056/NEJMoa0808455

18. Everson GW. Scorpions. *Encyclopedia of Toxicology.* 3rd ed. Academic Press 2014: 223–225. doi.org/10.1016/B978-0-12-386454-3.00784-3

19. Vázquez H, Chávez-Haro A, García-Ubbelohde W, et al. Pharmacokinetics of a F(ab')2 scorpion antivenom in healthy human volunteers. *Toxicon.* 2005;46(7):797–805. doi:10.1016/j.toxicon.2005.08.010

20. Drugs.com. Anascorp. Accessed August, 1, 2022. https://www.drugs.com/price-guide/anascorp.

21. Quan D, LoVecchio F, Bhattarai B, Flores M, Frechette A, Sinha M. Comparing clinical outcomes between two scorpion antivenom dosing strategies in children. *Clin Toxicol (Phila)*. 2019;57(9):760–764. doi:10.1080/15563650.2018.1551546
22. Hurst NB, Lipe DN, Karpen SR, et al. Centruroides sculpturatus envenomation in three adult patients requiring treatment with antivenom. *Clin Toxicol (Phila)*. 2018;56(4):294–296. doi:10.1080/15563650.2017.1371310

29 The Shy Widow: Black Widow Envenomations

Matthew Eisenstat

Case Presentation

A 3-year-old boy presents to the ED inconsolably crying. His parents report that he was playing outside 30 minutes prior to arrival. His parents heard crying and found him seated next to a tool shed in the backyard. Since that time, he has been crying constantly and reaching for his right thigh. After taking off his clothes his parents noticed a pair of small lesions surrounded by a circle of skin with red discoloration. You see that the child is crying, but overall appears well-perfused, with good skin color. You examine the child further and notice that there is a small patch of erythema surrounding two "pin-prick" lesions. The area is diaphoretic and the muscles of the anterior thigh are tight and contracted. His abdomen is rigid, although when you palpate his abdomen, he continues to reach for his leg. His heart rate is fast at 140 beats/min. The remainder of his vital signs are within normal limits for his age. The remainder of his exam is normal.

What Do You Do Now?

DISCUSSION

Background

"Black widow" is the colloquial name for spiders of the Latrodectus genus. Latrodectus species are found throughout the United States in all states except Alaska. Latrodectus species are known for their characteristic jet-black body and ventral red markings; however, depending on the specific species (there are five in the United States) and individual molting cycles, markings may differ greatly (Figure 29.1). The female spider has an overall larger body size and fang size, making envenomation in humans far more likely from the females of the Latrodectus species. Latrodectus often inhabit large, irregular webs found in dark areas such as sheds, garages, barns, attics, and basements. They are not aggressive, and most envenomation occurs to upper extremities when a person is reaching into an area where the spider is residing. There are an estimated 2,500 cases of envenomation reported to

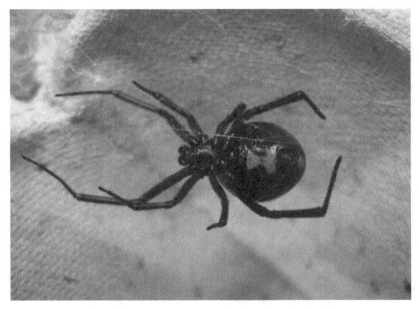

FIGURE 29.1 Typical appearance of a *Latrodectus* species in the United States.

https://commons.wikimedia.org/wiki/File:Adult_Female_Black_Widow.jpg

Author: Shenrich91, License: CC-BY-SA 3.0.

US poison centers each year, though this number likely underrepresents the true incidence as envenomation may be mild, not requiring medical attention, or providers may choose to treat a suspected envenomation without guidance from a local poison center.[1]

The physical bite of the black widow may be mild or unnoticed. The bite site, if visible, will generally only have mild erythema and fang marks and may or may not be obvious. The erythema may have an area of central clearing. Systemic symptoms if present generally occur within an hour. Symptoms include muscle cramping and pain, diaphoresis (local or systemic), abnormal vital signs (tachycardia and hypertension), nausea, vomiting, headache, and altered mental status. Symptoms generally progress proximally from the site of the envenomation, and more systemic involvement indicates more severe envenomation. Rarely, priapism, compartment syndrome, fetal distress in pregnant patients, and myocarditis have been reported in the literature. Few deaths have been reported in modern literature, though it is speculated that children and the elderly would be more at risk for severe outcomes.

Toxicology and Pathophysiology

Latrodectus venom contains seven known components although α-latrotoxin is the only known component to affect humans. The α-latrotoxin binds to neuronal presynaptic receptors, leading to an influx of calcium into the neuron. Calcium influx leads to exocytosis of neurotransmitters including norepinephrine, acetylcholine, gamma-aminobutyric acid (GABA), glutamate, and dopamine. Acetylcholine release leads to neuromuscular activation and thus cramping, pain, or rigidity of musculature. Norepinephrine leads to tachycardia and hypertension. GABA and glutamate can contribute to alterations in mental status. The broad range of symptoms can be explained by the neurotransmitters released and dose of venom delivered.

Workup and Diagnosis

Diagnosis of Latrodectus envenomation is predominately based on history and physical examination. Labs provide little utility in the diagnosis or management of this envenomation. If obtained, labs may indicate a nonspecific leukocytosis, elevated creatine kinase, and/or elevated lactate dehydrogenase. Imaging is not warranted in the evaluation of envenomation unless the diagnosis is unclear and other etiologies need to be excluded. For example, in cases of a suspected Latrodectus envenomation to the abdomen, alternative etiologies such as appendicitis, cholecystitis, or ovarian/uterine pathology may need to be ruled out with the preferred imaging method.

Treatment

As with any emergency, airway, breathing, and circulation take priority although life-threatening presentations are rare. Basic wound care is warranted, and tetanus prophylaxis should be updated. Wound debridement is generally not required as Latrodectus bites are not typically as destructive to local tissue as is the case in other arthropod envenomation, such as that of a brown recluse spider. Antibiotics are not needed prophylactically.

Pain management and supportive care are the mainstay of treatment. Mild envenomation can generally be treated with ice packs, NSAIDs, and/or acetaminophen. More severe envenomation may require IV opioids for pain and/or IV benzodiazepines for muscle cramping. Pain control should only be required for the initial duration of symptoms. After initial control of symptoms, oral opioids or benzodiazepines should not be needed as an outpatient.

Antivenom is available for Latrodectus envenomation. The current antivenom is an equine serum-derived whole immunoglobulin. Availability of antivenom is highly dependent on local practices and hospital purchasing. Regional poison centers may be able to assist with locating and acquiring antivenom if deemed appropriate. As with other equine-derived whole immunoglobulin antivenom products there is a considerable risk of anaphylaxis as well as serum sickness. Anaphylaxis generally would be seen immediately following antivenom administration and serum sickness associated with antivenoms occurs 5–10 days following administration. In case series, Latrodectus antivenom has been shown to shorten symptom duration and intensity. Indications for administration of antivenom include failure of supportive care (pain control), hypertensive emergency, priapism, or pregnancy with evidence of fetal distress. There has been one case of compartment syndrome associated with Latrodectus treated with antivenom alone; however this is not standard of care. Given that Latrodectus envenomation is rarely life-threatening, the use of the current whole immunoglobulin antivenom should be restricted to severe cases unless a practitioner familiar with the antidote is at bedside or under the explicit direction of a regional poison control center. Based on small retrospective studies, adverse events appear to be small (>10%); however, there have been two reported deaths attributed to antivenom reactions in the literature and no reported modern deaths attributed to envenomation in the United States. In one of those two cases, the antivenom was administered improperly with subsequent anaphylaxis and cardiac arrest.[2] In the other case, an individual with a history of asthma required resuscitation for severe anaphylaxis and died days later likely from complications of the resuscitation and severe illness.[3,4] A thorough history of previous allergies, atopy, and asthma should be obtained prior to administering immunoglobulin antivenom. Skin testing has been suggested by some prior to administration of antivenom. An urticarial wheal reaction after skin testing would theoretically indicate a patient is at risk for anaphylaxis. However, skin testing prior to antivenom administration has largely fallen out of favor. Studies of snake antivenom have shown little utility of skin testing, and medical decision-making and antivenom administration would be delayed as a result of skin testing.[5,6] The World Health Organization (WHO) recommends against skin testing prior to antivenom administration for snake envenomation. While the same evidence does not exist for Latrodectus antivenom, it can be inferred that spider antivenom skin testing would also lack usefulness. Anaphylaxis to antivenom is generally a reaction to animal protein or immunoglobulin components that would be the same throughout all antivenoms derived from that particular animal (equine, in this case). Therefore, it is safe to assume that spider antivenoms would likely show the same problems with skin testing.

While not currently commercially available $F(ab')_2$ Latrodectus antivenom has been developed and a randomized controlled trial (RCT) associated with a Phase 3 trial appeared to reduce the number of treatment failures though it failed to reach statistical difference.[7] In that trial, no adverse events occurred; however, the study was not powered to look for such events. Previous RCTs and experience with F(ab) redback (Latrodectus species) antivenom in Australia has been mixed in terms of pain reduction and resolution of systemic symptoms. Though it is likely based on experience with snake antivenom that F(ab) antivenoms that these newer products would have lower adverse event rates, efficacy for pain reduction and reduction of systemic symptoms has yet to be proved.

Previously used therapies such as calcium gluconate and dantrolene have not been shown to be effective in reducing pain or morbidity. These therapies should not be used for any envenomation.

Elevated blood pressure and tachycardia should generally not be treated with beta-blockers, calcium channel blockers, etc. If hypertensive emergency is suspected this would be a potential indication for antivenom, although this would more likely be an indication for more adequate pain control. If hypotension develops fluids and/or vasopressor agents would be indicated per provider preference. Dysrhythmias should be treated with standard advanced cardiac life support.

If anaphylaxis should occur following antivenom administration standard, anaphylaxis therapy such as epinephrine, antihistamines, H_2 blockers, and steroids should be used at the treating physicians' discretion.

Long-Term Concerns

There are little to any long-term concerns regarding Latrodectus envenomation. Patients appropriately treated with supportive care generally recover within 24–48 hours. Wound care for bites is generally minimal and should not require specialist care. If patients are given immunoglobulin antivenom they should be warned to look for symptoms of serum sickness (joint pain, rash, fever) 5–10 days following administration of antivenom.

CASE CONCLUSION

Your colleague initially presents the patient with concern for appendicitis and suggests imaging. Considering the acute onset of symptoms, and as an astute clinician, you recognize a syndrome consistent with Latrodectus envenomation. Despite several doses of opioid analgesia and ice packs to the site, the patient remains crying and in moderate distress. A dose of lorazepam calms him somewhat, and he is admitted overnight for pain control. He is discharged the next day in good condition.

- The bite site of a Latrodectus species may be mild or invisible to the eye.
- Systemic symptoms should be treated with supportive care.
- Abdominal rigidity can mimic a surgical abdomen.
- Failure of supportive care, hypertensive emergencies, pregnant patients with fetal distress, and priapism should be considered indications for the use of antivenom.

Further Reading

Repplinger DJ, Hahn I. Arthropods. In: Nelson LS, Howland M, Lewin NA, Smith SW, Goldfrank LR, Hoffman RS, eds. *Goldfrank's Toxicologic Emergencies.* 11th ed. McGraw Hill; 2019. Accessed March 16, 2022. https://accessem ergencymedicine.mhmedical.com/content.aspx?bookid=2569&sectionid= 210276505

Schneir A, Clark RF. Bites and stings. In: Tintinalli JE, Ma O, Yealy DM, Meckler GD, Stapczynski J, Cline DM, Thomas SH, eds. *Tintinalli's Emergency Medicine: A Comprehensive Study Guide.* 9th ed. McGraw Hill; 2020. Accessed March 16, 2022. https://demo-preview.mhmedical.com/content.aspx?bookid=2353&sectio nid=220746649

Walls RM, Hockberger RS, Gausche-Hill M. *Rosen's Emergency Medicine: Concepts and Clinical Practice.* 9th ed. Elsevier; 2018. Accessed March 16, 2022. https:// search-ebscohost-com.echo.louisville.edu/login.aspx?direct=true&db=cat073 99a&AN=ulh.ocn989157341&site=eds-live

References

1. Offerman S. The treatment of black widow spider envenomation with antivenin Latrodectus mactans: a case series. *Perm J.* 2011;15(3). doi:10.7812/tpp/10-136

2. Murphy CM, Hong JJ, Beuhler MC. Anaphylaxis with latrodectus antivenin resulting in cardiac arrest. *J Med Toxicol.* 2011;7(4):317–321. doi:10.1007/ s13181-011-0183-1

3. Clark RF. The safety and efficacy of antiven in latrodectus mactans. *J Toxicol: Clin Toxicol.* 2001;39(2):125–127. doi:10.1081/clt-100103827

4. Nordt SP, Clark RF, Lee A, Berk K, Lee Cantrell F. Examination of adverse events following black widow antivenom use in California. *Clin Toxicol.* 2011;50(1):70–73. doi:10.3109/15563650.2011.639714

5. Rojnuckarin P. Antivenom skin test: theory versus practice. *Acta Tropica.* 2009;109(1):86. doi:10.1016/j.actatropica.2008.09.004

6. Thiansookon A, Rojnuckarin P. Low incidence of early reactions to horse-derived F(ab')2 antivenom for snakebites in Thailand. *Acta Tropica*. 2008;105(2):203–205. doi:10.1016/j.actatropica.2007.09.007

7. Dart RC, Bush SP, Heard K, et al. The efficacy of antivenin latrodectus (black widow) equine immune F(ab')2 versus placebo in the treatment of latrodectism: a randomized, double-blind, placebo-controlled, clinical trial. *Ann Emerg Med*. Sep 2019;74(3):439–449. doi:10.1016/j.annemergmed.2019.02.007. Epub 2019 Mar 27. PMID: 30926190

30 Don't Get Washed Away in the Red Tide: Shellfish and Seafood-Related Toxins

Alyka Glor P. Fernandez and
Melissa H. Gittinger

Case Presentation

A 29-year-old man with a past medical history of seasonal allergies presents to the ED with a chief complaint of paresthesias, nausea, vomiting, and diarrhea that started shortly after dining at a sushi restaurant. He states that he was at an *omakase* dinner, which is multicourse meal in which every course is selected by the chef based on seasonality of ingredients. This *omakase* had 18 courses consisting of several types of fish and shellfish. His wife, who dined with him, also has complaints of paresthesia as well as a headache. The patient denies any history of food allergies. He denies any recent illnesses, including fevers or chills. On physical exam, an ill-appearing man is sitting up in bed with an emesis bag in hand. His vital signs are notable for tachycardia and mild tachypnea. He has no visible rashes, but he complains of numbness and tingling to his lips and tongue. His abdomen is soft and minimally tender in the epigastric region. He has signs of normal perfusion and normal mentation.

What Do You Do Now?

DISCUSSION

Background

In this patient presenting with GI and neurological symptoms shortly after consumption of seafood, the differential diagnosis should include illnesses caused by seafood-related toxins.

Seafood poisoning results from the ingestion of fish and shellfish that contain toxic substances. The incidence of seafood-related toxicity is unknown largely due to under-recognition and under-reporting. Coastal communities and travelers who consume seafood in the tropics and subtropics are at a heightened risk due to the geographic distribution of seafood-borne toxins. However, due to the globalization of seafood markets, clinicians in all parts of the world must be vigilant about marine toxins causing illnesses.

This chapter focuses on seafood toxins that are most often ingested as well as with those that are rarely encountered but can be lethal.

Toxicology and Pathophysiology

Shellfish Poisoning

While viral and bacterial causes such as *Vibrio* spp. have been associated with illness after shellfish ingestion, toxic shellfish poisoning causes illness due to the ingestion of shellfish contaminated with various toxins. There are several types of shellfish poisoning including paralytic, neurotoxic, diarrheic, and amnesic. Toxicity is not intrinsic to the shellfish themselves, but rather exogenous due to ingested dinoflagellates that produce toxins which ultimately lead to human toxicity. Dinoflagellates are one-celled aquatic organisms that can be the dominant members of phytoplankton (Table 30.1). They are particularly proliferative during the warm months of May through August.[1] These harmful algal blooms, which can last for a few weeks, have also been referred to as "the red tide" due to their ability to change the color of water.

Ciguatera Fish Poisoning

Ciguatera is endemic throughout tropical and subtropical regions of the IndoPacific and Caribbean regions. It is most prevalent from 35 degrees north (Georgia–North Carolina border) to 35 degrees south (just south of

TABLE 30.1 Overview of shellfish and seafood-related toxins

	Paralytic	Neurotoxic	Amnesic	Diarrheic
Geography	Most common in temperate waters: Pacific and Atlantic Coasts of North America The Philippines China Chile Scotland Ireland New Zealand Australia	Cases have been reported in: West coast of Florida North Carolina New Zealand	Only one human outbreak in Canada in 1987	Occurs worldwide
Toxin	Saxitoxin: Blocks entry of sodium into voltage-gated sodium channels Disrupts nerve conduction[4]	Brevetoxin: Enhances sodium entry into voltage-gated sodium channels leading to a neuroexcitatory effect[2]	Domoic acid: Acts similar to the neurotransmitter glutamic acid[4]	Okadaic acid: Inhibits serine/threonine protein phosphatases Disrupts intracellular processes Causes severe mucosal damage in the intestinal tract[3]
Associated marine organisms	Bivalve shellfish (i.e., mussels, oysters, clams)	Filter-feeding shellfish (i.e., clams, oysters, whelks, mussels, conch, coquinas)	Bivalve shellfish, crabs, and lobsters	Crabs, bivalve mollusks, especially blue mussels

Onset of symptoms	Within 30 minutes to 4 hours of ingestion			
Clinical effects	Mild cases present with paresthesia, dizziness, weakness, and ataxia. These patients recover within 2–3 days. Severe cases present with rapid onset of paralysis and acute respiratory failure. Death can occur within 12 hours.	Mild GI symptoms. Neurological effects, including paresthesia, dizziness, and ataxia.	Patients initially presented with GI symptoms. Within 48 hours, they developed unusual neurological symptoms: headaches, confusion, memory loss, seizures, and coma. Some patients had cardiovascular effects.	Patients present with abdominal pain, nausea, vomiting, diarrhea, headaches, and chills. Symptoms should resolve within 72 hours.
Management	Close observation, supportive care, and symptomatic treatment.			

Adelaide, Australia) in the months of May through August due to warmer water temperatures allowing the dinoflagellates to proliferate. The Pacific ciguatoxin-1 is 10 times more toxic than the more commonly encountered Caribbean ciguatoxin.[4] Ciguatera fish poisoning occurs due to ingestion of ciguatoxins, which accumulate in certain finfish. Marine dinoflagellates produce gambiertoxins, which are the precursors of ciguatoxins.[5] Fish that are herbivores feed on these organisms. Carnivorous fish then eat the smaller herbivores, which leads bioaccumulation of ciguatoxins to levels potentially toxic in humans who consume larger fish. Larger reef fish are the most common fish consumed by humans that may contain harmful levels of ciguatoxins (Box 30.1).

Ciguatoxin is a heat-stable toxin, which means that there is no type of preparation or cooking that can deactivate the toxin. Ciguatoxin activates voltage-sensitive sodium channels, which causes a hyperpolarization of the voltage dependence of the channel resulting in the sodium channels opening at resting membrane potentials, which leads to spontaneous firing of neurons.[4]

Ingestion of ciguatoxin can cause GI illness, neurological symptoms, and cardiovascular effects. GI illness can present as nausea, vomiting, diarrhea, and abdominal cramping. Neurological symptoms include diffuse myalgias and arthralgias, paresthesia, headache, dizziness, and cold allodynia. Paresthesia have been described as abnormal temperature sensation, loss of pinprick and vibration, and diminished light touch. Cold

---

BOX 30.1 Fish associated with ciguatera poisoning

Red bass
Snapper
Sea bass
Grouper
Cod
Mackerel
Tunas
Jacks
Barracuda
Moray eels

---

allodynia is the feeling of a burning sensation when touching a cold object, also referred to as "hot–cold temperature reversal." Cardiovascular effects are rare, but can include bradycardia, heart block, and hypotension. The onset of symptoms can range from within 1 hour of ingestion to up to 48 hours afterward.

Tetrodotoxin

Tetrodotoxin poisoning is the most common lethal marine poisoning, but the rates of death have decreased in recent years due to efforts to regulate the preparation and marketing of puffer fish.[4] While the puffer fish is the most well-known harbor of tetrodotoxin, other species have been found to contain this poison, such as triggerfish, horseshoe crabs, and certain species of octopus, as well as several species of salamander and flatworms (Box 30.2). In pufferfish, the highest concentration of the toxin is found in the liver, ovary, intestines, and skin.

Tetrodotoxin is a heat stable toxin. It binds to voltage-gated sodium channels in muscles and nerve tissues, which blocks the flow of ions through the channel.[5] Thus, it acts by preventing action potential generation and impulse conduction.

Symptoms develop rapidly and can be severe, with the most rapidly reported death occurring within 17 minutes of ingestion.[6] It has been observed that the severity of symptoms depends on the amount of toxin ingested. For mild poisoning, patients develop perioral and distal limb paresthesia, with others experiencing nausea and vomiting. These minor cases can resolve after a few hours. In those with moderate severity poisoning, weakness of the distal, bulbar, and facial muscles can precede dizziness, ataxia, and incoordination, which typically occur within 90 minutes. Patients with severe

---

BOX 30.2 **Fish associated with tetrodotoxin poisoning**

Puffer fish
Trigger fish
Horseshoe crabs
Certain species of octopi

---

poisoning can present with flaccid paralysis and respiratory failure but are fully conscious because tetrodotoxin does not lead to CNS depression. Life-threatening poisoning will feature devastating cardiovascular effects of bradycardia, hypotension, and dysrhythmia. If managed appropriately, minor cases can resolve within a few hours, but moderate to severe cases can take up to 5 days for full resolution of symptoms.[4]

Scombroid

Scombroid poisoning is not due to a toxic ingestion. Rather, it is due to mishandling and improper storage of seafood at the initial point of refrigeration after capture.[4] Gram-negative bacteria, such as *Escherichia coli*, *Morganella morganii*, *Pseudomonas aeruginosa*, and *Klebsiella* spp., convert histidine, normally found in dark fish meat, into histamine (Box 30.3).[7]

The accumulation of histamine during spoilage of the fish leads to consumption of a large amount of histamine. Thus, scombroid poisoning presents similarly to an allergic reaction. Symptoms can develop within 10 minutes to 2 hours of consumption. Patients can present with a rash, flushing, nausea, vomiting, diarrhea, abdominal pain, headache, dizziness, palpitations, perioral numbness, metallic taste, and respiratory distress.[1]

BOX 30.3 **Fish associated with scombroid poisoning**

Scombroid family
Tuna
Mackerel
Skipjack
Bonita
Suary
Seerfish
Bluefish
Mahi-Mahi
Herring
Sardines
Anchovies

From Ghafouri and Cantrell.

Palytoxin

Palytoxin and its analogs are potent marine toxins with high biological activity even at very low concentrations. It is a heat-stable toxin, so cooking will not inactivate the toxin. Additionally, it is stable in neutral solutions, but its toxicity is lost quickly under acidic and alkaline solutions. It acts through blockage of the Na^+/K^+-ATPase channel, which leads to a massive influx of Ca^{2+} that interferes with cell function and can lead to cell death.[8]

Palytoxin can affect several organ systems through ingestion, inhalation, and dermal contact. Poisoning from palytoxin has gained more attention due to the increasing popularity of keeping home aquariums as a hobby.[9] Handling of zoanthid corals while cleaning leads to aerosolization of the toxin, which has caused cases of respiratory illness in the aquarium hobbyist and those in the immediate vicinity.

Clupeotoxism is a poorly understood toxidrome that is now thought to be associated with consumption of palytoxin-containing clupeid fish.[10] Several symptoms are associated with palytoxin poisoning, including a bitter/metallic taste, abdominal cramps, nausea, vomiting, diarrhea, and paresthesia. The most reported complication is rhabdomyolysis, with severe cases leading to renal failure and disseminated intravascular coagulation (Box 30.4). Patients who present with cyanosis and respiratory distress are also at increased risk of fatal complications.[9]

BOX 30.4 **Marine life associated with palytoxin poisoning**

Xanthid crabs[10]
Demania reynaudii
Lophozozymus pictor
Demania alcalai
Clupeid fish[8]
Sardines
Herring
Anchovy
Epinephelus spp., a type of grouper
Scarus ovifrons, a blue humphead parrotfish
Zoanthid spp.[9]
Coral (i.e., *Palythoa toxica*)
Dinoflagellates (i.e., *Ostreopsis ovata*)

Workup and Diagnosis

The diagnosis of seafood-related toxicity relies on the clinical history, physical exam, and timing of ingestion. It is important for clinicians to keep marine toxins at the forefront of their mind when developing a differential diagnosis, especially when practicing in endemic areas. No specific tests to diagnose patients poisoned with these toxins are available in a clinically relevant timeframe.

Treatment

Treatment of marine-related poisoning is primarily supportive, with therapies directed at patients' specific symptoms. The toxins discussed in this chapter have no known antidotes. Mild symptoms resolve quickly, with GI illnesses requiring only vigilant hydration and treatment with antiemetics as needed. In more severe cases involving respiratory failure, airway management with intubation and mechanical ventilation may be required (Table 30.2).

Long-Term Concerns

Suspected cases of consumption of marine-borne food toxins should be immediately reported to public health authorities to prompt an investigation

TABLE 30.2 **Toxicology of marine organisms and treatment protocols**

Tetrodotoxin	Ciguatera	Scombroid	Palytoxin
Severe poisoning can be treated with gastric lavage depending upon the time of consumption and onset of illness.[11]	A controversial treatment previously suggested is the use of IV mannitol. However, a double-blind, randomized, controlled research study found no difference between the administration of mannitol and normal saline.[4]	Antihistamines are the agent of choice with H_1 antagonists and H_2 blockers. Epinephrine may be necessary in patients with respiratory distress, but corticosteroids are not indicated. In patients with hypotension, IV fluids may be given.[1]	Inhalation of palytoxin can lead to wheezing, which can be treated with nebulized albuterol. Patients presenting with hypoxia will require supplemental oxygen titrated to their needs.[9]

and limit further outbreaks of illness. Specifically, the local health department and the CDC can be notified by calling 1-800-232-4636. Patients should be advised to keep notes on what they ate and keep receipts from stores and restaurants to aid with reporting.

CASE CONCLUSION

The astute clinician recognized the importance of considering seafood toxins as the cause of this patient's illness. Given the patient is presenting with perioral paresthesia, the differential diagnosis includes tetrodotoxin poisoning and ciguatera toxin ingestion. On review of symptoms, the patient denied any symptoms of dizziness, ataxia, or other neurological symptoms. Thus, if his symptoms were due to the ingestion of tetrodotoxin and ciguatera, this would be a mild case. A quick phone call to the sushi restaurant confirmed that no puffer fish was served because their chef does not have the license required to prepare it. He also did not consume any clupeid fish that would alert the clinician to include palytoxin poisoning as a part of the differential diagnosis. However, tuna and mackerel were both served to the patient. He also ate oysters, blue mussels, and prawns. The patient's symptoms of vomiting and diarrhea can be due to diarrheic shellfish poisoning. Taken together, his presentation is mild with no electrolyte derangements. Ultimately, treatment required only IV antiemetics and fluid hydration. After a short period of observation and improvement in his vital signs and symptoms, he was discharged home with strict return precautions.

KEY POINTS TO REMEMBER

- Consider seafood poisoning as a cause of GI illness, especially when accompanied by neurological symptoms.
- Diagnosis relies on obtaining a thorough history.
- Treatment of seafood-related toxicity is largely supportive.
- Report foodborne illnesses to the local public health authorities to prevent further outbreaks.

References

1. Ghafouri N, Cantrell FL. Shellfish poisoning, paralytic. In: *Encyclopedia of Toxicology*. 2014:252–253. doi:10.1016/b978-0-12-386454-3.00785-5. Elsevier Inc https://www.sciencedirect.com/science/article/abs/pii/B9780123864543007855

2. Abraham A, Flewelling LJ, El Said KR, et al. An occurrence of neurotoxic shellfish poisoning by consumption of gastropods contaminated with brevetoxins. *Toxicon*. 2020;191:9–17. doi:10.1016/j.toxicon.2020.12.010

3. Corriere M, Soliño L, Costa PR. Effects of the marine biotoxins okadaic acid and Dinophysistoxins on fish. *J Mar Sci Eng*. 2021;9(3):293. doi:10.3390/jmse9030293

4. Isbister GK, Kiernan MC. Neurotoxic marine poisoning. *Lancet Neurol*. 2005;4(4):219–228. doi:10.1016/s1474-4422(05)70041-7

5. Özogul F, Hamed I. Marine-based toxins and their health risk. In: *Food Quality: Balancing Health and Disease*. 2018:109–144. doi:10.1016/b978-0-12-811442-1.00003-1. Academic Press https://www.sciencedirect.com/science/article/abs/pii/B9780128114421000031?via%3Dihub

6. Shoff W., Shepherd S. Scombroid, ciguatera, and other seafood intoxications. In: Ford MD, Delaney KA, Ling LJ, Erickson T, editors. *Clinical Toxicology*. Taylor & Francis: W.B. Saunders Company; 2001:959–968.

7. Hungerford JM. Scombroid poisoning: a review. *Toxicon*. 2010;56(2):231–243. doi:10.1016/j.toxicon.2010.02.006

8. Ramos V, Vasconcelos V. Palytoxin and analogs: biological and ecological effects. *Marine Drugs*. 2010;8(7):2021–2037. doi:10.3390/md8072021

9. Hall C, Levy D, Sattler S. A case of palytoxin poisoning in a home aquarium enthusiast and his family. *Case Rep Emerg Med*. 2015;2015:1–3. doi:10.1155/2015/621815

10. Deeds JR, Schwartz MD. Human risk associated with palytoxin exposure. *Toxicon*. 2009;56(2):150–162. doi:10.1016/j.toxicon.2009.05.035

11. Yang C-C. Tetrodotoxin. In: *Critical Care Toxicology*. 2017:2085–2099. doi:10.1007/978-3-319-17900-1_39

31 Acetylcholine Overload: Organophosphate and Carbamate Exposures

Luis Espinoza and Joshua da Silva

Case Presentation

You are working at a small hospital in rural Ohio when a 43-year-old man presents to the hospital complaining of difficulty breathing, profuse sweating, rhinorrhea, vomiting, and salivation. He also complains of abdominal cramps and states he has had multiple episodes of nonbloody diarrhea over the past couple of hours. He quickly becomes lightheaded and somnolent. His vital signs are heart rate 78 beats/min, respiratory rate 36 breaths/min, blood pressure 96/50 mm Hg, and SpO_2 88% on room air. The patient's wife states he is a farmer and applied insecticide to his crops about an hour prior to coming into the hospital. Auscultation of chest reveals coarse breath sounds, a regular heart rate, and no evidence of a murmur. ECG shows a QTc of 500 ms. Over the course of the next hour and a half, his respiratory status worsens, and he becomes progressively bradycardic.

What Do You Do Now?

DISCUSSION

The patient in this scenario is exhibiting cholinergic toxicity from orga-nophosphate poisoning, a syndrome characterized by a constellation of symptoms with varied clinical presentation highlighting the importance of a thorough history and physical exam. On a cellular level organophosphates block acetylcholinesterase (AChE) from metabolizing acetylcholine (ACh), leading to an excess of ACh and resulting in hazardous nicotinic and mus-carinic responses. Causes of drug-induced cholinergic crisis are carbamate acetylcholinesterase inhibitors (AChE-Is), which are used as treatment for myasthenia gravis as well as general anesthetic neuromuscular blocking agents and as insecticides, or organophosphorus AChE-I agents, which are used as pesticides and as the nerve agent class of chemical weapons of war.

Background

Pesticides and insecticides cause roughly 3 million poisonings and approx-imately 250,000 deaths worldwide every year.[1] Examples of these agents include organophosphates (malathion, parathion, famphur, and chlorpyr-ifos) and carbamates (carbofuran, aldicarb, carbaryl). They are commonly used in flea and tick powders, shampoos, sprays, and flea collars. They are also used commonly as garden and farm insecticides. These compounds are fat-soluble and are easily absorbed through the skin. As a result, accidental toxicities are common.[1,2]

These substances also have a well-documented history as agents of chem-ical warfare. One such agent is a nerve gas called sarin, made famous by terrorist attacks in Japan and Syria. On March 20, 1995, sarin was used by members of the Aum Shinrikyo cult to attack three Tokyo subway lines, causing more than 5,600 victims to report to the hospital in the hours fol-lowing the attack, 600 by ambulance and another 5,000 by private trans-portation.[3] During the Syrian Civil War in August 2013, sarin was also employed in Ghouta, causing anywhere from 300 to 1,800 fatalities with thousands of others critically injured.[4,5]

Toxicology and Pathophysiology

Muscarinic receptors are G-coupled protein receptors that almost ex-clusively work on the parasympathetic nervous system (except for sweat glands, which act on the sympathetic nervous system). There are five muscarinic receptor subtypes (M_1–M_5) which are activated by ACh, causing ligand bonding and leading to secondary messenger activation. M_2 and M_4 produce an inhibitory response and the remaining three are excitatory. These muscarinic receptors are found in the cerebral cortex, hippocampus, SA node, heart atria, pupils, detrusor muscle of the bladder, bronchi/airway smooth muscle, GI tract, blood vessels, and throughout the CNS.[1,6]

On the other hand, nicotinic receptors are chemically controlled (or ligand-gated) sodium channels that are found at skeletal neuromuscular junctions, autonomic ganglia, and the peripheral and central nervous systems.[7] A conformational change occurs in the nicotinic receptor when it is bound by ACh, causing an influx of positively charged sodium ions that triggers membrane depolarization. As a result of this nicotinic stimulation, the following reactions can be elicited: fasciculations, myotonic jerks, weakness, paralysis via stimulation of skeletal muscles at the neuromuscular junction, hypertension, mydriasis, diaphoresis, vomiting, hypersalivation, and other secretory processes due to activation at the central and peripheral nervous systems.[1,2,7]

ACh overload is driven by lack of AChE activity because AChE is a synaptic enzyme that breaks down synaptic ACh. With properly functioning AChE, the ACh breakdown byproducts are reabsorbed by the presynaptic neuron and recycled. AChE-Is effectively prevent AChE from hydrolyzing ACh, thereby leading to excessive muscarinic and nicotinic receptor stimulation. Muscarinic postsynaptic stimulation involves secretory glands and smooth muscles and causes a constellation of symptoms that includes miosis, bronchospasm, bronchorrhea, abdominal cramping, nausea, emesis, diarrhea, rhinorrhea, lacrimation, salivation, diaphoresis, and urination.[1–3,6] Nicotinic postsynaptic stimulation involves skeletal muscle and leads to muscle contractions, fasciculations, weakness, and flaccid paralysis. Centrally, this leads to neuronal overstimulation and seizures.[2,7] The combination of muscarinic and nicotinic overstimulation as well as excess acetylcholine in the CNS causes drowsiness, confusion, lightheadedness, headaches, delirium, and eventually leads to coma or even death.[2,4–6]

A mnemonic for remembering the muscarinic effects of ACh overload is DUMBBELLS:

D—Diaphoresis/diarrhea

U—Urination

M—Miosis

B—Bronchorrhea/Bronchoconstriction

B—Blurred vision/Bradycardia

E—Emesis

L—Laxation

L—Lacrimation

S—Salivation/Sialorrhea

A mnemonic for remembering the nicotinic effects of ACh overload uses the days of the week:

M—Muscle cramps/Mydriasis

T—Tachycardia

W—Weakness

tH—Hypertension

F—Fasciculations

S—Seizures

It is important to note that carbamates and organophosphate insecticides are not one and the same. While mechanistically similar, carbamates cause a carbamylation of AChE that is reversible, whereas organophosphates bind irreversibly via phosphorylation of AChE.[8] Carbamates can have a similar toxidrome, but duration is typically shorter than 36 hours due to the reversibility of the carbamylation. Despite their differences, lethal side effects, particularly bronchorrhea and bronchospasm, are present in both and should be treated promptly.[8]

Treatments for these side effects are aimed at controlling deadly side effects rather than acting as true reversal agents. Atropine competitively blocks the effects of ACh, thereby reducing secretions in the mouth and airway, reversing bronchoconstriction and bronchospasm, and increasing heart rate. Because it does not bind to nicotinic receptors in the neuromuscular junction, it will not improve muscle weakness, fasciculations, tremors, or paralysis, and it will not prevent seizures.[1,2,5]

The other medication used, pralidoxime (2-PAM), works to reactivate nicotinic AChEs by attaching to their anionic site near the bound organophosphate. This prompts the organophosphate to detach from the AChE enzyme and phosphorylate the 2-PAM with a higher affinity.[1,2,5] There is a time window within which 2-PAM must be administered for it to be effective. This is because the organophosphate molecules will eventually form an irreversible bond with AChE, a phenomenon known as "aging." Each agent has a different aging half-life, from only a few minutes after exposure to roughly 48 hours.[1,2] As a result, it is generally recommended that 2-PAM be administered as soon as possible, and definitively within 48 hours of a true organophosphate exposure.

Workup and Diagnosis

In suspected organophosphate exposures, obtaining a detailed history and performing a physical exam are extremely important since these features can overlap with numerous other toxidromes, such as the sympathomimetic toxidrome. Additionally, asking about exposures, occupation, medication history, allergies, and other components of the history can further delineate the presenting toxidrome and narrow down the differential diagnosis.

The presentation of an ACh overload/cholinergic crisis will inevitably vary from person to person, and is very dependent on which receptors are affected, the type of exposure, the nature of the offending agent, the amount and duration of exposure, the age of the patient (this can affect whether there is a predominantly muscarinic or nicotinic response), and the route of exposure (oral ingestion, inhalation, skin absorption). As discussed, ACh targets muscarinic and nicotinic receptors, with differing symptomatology between receptor activation. In the vignette, the patient was exhibiting muscarinic (blurred vision, diaphoresis, diarrhea, salivation), nicotinic (fasciculations [muscle "twitches"]), and CNS (restlessness, lightheadedness) effects.

The nicotinic effects of ACh overload include muscular fasciculations, fatigue, weakness, respiratory muscle weakness (tachypnea initially and then bradypnea), tachycardia (bradycardia is a later symptom), and hypertension. CNS effects include lightheadedness, dizziness, restlessness, anxiety/agitation, dysarthria, ataxia, confusion, delirium, seizures, coma, and death.[1,2,5,7] Often, there is a combination of nicotinic, muscarinic, and CNS effects.

Laboratory investigations include a complete blood count (establish a baseline, associated infections), comprehensive metabolic panel (electrolyte derangements and assess end-organ damage), ECG (observing the QTc and monitoring for ventricular arrhythmias), and chest X-ray (aspiration). If presenting with altered mentation, seizure, or mental status depression, a head CT scan without IV contrast is an important next step. A red blood cell cholinesterase activity level may also be obtained if capabilities exist, with a low value strongly indicating a likely diagnosis of a cholinergic toxidrome.[9] Despite the low levels of AChE in acute poisonings, chronic exposure to organophosphates or carbamates also leads to lower AChE levels. Patients gradually develop symptoms if the levels become low enough. Mildly symptomatic patients who continue to have exposures will eventually be hospitalized for ACh overload, mimicking symptoms in those hospitalized for acute toxicity.[1,2] Do not delay treatment for laboratory testing because results may not be available for several days. The diagnosis is mainly clinical, and the above-discussed red blood cell cholinesterase and AChE levels are almost always send-out labs that will not result in a clinically actionable timeframe.[9]

Treatment

Upon arrival in the ED, stabilization of the airway, breathing, and circulation is critical. Ensure that the patient is responsive and breathing spontaneously. Alarm signs and symptoms include secretions that might compromise the airway, a Glasgow Coma Scale of 8 or less, and hemodynamic instability.[1-5] It is vital that healthcare professionals don personal protective equipment during the initial resuscitation—including gloves, gowns, masks, and face shields—and always avoid dermal and inhalational contact. Aggressive decontamination should be done as soon as possible, which entails removing clothing, jewelry, and other objects that may have been exposed to the insecticide/pesticide because the offending agent can still be absorbed through the skin. Additionally, the skin and eyes should be washed and irrigated, respectively, to prevent continued absorption of the offending agent. Regardless of symptom severity, all patients should be decontaminated.[1-5] If the patient arrives and is not critical, care should start with thorough decontamination. After decontamination and ensuring the airway is secure, focus should be on prompt administration of cholinergic antidotes, especially if the patient exhibits the "Killer B's" (bronchospasm, bronchorrhea, and bradycardia), which are cited as the main cause of death in patients with ACh overload.[1-3,5] Atropine is a competitive inhibitor of ACh at muscarinic receptors and works to temporize dangerous toxic effects of ACh overload. The goal of atropine is not to treat bradycardia but to dry secretions that could compromise the airway and lead to cardiopulmonary arrest. Because atropine crosses the blood–brain barrier, it will also target CNS postsynaptic ACh receptors, alleviating extrapyramidal symptoms such as restlessness, agitation, and other CNS symptoms. However, fasciculations, muscular or respiratory weakness, seizures, and other nicotinic symptoms will not be affected by atropine because atropine has no effect on nicotinic receptors.[1-3,5,8] The recommended dose of intravenous atropine is 2–5 mg in adults and 0.05 mg/kg in children, with a doubling of the dose every 5 minutes until bronchorrhea/bronchospasm improve.[1,2]

Patients with organophosphate poisoning will normally require large amounts of atropine. As a result, the pharmacy should be made aware ahead of time of the need for extra supplies of atropine. Typically, less atropine is needed for nerve agents as these mainly target nicotinic receptors, which atropine does not affect. Glycopyrrolate can be used for continued treatment of secretions, as well as anticholinergic eye drops if nothing else is available.[1,2] Treatment of nicotinic symptoms is focused on salvaging AChE that has been inactivated by organophosphates using a class of medications called "oximes." These compounds include 2-PAM and obidoxime, with 2-PAM being more readily available in the United States. 2-PAM works on AChE by dissociating organophosphate molecules and regenerating AChE, thereby restoring ACh metabolism. The goal of 2-PAM is improvement in muscular or respiratory weakness and resolution of muscle fasciculations.[1,2,5,8] An important caveat with administration of 2-PAM is that no more than three injections should be given as an initial dose due to toxicity at higher doses. CNS effects, such as agitation and seizures, are treated with seizure precautions and benzodiazepines, mainly diazepam. While any benzodiazepine or GABAergic agent will help with seizures, antiepileptic medications that are sodium channel blockers are to be avoided.[1,2] Both a toxicologist and an intensivist should be consulted immediately when the diagnosis of cholinergic crisis is suspected or confirmed.

On February 5, 2003, the US Food and Drug Administration approved pyridostigmine bromide as a "pretreatment" for nerve gas poisoning, particularly for use by US military personnel with potential exposure to these agents. Pyridostigmine is a reversible carbamate AChE inhibitor that has been used since 1955 in the treatment of myasthenia gravis. Several studies were conducted and showed that administration of pyridostigmine prior to exposure to soman—the AChE-I with the shortest half-life (only 5 minutes)—coupled with post-exposure treatment with atropine and 2-PAM effectively increased survival.[10] US military troops facing the threat of exposure to soman are to take pyridostigmine every 8 hours prior to the expected soman exposure. The hypothesis is that some AChE-Is are shielded from soman because they will be bound to pyridostigmine, preventing all the AChE-Is from undergoing rapid aging and increasing the time 2-PAM can be administered. This pretreatment with pyridostigmine has been considered for farmers, agriculturalists, and other people who face possible exposure to these harmful agents.[10]

The mortality rate in organophosphate toxicity is anywhere from 3% to 25%. Cardiac arrest and death are typically secondary to respiratory failure, which overwhelmingly occurs due to the "killer B's" previously described. Despite being extremely uncommon, other causes of death to note include sepsis resulting from aspiration pneumonia (bronchorrhea/excessive sialorrhea/bronchospasm refractory to both atropine and 2-PAM) shock, arrhythmias, status epilepticus, and severe electrolyte losses from the copious secretions and diarrhea. Some studies have shown that as many as 40% of patients require mechanical ventilation, with a mean hospitalization of 7 days for those who survive long enough to be discharged from the hospital.[1,2,5,8]

Long-Term Concerns

Long-term prognosis for those who recover is generally good, especially if the exposure was of short duration. However, repeated or prolonged exposures can cause effects on long-term memory, concentration, coordination, respiration, vision, and the GI and cardiovascular systems (manifesting as arrhythmias, labile blood pressures, hypertension). Three notable long-term syndromes have been well-documented in the literature: Intermediate Syndrome (IS), Gulf War Illness (GWI), and organophosphate-induced delayed polyneuropathy (OPIDP).

IS manifests as delayed neurological symptoms beginning 24–96 hours following exposure and lasting anywhere from 2 to 40 days. Symptoms include neck flexor weakness and cranial nerve palsies and can lead to mechanical ventilation due to respiratory muscle involvement. Unfortunately, 2-PAM, atropine, and other ACh overload antidotes have not been shown to be effective treatments for IS, and management is mainly supportive.[11]

GWI refers to symptoms experienced by tens of thousands of US military personnel who were deployed to the Kuwaiti Theater of Operations for a 6-week assignment. After returning home, these personnel developed insomnia, diarrhea or constipation, extremity paresthesias and numbness, fatigue, word-finding difficulty, memory impairment, ataxia, difficulty with balance, vertigo, and nonspecific severe physical symptoms such as stomach cramping and myalgias.[12] The cause was thought to be prolonged exposure to low levels of organophosphates. Scientists eventually concluded that the Q isoensyme of the paraoxonase-1 (PON1) gene was at play insofar as those with lower levels of this gene had decreased ability to hydrolyze substrate molecules within the organophosphates. Ultimately, the neurocognitive and somatic long-term side effects seen were likened to those experienced by survivors of the Japan sarin attacks of 1994–1995.[12] As with IS, treatment of GWI is mainly symptomatic and supportive, with symptoms lasting into the present day for many of those affected.

Last, OPIDP is an extremely rare syndrome seen with single or short-term exposures. Symptoms begin 1–4 weeks after exposure and include lower extremity cramping, paresthesias, and complete loss of sensation after which patients may develop progressive ascending weakness, dampened deep tendon reflexes in the lower extremities, and, in very rare cases, weakened deep tendon reflexes and sensory changes of the upper extremities.[13] What starts out as bilateral foot drop can progress to complete quadriplegia in severe cases. Recovery of peripheral nerve function is highly dependent on the degree of pyramidal involvement, with severe cases having spastic ataxia permanently. Pediatric patients have been shown to have a much better prognosis than older adults. Treatment is symptomatic. Physical and occupational therapy are mainstays in recovery of peripheral nerve function and conditioning. Though the name OPIDP implies that organophosphates are the sole causative agents, this syndrome has also been seen after exposures to triaryl phosphates used as hydraulic fluids and lubricants.[13]

CASE CONCLUSION

The patient discussed in this case was promptly decontaminated. Afterwards, he was treated symptomatically with a couple of liters of lactated ringers for hypotension presumed to be from his fluid losses as well as oxygen via BiPAP for his hypoxia and worsening respiratory status. Ultimately, he was admitted to the ICU for a presumptive cholinergic toxicity, where he was started on atropine and 2-PAM. Chest X-ray also revealed an aspiration pneumonia. Over the course of the next two days, his hypersecretory status improved significantly and his supplemental oxygen was weaned to 4L via nasal cannula. On the third day of his ICU stay he was transferred out to the med-surg floor due to clinical and hemodynamic improvement. Over the next four days he was treated with antibiotics for his aspiration pneumonia and was weaned off oxygen altogether. He was discharged in stable condition on day seven of his hospitalization.

KEY POINTS TO REMEMBER

- A large portion of the insecticide/pesticide poisoning population includes farmers and people who live in rural areas who present with accidental overexposures. However, always consider nonaccidental exposures.
- Obtaining a detailed history and physical examination are key to delineating the presenting toxidrome; early decontamination should be started on every patient regardless of symptom severity, and treatment should be initiated with atropine and 2-PAM if organophosphate/carbamate exposure is suspected.
- These patients often require monitoring in the ICU, and upward of 40% will potentially require intubation, with the average length of hospitalization being 5–9 days for those who survive long enough for extubation and discharge.
- Long-term effects are seen in repeated overexposures, so preventive measures, including proper work apparel and face masks, are essential in preventing further poisonings.

References

1. Hulse EJ, Haslam JD, Emmett SR, Woolley T. Organophosphorus nerve agent poisoning: managing the poisoned patient. *Br J Anaesth*. 2019;123(4):457–463. doi:10.1016/j.bja.2019.04.061

2. Eddleston M, Buckley NA, Eyer P, Dawson AH. Management of acute organophosphorus pesticide poisoning. *Lancet*. 2008;371(9612):597–607. doi:10.1016/S0140-6736 (07) 61202-1

3. Okumura T, Takasu N, Ishimatsu S, et al. Report on 640 victims of the Tokyo subway sarin attack. *Ann Emerg Med*. 1996;28(2):129–135. doi:10.1016/s0196-0644 (96) 70052-5

4. Rosman Y, Eisenkraft A, Milk N, et al. Lessons learned from the Syrian sarin attack: evaluation of a clinical syndrome through social media. *Ann Intern Med*. 2014;160(9):644–648. doi:10.7326/M13-2799

5. Reddy DS, Colman E. A comparative toxidrome analysis of human organophosphate and nerve agent poisonings using social media. *Clin Transl Sci*. 2017;10(3):225–230. doi:10.1111/cts.12435

6. Haga T. Molecular properties of muscarinic acetylcholine receptors. *Proc Jpn Acad Ser B Phys Biol Sci*. 2013;89(6):226–256. doi:10.2183/pjab.89.226

7. Hogg RC, Raggenbass M, Bertrand D. Nicotinic acetylcholine receptors: from structure to brain function. *Rev Physiol Biochem Pharmacol*. 2003;147:1–46. doi:10.1007/s10254-003-0005-1. Epub 2003 Mar 20. PMID: 12783266

8. King AM, Aaron CK. Organophosphate and carbamate poisoning. *Emerg Med Clin North Am*. 2015;33(1):133–151. doi:10.1016/j.emc.2014.09.010

9. Lutovac M, Popova OV, Jovanovic Z, et al. Management, diagnostic and prognostic significance of acetylcholinesterase as a biomarker of the toxic effects of pesticides in people occupationally exposed. *Open Access Maced J Med Sci*. 2017;5(7):1021–1027. doi:10.3889/oamjms.2017.200

10. Layish I, Krivoy A, Rotman E, Finkelstein A, Tashma Z, Yehezkelli Y. Pharmacologic prophylaxis against nerve agent poisoning. *Isr Med Assoc J*. 2005;7(3):182–187.

11. Ralston SA, Murray BP, Vela-Duarte D, Orjuela KD, Pastula DM. Neuroterrorism preparedness for the neurohospitalist. *Neurohospitalist*. 2018;9.

12. Haley RW, Kramer G, Xiao J, Dever JA, Teiber JF. Evaluation of a gene–environment interaction of PON1 and low-level nerve agent exposure with Gulf War illness: a prevalence case–control study drawn from the US military health survey's national population sample. *Environ Health Perspect*. May 11, 2022;130(5):057001.

13. Lotti M, Moretto A. Organophosphate-induced delayed polyneuropathy. *Toxicol Rev*. 2005;24(1):37–49. doi:10.2165/00139709-200524010-00003

32 Redox Cycling Out of Control: Herbicide Ingestions

Nicholas Titelbaum

Case Presentation

A 21-year-old man with unknown past medical history presents to the ED by EMS with a chief complaint of seizures at home after applying a weed killer in the field behind his house. On arrival to the ED, he has another seizure. Initial vital signs are heart rate 116 beats/min, blood pressure 163/102 mm Hg, respiratory rate 20 breaths/min, temperature 96.8°F/36.0°C, SpO_2 95% on room air. You find him to be confused and somnolent and notice blue stains on his fingers and earlobe. Initial bloodwork is notable for pH 7.0, pCO_2 36 mmHg, HCO_3- 18 mEq/L, blood urea nitrogen 88 mg/dL, and creatinine 14.3 mg/dL.

What Do You Do Now?

DISCUSSION

Background

The patient in this clinical vignette presents with seizures, respiratory acidosis, and acute renal failure in the setting of exposure to a herbicide. The term "herbicide" is used to refer to any xenobiotic that impairs plant growth. The first chemical herbicide, 2,4-dichlorphenoxyacetic acid (2,4-D) was developed in the 1940s during World War II. Since that time, hundreds of herbicides have been developed and now constitute a multibillion-dollar industry. In 2012, herbicides made up 58% of the US pesticide market and 44% of the world pesticide market, with four of the five most widely used pesticides being the herbicides glyphosate, atrazine, metolachlor-S, and 2,4-D.[1]

Herbicides work to restrict plant growth through a variety of mechanisms including amino acid inhibition, photosynthesis inhibition, growth regulation, and cell division inhibition.[2] Given the variety of mechanisms by which herbicides work, many commercial products contain combinations of herbicides. The human toxicities for each herbicide are highly variable and different from the effects they have on plants. The geographic incidence of individual herbicide poisoning largely depends on their availability. Organizations such as the Environmental Protection Agency (EPA) have enacted measures to regulate and restrict the use of some of the more dangerous herbicides, including paraquat. Therefore, poisonings and deaths from the more widely available glyphosate have increased as those from paraquat have decreased.

The 2020 Annual Report of the American Association of Poison Control Centers' National Poison Data System (NPDS) noted more than 75,000 human exposures to pesticides, although the data for herbicides specifically was not available in the report.[3] Herbicide exposure accounted for 17 of the 26 deaths attributed to pesticides, with all identifiable herbicide-related deaths due to exposure to glyphosate, paraquat, diquat, or dinitrophenol (DNP). Additionally, accidental ingestions of herbicides placed in secondary containers such as water or soft drink bottles have been associated with relatively high morbidity and mortality.[4] Due to the wide variety of herbicides that are capable of producing toxicity, we will restrict our discussion to some of the most toxic and most widely available substances: paraquat, diquat, and glyphosate.

Toxicology and Pathophysiology

Paraquat and Diquat

Paraquat (1,1'-dimethyl-4,4'bipyridinium) and diquat (1,1'-ethylene-2,2'-bipyridyldiylium) are both nonselective contact pesticides, harming all plants they contact.[5] The human lethal dose (LD50) of paraquat is 3–5 mg/kg, or approximately 10–15 mL of a 20% solution.[6] The overall mortality rate of paraquat poisoning is 50–90% but approaches 100% when considering cases of intentional self-poisoning with concentrated formulations.[7,8]. Acute paraquat toxicity in humans typically follows ingestion. However, people can also be exposed to paraquat via inhalation and dermal absorption. Farmworkers may be particularly vulnerable to toxic effects from dermal absorption.[9,10] Less data are available regarding diquat poisoning compared with paraquat.

Both paraquat and diquat are irritating and corrosive. They generate free radicals that cause oxidative damage to cellular lipid membranes, leading to cellular injury and death.[11,12] Once inside cells, paraquat and diquat undergo redox cycling, alternating between reduced and oxidized states, and generate reactive oxygen species which leads to cytotoxicity.[13,14] Redox cycling continues so long as nicotinamide adenine dinucleotide phosphate (NADPH) and oxygen are available. In large exposures, NADPH and protective enzymes such as glutathione, superoxide dismutase, and catalase may be depleted or overwhelmed.[15] The resultant cell death leads to an influx of macrophages and neutrophils, contributing to an inflammatory response that over several days may lead to fibrosis and destruction of normal organ tissue structure.[16] Paraquat and diquat are not metabolized and primarily undergo renal excretion.[17] Renal injury is common in poisoning and may prolong the toxic effects.[18]

Lung injury represents the most lethal and most difficult to treat effect of paraquat toxicity. Pneumocytes selectively accumulate paraquat, and the resultant tissue damage can lead to pulmonary edema, acute respiratory distress syndrome (ARDS), and pulmonary fibrosis.[19] Pulmonary fibrosis usually develops 7–14 days after ingestion and is the most common cause of death from paraquat toxicity.[20]

Paraquat can cause GI irritation resulting in nausea, vomiting, and pain in the mouth and abdomen. Damage to the oral mucosa can cause pseudodiphtheria and ulcers.[21] Esophageal injury can result in rupture, pneumomediastinum, mediastinitis, and pneumothorax.[22] Acute kidney injury may be seen 5 days after ingestion and typically resolves in 3 weeks among those who survive paraquat poisoning.[23] Other effects related to end-organ damage include myocardial necrosis, cardiovascular collapse, liver injury, pancreatitis, hemolytic anemia, cerebral edema, and skeletal muscle necrosis.[12,24]

Although uncommon, paraquat can also cause neurotoxicity, which may be manifested as seizures, altered mental status, cerebral edema, and neuronal injury. The precise mechanism is unknown, but several proposed mechanisms include anoxia, free radical damage, and induction of apoptosis.[12,25]

In contrast to paraquat, diquat does not as readily accumulate in the pneumocytes, and ARDS is less severe if it develops. Neurotoxicity is more prominent with diquat poisoning compared with paraquat. Patients may have mood changes including increased confusion, irritability, disorientation, and combativeness as well as diminished reflexes and seizures.[2,26] Diquat can cause acute kidney injury, GI damage, and end-organ damage otherwise similar to paraquat.

Glyphosate

As of 2012, glyphosate was the most widely used herbicide and pesticide in the United States.[1] Glyphosate is a nonselective postemergence herbicide that can kill plants that have already sprouted. In humans, glyphosate is an irritant of the GI tract. However, glyphosate itself is thought to be minimally toxic, with surfactant coformulants likely the more toxic component of glyphosate herbicides.[27,28] In the majority of acute exposures, patients may experience nausea, vomiting, diarrhea, and/or diarrhea. In more severe cases, patients may develop GI hemorrhage, multiorgan failure with hypotension, cardiac dysrhythmias, ARDS, renal and hepatic injury, pancreatitis, hyperkalemia, metabolic acidosis, encephalopathy, and seizures.[29–32] Symptoms may progress to refractory shock, respiratory failure, and death.

Workup and Diagnosis

The diagnosis of herbicide poisoning relies on taking a detailed history and maintaining a high index of suspicion because herbicide poisonings are infrequent in many areas. Important considerations include the type of herbicide, the amount and route of exposure, the timing of exposure, and the patient's symptoms. To determine which herbicide xenobiotics a patient was exposed to, it is essential to identify both the exact brand and the formulation, as many brands produce several distinct herbicide formulations.

Paraquat and Diquat

Quantitative tests for paraquat and diquat are not immediately available. A urinary dithionite test is a simple and rapid method for evaluating for paraquat or diquat poisoning. Several protocols have been described for performing this test, with one calling for the addition of 2 g sodium bicarbonate and 1 g sodium dithionite to 10 mL of urine and another performed by adding 10 mL of urine to 2 mL of a freshly mixed 1% sodium dithionite solution in 1 M sodium hydroxide.[19,33] A color change to blue or green confirms ingestion of paraquat or diquat, respectively. When the urinary dithionite test is performed within 24 hours of paraquat exposure, the intensity of the color may provide prognostic value: a clear to light blue result indicates a paraquat concentration of less than 1 mg/L and is predictive of survival, while a navy to dark blue result represents a paraquat concentration greater than 1 mg/L and is suggestive of a fatal outcome.[12] A plasma dithionite test performed by adding 200 mcL of 1% sodium dithionite in a 2 M sodium hydroxide solution to 2 mL of the patient's plasma has also been described, with a positive test associated with 100% mortality and a negative or equivocal test with 68% survival rate.[34]

If a quantitative plasma paraquat level can be obtained in a patient exposed at a known time, several nomograms and a Severity Index of Paraquat Poisoning (SIPP) score can be used to predict survival.[35-37] The SIPP score is calculated by multiplying the plasma paraquat concentration (mg/L) by the time since ingestion (hours), with a score lower than 10 predictive of survival, 10–50 predictive of death from respiratory failure, and greater than 50 suggestive of death from circulatory failure.[37]

Other important tests in the evaluation of a patient with concern for paraquat or diquat poisoning include serial testing of blood gas, complete blood count, electrolytes, kidney function, liver function, lipase, ECG, and chest X-ray. The rate of creatinine concentration increase is another prognostic indicator, with an increase of less than 0.03 mg/dL/h over 5 hours predictive of survival and of greater than 0.05 mg/dL/h over 12 hours predictive of death.[38,39]

High-resolution CT of the lungs should also be obtained, with several studies showing that a greater amount and persistence of ground-glass opacities correlated with higher likelihood of death.[40,41] CT findings may progress over several days to pulmonary fibrosis, pleural effusion, and consolidation.

Glyphosate

The diagnosis of glyphosate poisoning is made by a thorough history and clinical findings consistent with glyphosate exposure. Quantitative glyphosate testing is not widely available. Useful laboratory testing in the evaluation of such patients includes blood gas, chemistry with particular attention to the potassium level, kidney function, liver function, lipase, ECG, and chest X-ray. As glyphosate is corrosive to the GI tract, an endoscopy can be considered to assess for injury, but the risk of perforation should be considered.[42]

Treatment

The general management for all herbicide poisonings involves standard assessment and management of airway, breathing, and circulation with supportive care as indicated. Nausea, vomiting, and diarrhea are common findings after many herbicide ingestions and should be treated with IV fluids and antiemetics. Patients with dermal exposures should be decontaminated by irrigation with soap and water along with removal and safe disposal of potentially contaminated clothing and apparel. If there are no concerns for airway compromise, oral activated charcoal can be considered. All patients presenting after acute herbicide ingestion should be observed for at least 6 hours, and people presenting after intentional ingestions or with GI symptoms should be observed for at least 24 hours.[11]

Paraquat and Diquat

Given the severity of paraquat ingestions, many treatment modalities have been utilized, but efficacy data are poor. Palliative care should be strongly considered in cases of paraquat ingestions with strongly positive urinary dithionite tests, hemodynamic instability, or worsening lung injury.[8,11]

An adsorbent should be administered as quickly as possible to patients presenting after ingestion of paraquat or diquat if the airway is protected. Activated charcoal, Fuller's earth, and bentonite are all equally effective, but activated charcoal is the most widely available.[43]

The administration of oxygen may increase the redox cycling caused by paraquat and diquat and thereby worsen pulmonary toxicity. Therefore, supplemental oxygen should only be administered if the patient has severe hypoxia and should be targeted toward maintaining the minimum tolerable oxygenation status, usually an oxygen saturation of 88–92%. Intubation and ventilatory support may be required.

IV fluids should be administered to minimize acute kidney injury and augment the renal clearance of paraquat and diquat. If renal failure occurs, IV fluids should be stopped and hemodialysis should be considered. Hemodialysis and hemoperfusion are both able to remove paraquat and diquat, but their utility in reducing mortality is likely limited for several reasons. Endogenous clearance of paraquat is quick, with most eliminated within 6–12 hours. Therefore, unless initiated soon after ingestion, enhanced elimination is unlikely to hasten removal. Additionally, paraquat distributes to the lungs rapidly, and a dog model demonstrated hemoperfusion was only effective at reducing lung exposure if initiated within 2 hours postingestion.[8,44] Paraquat fatality rates are comparable at facilities that routinely utilize hemoperfusion or hemodialysis compared to those that do not.[45–47] Similarly, limited reports of extracorporeal membrane oxygenation (ECMO) in severe paraquat toxicity did not prevent mortality.[48,49] There is a report of ECMO being used as a bridge to lung transplantation, but there is high mortality for patients who receive lung transplantation after paraquat poisoning.[50–52].

A variety of antidotes attempting to impair the pathways resulting in paraquat and diquat toxicity have been investigated, but none has been proved to reduce mortality in humans.[19,53–55] At this time, there is insufficient evidence to recommend their routine administration. These antidotes may be administered upon the recommendation of a medical toxicologist on a case-by-case basis.

Diquat toxicity is understudied compared with paraquat toxicity. In general, management should be similar to that of paraquat poisoning.[56] Diquat-related seizures should be managed similarly to all toxicant-induced seizures, with benzodiazepines or barbiturates as first-line treatments.

Glyphosate

The management of glyphosate poisoning is primarily standard supportive measures as outlined at the beginning of this section. If patients develop acute kidney injury, hemodialysis can be considered. ECMO may be helpful in cases of severe glyphosate toxicity with respiratory or cardiovascular failure. There is no known antidote.

Long-Term Concerns

Among survivors, paraquat-induced pulmonary fibrosis may resolve gradually over months to years.[57] Additional long-term effects of paraquat poisoning include renal failure, heart failure, and esophageal strictures.[58]

Glyphosate's potential for carcinogenicity is controversial. In 2015, the International Agency for Research on Cancer (IARC) classified glyphosate as "probably carcinogenic to humans."[59] However, the EPA determined it to not likely be carcinogenic in humans in 2017 and reaffirmed its decision in 2020.[60,61]

CASE CONCLUSION

The patient underwent hemodialysis followed by continuous renal replacement therapy with slight improvement of his kidney function. He also developed elevated serum transaminase levels and was treated with N-acetylcysteine. After 2 weeks in the hospital, he was discharged with arrangements made for long-term hemodialysis.

$$H_3C-N^+=\!\!\!\langle\rangle\!\!-\!\!\langle\rangle\!\!=N^+-CH_3$$
$$Cl^- \qquad\qquad Cl^-$$

Paraquat.
(Author: Calvero. Public domain. https://commons.wikimedia.org/wiki/File:Paraquat.svg)

Diquat. (Author: Dschanz. Public domain. https://commons.wikimedia.org/wiki/File:Diquat_dibromide.svg)

Glyphosate. (Author: Yikrazuul. Public domain. https://commons.wikimedia.org/wiki/File:Glyphosate.svg)

KEY POINTS TO REMEMBER

- The term "herbicide" refers to hundreds of xenobiotics with a wide range of toxicity in humans. When assessing a patient with concern for herbicide poisoning, an effort should be made to identify both the brand and formulation.
- Both paraquat and diquat poisoning result in redox cycling, with the generation of free radicals contributing to multiorgan injury.
- Paraquat preferentially accumulates in the lungs, and pulmonary effects are a prominent feature of paraquat toxicity. Diquat poisoning is more characterized by neurotoxicity.
- Glyphosate is the most commonly used herbicide and pesticide in the United States. Toxicity is thought to primarily be a result of the surfactant it is formulated with.
- The mainstay of management for most herbicide poisonings is standard supportive care. However, oxygen should only be used for severe hypoxia following paraquat or diquat exposure because oxygen may worsen redox cycling.

Further Reading

Center for Disease Control and Prevention. Facts about paraquat. 2018. Accessed
     March 4, 2022 https://emergency.cdc.gov/agent/paraquat/basics/facts.asp.
Fortenberry GZ, Beckman J, Schwartz A, et al. Magnitude and characteristics of
     acute paraquat- and diquat-related illnesses in the US: 1998–2013. *Environ Res.*
     2016;146:191–199. doi:10.1016/j.envres.2016.01.003
Magalhães N, Carvalho F, Dinis-Oliveira RJ. Human and experimental toxicology of
     diquat poisoning: toxicokinetics, mechanisms of toxicity, clinical features, and
     treatment. *Hum Exp Toxicol.* 2018;37(11):1131–1160. doi:10.1177/0960327118765330
Singh S, Kumar V, Gill JPK, et al. Herbicide glyphosate: toxicity and microbial
     degradation. *Int J Environ Res Public Health.* 2020;17(20):7519. doi:10.3390/
     ijerph17207519

References

1. Atwood D, Paisley-Jones C. 2017. *Pesticides Industry Sales and Usage 2008–2012
   Market Estimates.* U.S. Environmental Protection Agency. Accessed March 4,
   2022. https://www.epa.gov/sites/default/files/2017-01/documents/pesticides-indus
   try-sales-usage-2016_0.pdf.

2. Todd B, Suter II G. *Causal Analysis/Diagnosis Decision Information System
   (CADDIS) Volume 2: Herbicides.* U.S. Environmental Protection Agency. 2017.
   Accessed 4 March 2022. https://www.epa.gov/caddis-vol2/caddis-volume-2-sour
   ces-stressors-responses-herbicides.

3. Gummin DD, Mowry JB, Beuhler MC, et al. 2020 Annual report of the
   American Association of Poison Control Centers' National Poison Data System
   (NPDS): 38th annual report. *Clin Toxicol.* 2021;59(12):1282–1501. doi:10.1080/
   15563650.2021.1989785.

4. Carpenter JE, Murray BP, Moran TP, Dunkley CA, Layer MR, Geller RJ. Poisonings
   due to storage in a secondary container reported to the National Poison
   Data System, 2007–2017. *Clin Toxicol (Phila).* 2021;59(6):521–527. doi:10.1080/
   15563650.2020.1833026

5. Fortenberry GZ, Beckman J, Schwartz A, et al. Magnitude and characteristics of
   acute paraquat- and diquat-related illnesses in the US: 1998–2013. *Environ Res.*
   2016;146:191–199. doi:10.1016/j.envres.2016.01.003

6. Giulivi C, Lavagno CC, Lucesoli F, Bermúdez MJ, Boveris A. Lung damage in
   paraquat poisoning and hyperbaric oxygen exposure: superoxide-mediated
   inhibition of phospholipase A2. Free Radic Biol Med. 1995;18(2):203–213.
   doi:10.1016/0891-5849(94)00111-v

7. Delirrad M, Majidi M, Boushehri B. Clinical features and prognosis of paraquat
   poisoning: a review of 41 cases. *Int J Clin Exp Med.* 2015;8(5):8122–8128.

8. Gawarammana IB, Buckley NA. Medical management of paraquat ingestion. *Br J
   Clin Pharmacol.* 2011;72(5):745–757. doi:10.1111/j.1365-2125.2011.04026.x

9. Lee K, Park EK, Stoecklin-Marois M, et al. Occupational paraquat exposure of agricultural workers in large Costa Rican farms. *Int Arch Occup Environ Health*. 2009;82(4):455–462. doi:10.1007/s00420-008-0356-7

10. Levin PJ, Klaff LJ, Rose AG, Ferguson AD. Pulmonary effects of contact exposure to paraquat: a clinical and experimental study. *Thorax*. 1979;34(2):150–160. doi:10.1136/thx.34.2.150

11. Robert, D. Herbicides. In: LS Nelson, MA Howland, NA Lewin, SW Smith, LR Goldfrank and RS Hoffman, eds., *Goldfrank's Toxicologic Emergencies*. 11th ed. McGraw-Hill Education; 2019:1466–1485.

12. Reigart JR, Roberts JR, eds. Paraquat and diquat. In: *Recognition and Management of Pesticide Poisonings*, 6th ed. U.S. Environmental Protection Agency; 2013:110–117. Accessed March 4, 2022. http://npic.orst.edu/RMPP/rmpp_main2a.pdf.

13. Bonneh-Barkay D, Reaney SH, Langston WJ, Di Monte DA. Redox cycling of the herbicide paraquat in microglial cultures. *Brain Res Mol Brain Res*. 2005;134(1):52–56. doi:10.1016/j.molbrainres.2004.11.005

14. Fussell KC, Udasin RG, Gray JP, et al. Redox cycling and increased oxygen utilization contribute to diquat-induced oxidative stress and cytotoxicity in Chinese hamster ovary cells overexpressing NADPH-cytochrome P450 reductase. *Free Radic Biol Med*. 2011;50(7):874–882. doi:10.1016/j.freeradbiomed.2010.12.035

15. Smith LL. Paraquat toxicity. *Philos Trans R Soc Lond B Biol Sci*. 1985;311(1152):647–657. doi:10.1098/rstb.1985.0170

16. Huang J, Ning N, Zhang W. Effects of paraquat on IL-6 and TNF-α in macrophages. *Exp Ther Med*. 2019;17(3):1783–1789. doi:10.3892/etm.2018.7099

17. Chan BS, Lazzaro VA, Seale JP, Duggin GG. The renal excretory mechanisms and the role of organic cations in modulating the renal handling of paraquat. *Pharmacol Ther*. 1998;79(3):193–203. doi:10.1016/s0163-7258(98)00015-1

18. Vaziri ND, Ness RL, Fairshter RD, Smith WR, Rosen SM. Nephrotoxicity of paraquat in man. *Arch Intern Med*. 1979;139(2):172–174

19. Dinis-Oliveira RJ, Duarte JA, Sánchez-Navarro A, Remião F, Bastos ML, Carvalho F. Paraquat poisonings: mechanisms of lung toxicity, clinical features, and treatment. Crit Rev Toxicol. 2008;38(1):13–71. doi:10.1080/10408440701669959

20. Bismuth C, Garnier R, Dally S, Fournier PE, Scherrmann JM. Prognosis and treatment of paraquat poisoning: a review of 28 cases. *J Toxicol Clin Toxicol*. 1982;19(5):461–474. doi:10.3109/15563658208992501

21. Stephens DS, Walker DH, Schaffner W, et al. Pseudodiphtheria: prominent pharyngeal membrane associated with fatal paraquat ingestion. *Ann Intern Med*. 1981;94(2):202–204. doi:10.7326/0003-4819-94-2-202

22. Chen KW, Wu MH, Huang JJ, Yu CY. Bilateral spontaneous pneumothoraces, pneumopericardium, pneumomediastinum, and subcutaneous emphysema: a

rare presentation of paraquat intoxication. *Ann Emerg Med.* 1994;23(5):1132–1134. doi:10.1016/s0196-0644(94)70116-4

23. Kim SJ, Gil HW, Yang JO, Lee EY, Hong SY. The clinical features of acute kidney injury in patients with acute paraquat intoxication. *Nephrol Dial Transplant.* 2009;24(4):1226–1232. doi:10.1093/ndt/gfn615

24. Newstead CG. Cyclophosphamide treatment of paraquat poisoning. *Thorax.* 1996;51(7):659–660. doi:10.1136/thx.51.7.659

25. Huang C, Zhang X, Jiang Y, et al. Paraquat-induced convulsion and death: a report of five cases. *Toxicol Ind Health.* 2013;29(8):722–727. doi:10.1177/0748233712442712

26. Schmidt DM, Neale J, Olson KR. Clinical course of a fatal ingestion of diquat. *J Toxicol Clin Toxicol.* 1999;37(7):881–884. doi:10.1081/clt-100102471

27. Mesnage R, Benbrook C, Antoniou MN. Insight into the confusion over surfactant co-formulants in glyphosate-based herbicides. *Food Chem Toxicol.* 2019;128:137–145. doi:10.1016/j.fct.2019.03.053

28. Mahendrakar K, Venkategowda PM, Rao SM, Mutkule DP. Glyphosate surfactant herbicide poisoning and management. *Indian J Crit Care Med.* 2014;18(5):328–330. doi:10.4103/0972-5229.132508

29. Picetti E, Generali M, Mensi F, et al. Glyphosate ingestion causing multiple organ failure: a near-fatal case report. *Acta Biomed.* 2018;88(4):533–537. doi:10.23750/abm.v88i4.6322

30. Singh S, Kumar V, Gill JPK, et al. Herbicide glyphosate: toxicity and microbial degradation. *Int J Environ Res Public Health.* 2020;17(20):7519. doi:10.3390/ijerph17207519

31. Zouaoui K, Dulaurent S, Gaulier JM, Moesch C, Lachâtre G. Determination of glyphosate and AMPA in blood and urine from humans: about 13 cases of acute intoxication. *Forensic Sci Int.* 2013;226(1-3):e20–e25. doi:10.1016/j.forsciint.2012.12.010

32. Moon JM, Chun BJ. Predicting acute complicated glyphosate intoxication in the emergency department. *Clin Toxicol (Phila).* 2010;48(7):718–724. doi:10.3109/15563650.2010.488640

33. Seok S, Kim YH, Gil HW, Song HY, Hong SY. The time between paraquat ingestion and a negative dithionite urine test in an independent risk factor for death and organ failure in acute paraquat intoxication. *J Korean Med Sci.* 2012;27(9):993–998. doi:10.3346/jkms.2012.27.9.993

34. Koo JR, Yoon JW, Han SJ, et al. Rapid analysis of plasma paraquat using sodium dithionite as a predictor of outcome in acute paraquat poisoning. *Am J Med Sci.* 2009;338(5):373–377. doi:10.1097/MAJ.0b013e3181b4deee

35. Senarathna L, Eddleston M, Wilks MF, et al. Prediction of outcome after paraquat poisoning by measurement of the plasma paraquat concentration. *QJM.* 2009;102(4):251–259. doi:10.1093/qjmed/hcp006

36. Eddleston M, Wilks MF, Buckley NA. Prospects for treatment of paraquat-induced lung fibrosis with immunosuppressive drugs and the need for better prediction of outcome: a systematic review. *QJM*. 2003;96(11):809–824. doi:10.1093/qjmed/hcg137

37. Sawada Y, Yamamoto I, Hirokane T, Nagai Y, Satoh Y, Ueyama M. Severity index of paraquat poisoning. *Lancet*. 1988;1(8598):1333. doi:10.1016/s0140-6736(88)92143-5

38. Ragoucy-Sengler C, Pileire B. A biological index to predict patient outcome in paraquat poisoning. *Hum Exp Toxicol*. 1996;15(3):265–268. doi:10.1177/096032719601500315

39. Roberts DM, Wilks MF, Roberts MS, et al. Changes in the concentrations of creatinine, cystatin C, and NGAL in patients with acute paraquat self-poisoning. *Toxicol Lett*. 2011;202(1):69–74. doi:10.1016/j.toxlet.2011.01.024

40. Kim YT, Jou SS, Lee HS, et al. The area of ground glass opacities of the lungs as a predictive factor in acute paraquat intoxication. *J Korean Med Sci*. 2009;24(4):636–640. doi:10.3346/jkms.2009.24.4.636

41. Kang X, Hu DY, Li CB, et al. The volume ratio of ground glass opacity in early lung CT predicts mortality in acute paraquat poisoning. *PLoS One*. 2015;10(4):e0121691. doi:10.1371/journal.pone.0121691

42. Chen HH, Lin JL, Huang WH, et al. Spectrum of corrosive esophageal injury after intentional paraquat or glyphosate-surfactant herbicide ingestion. *Int J Gen Med*. 2013;6:677–683. doi:10.2147/IJGM.S48273

43. Okonek S, Setyadharma H, Borchert A, Krienke EG. Activated charcoal is as effective as fuller's earth or bentonite in paraquat poisoning. *Klin Wochenschr*. 1982;60(4):207–210. doi:10.1007/BF01715588

44. Pond SM, Rivory LP, Hampson EC, Roberts MS. Kinetics of toxic doses of paraquat and the effects of hemoperfusion in the dog. *J Toxicol Clin Toxicol*. 1993;31(2):229–246. doi:10.3109/15563659309000391

45. Koo JR, Kim JC, Yoon JW, et al. Failure of continuous venovenous hemofiltration to prevent death in paraquat poisoning. *Am J Kidney Dis*. 2002;39(1):55–59. doi:10.1053/ajkd.2002.29880

46. Hong SY, Yang JO, Lee EY, Kim SH. Effect of haemoperfusion on plasma paraquat concentration in vitro and in vivo. *Toxicol Ind Health*. 2003;19(1):17–23. doi:10.1191/0748233703th171oa

47. Wilks MF, Fernando R, Ariyananda PL, et al. Improvement in survival after paraquat ingestion following introduction of a new formulation in Sri Lanka. *PLoS Med*. 2008;5(2):e49. doi:10.1371/journal.pmed.0050049

48. Feng MX, Lu YQ. Performance of extracorporeal membrane oxygenation in patients with fatal paraquat poisoning: grasp for straws? *World J Emerg Med*. 2021;12(3):232–234. doi:10.5847/wjem.j.1920-8642.2021.03.013

49. Bertram A, Haenel SS, Hadem J, et al. Tissue concentration of paraquat on day 32 after intoxication and failed bridge to transplantation by extracorporeal

membrane oxygenation therapy. *BMC Pharmacol Toxicol*. 2013;14:45. doi:10.1186/2050-6511-14-45

50. Tang X, Sun B, He H, et al. Successful extracorporeal membrane oxygenation therapy as a bridge to sequential bilateral lung transplantation for a patient after severe paraquat poisoning. *Clin Toxicol (Phila)*. 2015;53(9):908–913. doi:10.3109/15563650.2015.1082183

51. Sequential bilateral lung transplantation for paraquat poisoning. A case report. The Toronto Lung Transplant group. *J Thorac Cardiovasc Surg*. 1985;89(5):734–742.

52. Jiang WZ, Chen YQ, Zhang YL, Zhang TT, Liu YM, Xu X. Lung transplantation in patients with paraquat poisoning: a case report and literature review. *Zhonghua Lao Dong Wei Sheng Zhi Ye Bing Za Zhi*. 2019;37(4):292–296. doi:10.3760/cma.j.issn.1001-9391.2019.04.013

53. Li LR, Chaudhary B, You C, Dennis JA, Wakeford H. Glucocorticoid with cyclophosphamide for oral paraquat poisoning. *Cochrane Database Syst Rev*. 2021;6(6):CD008084. doi:10.1002/14651858.CD008084.pub5

54. Gawarammana I, Buckley NA, Mohamed F, et al. High-dose immunosuppression to prevent death after paraquat self-poisoning: a randomised controlled trial. *Clin Toxicol (Phila)*. 2018;56(7):633–639. doi:10.1080/15563650.2017.1394465

55. Yang JO, Gil HW, Kang MS, Lee EY, Hong SY. Serum total antioxidant statuses of survivors and nonsurvivors after acute paraquat poisoning. *Clin Toxicol (Phila)*. 2009;47(3):226–229. doi:10.1080/15563650802269901

56. Magalhães N, Carvalho F, Dinis-Oliveira RJ. Human and experimental toxicology of diquat poisoning: toxicokinetics, mechanisms of toxicity, clinical features, and treatment. *Hum Exp Toxicol*. 2018;37(11):1131–1160. doi:10.1177/0960327118765330

57. Lee KH, Gil HW, Kim YT, Yang JO, Lee EY, Hong SY. Marked recovery from paraquat-induced lung injury during long-term follow-up. *Korean J Intern Med*. 2009;24(2):95–100. doi:10.3904/kjim.2009.24.2.95

58. Center for Disease Control and Prevention. *Facts About Paraquat*. 2018. Accessed March 4, 2022. https://emergency.cdc.gov/agent/paraquat/basics/facts.asp.

59. Glyphosate. In: *Some Organophosphate Insecticides and Herbicides*. Vol 112. International Agency for Research on Cancer; 2013:321–412. https://monographs.iarc.who.int/wp-content/uploads/2018/07/mono112.pdf

60. US EPA. Glyphosate. 2022. Accessed March 4, 2022. https://www.epa.gov/ingredients-used-pesticide-products/glyphosate.

61. Benbrook CM. How did the US EPA and IARC reach diametrically opposed conclusions on the genotoxicity of glyphosate-based herbicides? *Environ Sci Eur*. 2019;31:2. https://doi.org/10.1186/s12302-018-0184-7

33 I Am All Choked Up Over Chlorine: Chlorine and Other Pulmonary Irritants

Emily Kiernan

Case Presentation

A 60-year-old man presented to the ED with difficulty breathing for 2 hours. The dyspnea began suddenly and was described as burning and wheezing. Upon questioning, he also reports tightness in his chest, with no radiation to his neck, arms, or back. He denies nausea or vomiting. The dyspnea was progressive but is unchanged. He denies exertional dyspnea, orthopnea, or leg swelling. Earlier that day, he reports that he was at the high school athletic facility where he works as a maintenance professional. He has a past medical history of hypertension and hyperlipidemia. His home medications are lisinopril and atorvastatin. He does not use tobacco products or illicit drugs. His physician has not made any changes to his medication regimen. His heart rate is 100 beats/min and regular, his blood pressure is 140/90 mm Hg, and his oxygen saturation is 97% on room air. His physical examination is notable for diffuse wheezing in all anterior and posterior lung fields. Ultrasound of the heart and lungs does not reveal a pericardial effusion or B-lines, and lung sliding is present in all lung views.

DISCUSSION

Background

An elderly male with cardiac risk factors and shortness of breath is a medically complex case with an extensive differential diagnosis ranging from a benign musculoskeletal strain to life-threatening causes that require immediate intervention. The emergency medicine practitioner must be vigilant and comprehensive during their evaluation as to not miss a life-threatening cause of this presentation. A patient with new onset of respiratory distress and wheezing but no history of obstructive or restrictive lung disease should be carefully evaluated for environmental and occupational exposures. In this case, new-onset wheezing after returning from work at an athletic facility should prompt further history from the patient. When the emergency medicine practitioner inquires about the patient's job, he reveals that he was tasked to add chlorine tablets to the indoor pool. However, his boss gave him the wrong amount, and he added 10 times the recommended amount of chlorine. He noticed that his eyes and mouth started to burn after about 30 minutes, so he finished the task and left the area. A few hours later, he started to have difficulty breathing.

Toxicology and Pathophysiology

Irritant gases, including chlorine, are a heterogenous group of chemicals that are found in a variety of industrial and occupational settings.[1,2] When an irritant chemical enters the respiratory tract, it can cause local tissue damage, which precipitates a host inflammatory response.[1,2] The combination of local tissue damage with excessive cellular debris and exudates can cause acute respiratory distress syndrome (ARDS). The exact mechanism of initial cellular damage varies by irritant gas, but many require dissolution in lung water to liberate an acid or the creation of oxygen or nitrogen free radicals. The specific mechanism of action should be considered when evaluating a patient with an irritant gas exposure.

When discussing irritant gases, the water solubility, or how well a chemical can dissolve in water, is an important property that determines the clinical effect.[2] A highly water-soluble irritant gas primary affects mucous membranes in the upper airways, eyes, and nasal passages since it will dissolve in mucosal secretions before being able to penetrate more deeply into the airway tract. The patient will experience immediate symptoms that are considered a "warning sign" to leave the area. Intermediately water-soluble irritant gases primarily affect the upper airway but can also cause irritation deep into the alveoli. The patient may experience some warning signs including airway irritation and breathing difficulty, but this may be a delayed effect. Slightly water-soluble irritant gases primarily affect the alveolar-capillary membrane. These chemicals will typically cause a delayed onset of symptoms and do not provide adequate warning for the patient to leave the area, leading to prolonged exposure and the risk of severe a delayed onset of symptoms.

Workup and Diagnosis

Time since exposure and duration of exposure, water solubility, and concentration of the irritant gas will help to predict the onset of symptoms (Table 33.1). However, the identification of the specific irritant gas is not as important because the clinical presentation will be similar due to the final common pathway of cellular damage and fluid accumulation in the alveoli.

Highly Water-Soluble Irritant Gases

Highly water-soluble irritant gases cause immediate onset of mucosal membrane and skin irritation. This can result in skin discomfort, conjunctival irritation, chemosis, nasal or oropharyngeal pain, drooling, mucosal edema, cough, and/or stridor. Since the patient has a warning to remove themselves from the exposure, this typically does not lead to a significant progression of

TABLE 33.1 **Irritant gases by water-solubility**

Highly water-soluble	Moderately water-soluble	Low water-soluble
Ammonia (NH$_3$)	Chlorine	Phosgene (carbonyl chloride)
Chloramines	Chlorine dioxide	Nitrogen dioxide
Formaldehyde	Hydrogen sulfide	
Hydrogen chloride		
Hydrogen fluoride		
Sulfur dioxide		

worsening signs and symptoms. However, if the patient is exposed to highly concentrated gas, they may develop early signs and symptoms despite the warning properties.

Moderately Water-Soluble Irritant Gases

Moderately water-soluble irritant gases can cause a delayed onset of mucosal membrane and skin irritation when compared with the highly water-soluble irritant gases. This can result in skin discomfort, conjunctival irritation, chemosis, nasal or oropharyngeal pain, drooling, mucosal edema, cough, and stridor.

Low Water-Soluble Irritant Gases

Low water-soluble irritant gases do not typically produce mucosal membrane or skin irritation. Because of this, these gases do not typically provide an adequate warning signal, allowing the patient to have a prolonged exposure and allowing the irritant gas to enter the lower respiratory tract and bronchopulmonary system. Clinically, this can lead to a delayed onset of tracheobronchitis, bronchiolitis, bronchospasm, and ARDS.

If a patient had a significant (high concentration, prolonged exposure) irritant gas exposure, regardless of the water solubility, they could progress to ARDS. ARDS is an acute, nonspecific syndrome that is not attributed to another cause, like congestive heart failure and that has clinical, physiological, and radiographic abnormalities caused by pulmonary inflammation and alveolar filling.[3,4] Patients with ARDS typically present with dyspnea, chest tightness, chest pain, cough, frothy sputum, wheezing or crackles, and hypoxemia. Chest radiographic abnormalities may include bilateral pulmonary infiltrates with an alveolar filling pattern and a normal cardiac silhouette.

Chlorine Gas

Chlorine is a greenish-yellow gas that is a widely used oxidizing agent with various industrial uses including bleaching operations, sewage treatment, swimming pool chlorination tablets, and chemical warfare.[1] Occupational exposure is common, but household exposures can be seen when bleach is mixed with other acid-based cleaning products, which can liberate chlorine gas. Exposure to chlorine gas may only result in mild symptoms initially because of its intermediate solubility. Given the ability to manifest mild "warning signs," there may be a substantial time delay before the patient is removed from the exposure. Clinical symptoms typically manifest after several hours. Chlorine dissolution into the water of the lungs[1,2] will generate HCl and hypochlorous acids. Hypochlorous acid rapidly decomposes into HCl and an oxygen atom. Pulmonary damage is caused by local tissue damage from the acid species as well as the free radical oxygen atom. Additionally, dermal injuries can occur. Since chlorine is one of the most highly produced and used chemicals around the world, it is frequently transported, as a liquid, at temperatures below −30°F/−34°C or at higher pressure. Contact with this very cold liquid can cause frostbite injuries.[5]

Treatment

In this case, the patient has no history of tobacco use or underlying lung disease but presents with wheezing and shortness of breath. You assess airway, breathing, and circulation and determine that the patient can protect his own airway and, despite mild mucous membrane irritation, does not have evidence of upper airway edema. Additionally, the patient has diffuse wheezing and tachypnea, so you initiate nebulizer beta-2 agonist treatment. You inform the patient about the presumed diagnosis, the plan for treatment, and further evaluation in the ED.

On arrival to the ED, always consider decontamination after a chemical exposure. Most gas exposures will not require significant decontamination but consider removing the clothing and washing the skin if irritation is present.[2,3]

Management of patients with exposure to irritant gas begins with careful inspection of the airway to ensure patency, assessment of bronchial and pulmonary secretions, and monitoring the patient's ability to maintain normal oxygenation. Several therapies have been evaluated, but there is no specific antidote for irritant gas exposure. Symptomatic and supportive care remains the cornerstone of therapy, including supplemental oxygen, bronchodilators, and airway suctioning, as needed.[3] Supplemental oxygen should be avoided in patients who are not hypoxic due to the risk of worsening oxidative stress and free radical formation.

If the patient has ocular irritation, examine for eye injuries, flush the eyes extensively, and refer to an ophthalmologist as soon as possible.[6]

Although irritant gases do not typically cause primary end-organ dysfunction or hypoxia, direct damage to the lungs or resultant hypoxia and increased stress on the body can lead to further complications. In a patient with underlying hypertension and hyperlipidemia, it would be important to consider other etiologies of the presentation, including acute coronary syndrome, pulmonary embolism, aortic insufficiency. A rapid bedside ECG and point-of-care ultrasound (POCUS) are important in this scenario. Additionally, laboratory assessment to evaluate for symptomatic anemia, acute heart failure, or acute myocardial infarction can be considered in the right clinical scenario. However, in an otherwise healthy patient with a strong history of irritant gas exposure, no further diagnostic testing may be required.

The use of inhaled or nebulized bronchodilators, including beta-2 agonists, is recommended in patients who present with evidence of bronchoconstriction or increased airway resistance on exam after exposure to an irritant gas. Most patients will improve with this therapy alone, but the addition of ipratropium bromine can also be considered.[3,7]

Bicarbonate therapy has historically been contraindicated in acid exposure because of the potential exothermic reaction during neutralization and subsequent heat generation. However, the theoretical risk after an acid-based irritant gas exposure would likely lead to dissipation of heat and gas generated during neutralization given the large surface area of the lungs and open body cavity.[2,8] Based on the available human data, there does not appear to be a specific benefit for nebulized bicarbonate but this may be a reasonable approach in a patient with persistent symptoms after inhaled bronchodilators.[3,7,8] The sodium bicarbonate solution can be administered as 3 mL sterile water mixed with 1 mL of 7.5% or 8.4% sodium bicarbonate solution (resulting in an ~2% solution for nebulization).

Systemic or inhaled corticosteroid therapy is controversial in the treatment irritant gas exposure. Clinical data on the efficacy after human exposure are inconclusive, and there have not been any human randomized control studies. However, the use of corticosteroid therapy in a patient with ARDS from other causes shows a potential benefit and can be considered, via inhalation or IV routes, according to your institutional protocol. However, corticosteroids are not routinely indicated for patients with mild signs or symptoms of irritant gas toxicity.[3,7,9]

Extracorporeal membrane oxygenation (ECMO) is a treatment option in cases where other advanced oxygenation and ventilation strategies have failed. ECMO has been successfully used in cases of toxic inhalation-induced lung injury, as in cases with severe chlorine gas exposure.[10]

Long-Term Concerns

After an acute irritant gas exposure, some patients develop reactive airways dysfunction syndrome (RADS) (also referred to as irritant induced asthma or occupational asthma without latency). This is possible with almost any irritant gas, including chlorine.[11] Patients who develop RADS tend to have a lower incidence of atopy and are exposed to agents not typically considered to be immunologically sensitizing, when compared to those with the diagnosis of occupational asthma. Patients with RADS tend to have significant improvement in airflow after administration of a beta2 adrenergic agonist treatment. Recovery can take months, especially if the patient continues to have ongoing exposure to the irritant gas. Patients can be referred to their primary care physicians or a pulmonologist if they have persistent symptoms after an irritant gas exposure.[11]

CASE CONCLUSION

After providing a bronchodilator via nebulizer, your patient feels significantly better, and his breath sounds are clear in all lung fields. You observe the patient for 4–6 hours in case of recurrent symptoms, and he continues to do well. The patient is discharged from the ED. You discuss the need for proper personal protective equipment (PPE) while handing any chemical and that chemical-specific PPE should be available from his employer. You encourage your patient to follow-up with his primary care physician and discuss any concerns for possible RADS if he develops a recurrence of symptoms. You follow-up with the patient a week later; he is doing well with no complaints.

KEY POINTS TO REMEMBER

- Any patient with new onset of respiratory distress and wheezing and no history of obstructive or restrictive lung disease should be carefully evaluated for environmental and occupational exposures.
- Irritant gas exposure can lead to a range of presentations from mucous membrane irritation to ARDS based on water solubility, duration of exposure, and concentration of the chemical.
- Management of patients with exposure to irritant gas begins with careful inspection of the ABCs, focusing on airway patency and breathing.
- While there is no specific antidote, symptomatic and supportive care with supplemental oxygen, bronchodilators, and airway suctioning are the cornerstone of therapy.
- Irritant gas exposure can lead to reactive airways dysfunction syndrome (RADS). Patients should stop the exposure and be evaluated by a PCP or pulmonologist.

Further Reading

Achanta S, Jordt SE. Toxic effects of chlorine gas and potential treatments: a literature review. *Toxicology Mechanisms and Methods*. 2021 May 4;31(4):244–256.

Zellner T, Eyer F. Choking agents and chlorine gas–history, pathophysiology, clinical effects, and treatment. *Toxicol Lett*. Mar 1, 2020;320:73–79.

References

1. Nelson LS, Odujebe OA. *Goldfrank's Toxicologic Emergencies*. 11th ed. McGraw-Hill Education; 2019.
2. Maddry JK. *Critical Care Toxicology*. 2nd ed. Springer International Publishing AG; 2017.
3. Huynh Tuong A, Despréaux T, Loeb T, Salomon J, Mégarbane B, Descatha A. Emergency management of chlorine gas exposure—a systematic review. *Clin Toxicol*. Feb 1, 2019;57(2):77–98.
4. Ferguson ND, Fan E, Camporota L, et al. The Berlin definition of ARDS: an expanded rationale, justification, and supplementary material. *Intensive Care Med*. Oct 2012;38(10):1573–1582.

5. Centers for Disease Control and Prevention. *Facts about Chlorine*. Centers for Disease Control and Prevention. April 4, 2018. Accessed July 10, 2022.https://emergency.cdc.gov/agent/chlorine/basics/facts.asp.

6. Levy DM, Divertie MB, Litzow TJ, Henderson JW. Ammonia burns of the face and respiratory tract. *JAMA*. 1964;190:873–876.

7. Govier P, Coulson JM. Civilian exposure to chlorine gas: a systematic review. *Toxicol Lett*. Sep 1, 2018;293:249–252.

8. Chisholm CD, Singeltary EM, Okerberg CV, et al. Inhaled sodium bicarbonate therapy for chlorine inhalation injuries. *Ann Emerg Med*. 1989;18:466.

9. de Lange DW, Meulenbelt J. Do corticosteroids have a role in preventing or reducing acute toxic lung injury caused by inhalation of chemical agents? *Clin Toxicol*. Feb 1, 2011;49(2):61–71.

10. Paul S, Campbell B, Meltzer EC, Sedrakyan A. ECMO as an emergency medical countermeasure. *Lancet Respir Med*. Sep 1, 2014;2(9):685–687.

11. Shakeri MS, Dick FG, Ayres JG. Which agents cause reactive airways dysfunction syndrome (RADS)? A systematic review. *Occup Med (Lond)*. 2008;58:205–211.

34 You Are Getting Chernobyl Close to Home: Acute Radiation Syndrome and Cutaneous Radiation Syndrome

Girgis Fahmy and Ziad Kazzi

Case Presentation

A 42-year-old man with history of hypertension, hyperlipidemia, and type 2 diabetes mellitus is brought to the ED by EMS due to a right index finger injury, headache, and nausea that started shortly after he had an accident at work. He is a nuclear medicine technologist at an outpatient medical center where they perform cardiac stress testing and thyroid disease diagnostic tests and treatments. The patient reports that he broke a glass container that contained radioactive iodine I-131 and that his hands, arms, and shirt were splashed with the liquid. He has a deep cut to his right index finger and the bleeding has been controlled with direct pressure. The patient adds that although he was wearing reading glasses, he was not using a mask or gloves. The patient's medications are metformin, lisinopril, and atorvastatin.

Vital signs are heart rate 110 beats/min, blood pressure 112/52 mm Hg, respiratory rate 20 breaths/min, temperature 100.2°F/38.0°C. On physical exam, the patient appears anxious and is holding his right index finger wrapped with gauze.

What Do You Do Now?

DISCUSSION

A middle-aged man presents to the ED after having direct contact with a radioactive liquid solution of iodine-131 with contamination to his hands and clothes. In addition to the direct external contamination, there is also a risk of inhaling radioactive iodine that could have existed in gaseous form and a risk of contamination of the mucous membranes of his eyes. Iodine could have also become internalized through his right finger wound. He has an injury to his hand that needs repair and nonspecific complaints (headache and nausea) which can occur in patients with the prodromal stage of the acute radiation syndrome (ARS). Although other diseases present similarly and must be considered in a patient with this symptomatology, the focus here will be external and internal contamination with radioactive material and on the risk of developing ARS.

Background

ARS is the acute illness that is caused by exposure of the whole body, or most of the body, to a high dose (>2 Gy) of penetrating radiation (e.g., gamma rays or X-rays) during a short period of time (e.g., minutes to several hours).[1] Radiation can be divided into two types: ionizing and nonionizing. *Ionizing radiation* has sufficient energy to remove an electron from an atom or molecule.[2,3] This disruption leads to direct damage to the DNA or alteration of chemical bonds and formation of free radicals, which then cause cellular or DNA damage. Examples of ionizing radiation include gamma rays and X-rays. Particulate forms of ionizing radiation include alpha particles, beta particles, and neutrons. Ionizing radiation is emitted from radioactive atoms such as iodine-131, cesium-137, strontium-90, polonium-210, and uranium-238.[4] *Nonionizing radiation* does not have the ability to disrupt atoms that it encounters. Its only known biological effect is due to the heat it transmits to the cell. Examples of nonionizing radiation include radio waves, infrared waves, microwaves, and ultraviolet radiation.[5]

Ionizing radiation is emitted from naturally occurring or man-made sources such as CT scanners, plain radiography, and nuclear medicine scans. Natural radiation consists of cosmic rays or of ionizing radiation that originates from different radioactive atoms that are found in the Earth's crust, such as radon. This means that natural background radiation varies by location and elevation, with higher levels measured at high altitudes and in certain locations.

Toxicology and Pathophysiology

ARS progresses through four stages: prodromal, latent, manifest illness, and recovery or death.[3] The prodromal phase typically occurs within 48 hours of exposure. This phase is characterized by nonspecific signs and symptoms including anorexia, apathy, asthenia, nausea, vomiting, diarrhea, fever, and tachycardia.[3,6] The time to onset of various symptoms, their severity, and the duration of each stage are related to the dose of radiation exposure. The prodromal phase is followed by the latent phase, which is characterized by an improvement in initial symptoms. This transient period is followed by the manifest illness stage. During this stage the patient exhibits symptoms of the four sub-syndromes previously mentioned. At this stage, the patient may develop neutropenia, thrombocytopenia, anemia, GI mucosal damage or hemorrhage, and electrolyte abnormalities. The course can become complicated by infections, sepsis, and bleeding. The manifest illness stage can last several weeks depending on the dose received and the resulting complications. If the patient survives this stage, recovery may occur over several weeks to months, during the which the patient may develop delayed effects of acute radiation exposure (i.e., DEARE) such as pulmonary fibrosis or cataracts.

ARS sub-syndromes can occur individually or in combination depending on the severity of the exposure. There is an inverse relationship between the radiation dose received by the patient and time to onset of clinical manifestation of various ARS sub-syndromes.

The cutaneous sub-syndrome is the manifestation of radiation exposure to the skin which can vary from hair loss at lower exposures (>2 Gy) to necrosis at higher doses (>20 Gy).[7] Clinical manifestations include erythema, pruritis, nonspecific swelling or edema, desquamation, and ulceration. Typically, after exposure, patients will have transient erythema or pruritis, eventually progressing to blistering and ulceration that can evolve in 3 weeks or even a few years after exposure.[3]

The hematopoietic sub-syndrome is the manifestation of radiation exposure to the bone marrow after an absorbed whole-body dose between 2 and

6 Gy.[4] The earliest laboratory finding is a fall in the absolute lymphocyte count followed by falling absolute neutrophil, platelet, and red blood cell counts.[4] During this manifest illness phase, the patient is prone to developing infections and GI bleeding (at the higher side of the dose range). Recovery can occur if there are remaining bone marrow stem cells that can regenerate the blood cell lines. There is a direct correlation between the radiation dose received and the rate of decline of the absolute lymphocyte count.[8] Mortality in these patients is typically due to infections, sepsis, bleeding, and poor wound healing in the setting of pancytopenia (Figure 34.1).[4]

Damage from radiation to the mucosal lining of the GI tract along with loss of proliferative epithelial cells causes the GI sub-syndrome. This syndrome manifests after exposure to a whole-body dose of 6–10 Gy and carries a very poor prognosis due to infections and GI bleeding.[4] Thrombocytopenia exacerbates GI bleeding that may occur, and the

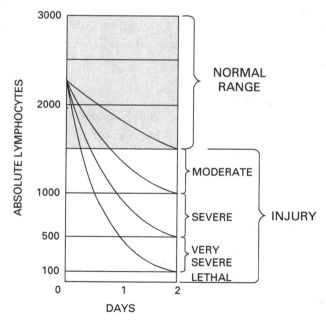

FIGURE 34.1 Andrew lymphocyte nomogram.

Image acquired from CDC Website.

lymphocytopenia along with disruption of the mucosal lining contributes to increased risk for sepsis.

The neurovascular sub-syndrome is the manifestation of radiation injury in the cerebrovascular system. This sub-syndrome is poorly characterized given limited data.[4] Previous reports have demonstrated altered mental status, seizures, and coma at doses of greater than 30 Gy,[4] while other reports have demonstrated severe symptoms progressing to death at doses of greater than 10 Gy.[7] Clinically, patients typically have a brief latency period lasting several hours followed by cerebral edema and increased intracranial pressure, progressing to coma and death within 48 hours.[9]

Victims who recover from ARS may still develop long-term complications and delayed-onset clinical illnesses. After the bombing of Nagasaki and Hiroshima, those exposed to even low levels of radiation had an increased incidence of cataracts compared to the general population. This risk existed between 6 months and 35 years after exposure.[9] In addition, patient who received a dose of greater than 8 Gy to the thorax developed pulmonary disease, progressing to pneumonitis and pulmonary fibrosis.[4] Low doses of radiation, as little as 1 Gy, can have an impact on male and female fertility. This effect is usually temporary, but is variable depending on age, gender, and dose.[4]

Workup and Diagnosis

Appropriate triage and initial assessment of patients exposed to radiation are crucial to patient outcomes. In this case, the patient has an injured finger without an exsanguinating hemorrhage and therefore does not have a life-threatening emergency and does not require a life-saving intervention. Due to the possibility of external contamination with radioactive materials, he will need to be surveyed with a Geiger-Muller counter followed by decontamination with soap and water. These steps can be performed at the nuclear medicine clinic or by prehospital personnel. However, ED staff should be expected to repeat the assessment or conduct de novo upon the arrival to the ED. Staff should wear surgical scrubs, gowns, surgical caps, masks, shoe covers, and face shields. Two sets of gloves should be worn, and the gloves and shoe covers should be taped to the gown. Respiratory protection with an N95 or elastomeric mask is preferred but surgical masks are suitable alternatives when the former are not available.[3]

Treatment

If a patient has an acute traumatic injury or impending cardiopulmonary arrest, this should be addressed immediately by medical providers. Based on previous historical incidents, medical personnel are unlikely to receive significant acute radiation doses when caring for patients who are externally or internally contaminated radioactive material.[3] Initial evaluation of patients includes standard ED procedures which includes an evaluation of a patient's airway, breathing, and circulation with appropriate intervention as needed. If a patient requires emergent surgery, it is recommended that this happens during the initial 24 hours, given expected difficulty in wound healing associated with hematopoietic dysfunction. Once the primary and secondary surveys are complete, the most important components of a patient history include location during the incident, duration of potential exposure, time between exposure and presentation, occupation, and any other recent radiation exposures (e.g., recent nuclear medicine procedure).[3] Physical examination of these patients should be consistent with advanced trauma life support (ATLS) algorithms. The time elapsed between exposure and the onset of prodromal manifestations like diarrhea and vomiting can be used to estimate the dose of radiation received by the patient. This can assist providers in their severity assessment and disposition decisions in scarce resource settings.

Initial laboratory studies in patients who have been exposed to radiation should include a complete blood count with differential (with repeat values every 6 hours to trend the absolute lymphocyte count) and comprehensive metabolic panels including liver function tests, prothrombin time with INR, type and screen, and serum amylase (salivary gland inflammation can demonstrate increased values upon exposure of the head to penetrating forms of ionizing radiation like gamma rays). In addition to the laboratory tests that can be done in the ED, specialized cytogenetic testing for dicentric chromosomes can be requested from the Radiation Emergency Assistance Center and Training Site (REAC/TS) in Oak Ridge, Tennessee. Assessment of internal contamination with radioactive material can be done using indirect biological assays of urine or feces (depending on the specific radionuclide and exposure scenario) or direct assessments using radiation detection devices. This latter technique can be used when the radioactive material emits gamma rays and after the skin surface is deemed clean from any external contamination. Patients who are at high risk for severe hematopoietic sub-syndrome may require stem cell transplantation, for which a blood sample should be sent for human leukocyte antigen (HLA) typing.[3]

The mainstay of initial treatment of ARS is supportive care including antiemetics, antidiarrheals, prevention and treatment of infections, and blood products. Additionally, cytokines (e.g., FDA-approved colony stimulating factors such as filgrastim, sargramostim, pegylated-filgrastim, and romiplostim) are used to stimulate the recovery of the bone marrow function by stimulating surviving stem cells. In refractory cases, stem cell transplant may be performed depending on several conditions that are assessed by the transplant professional. In these cases, the Radiation Injury Treatment Network (RITN) serves as a national resource through its network of stem cell transplant centers.[4] Arguably equally important is the incorporation of a multidisciplinary team including a burn specialist, hematologist, gastroenterologist, medical toxicologist, infectious disease specialist, and trauma surgeon, depending on the injury complex.[4] Patients who have received 2 Gy or greater dose of radiation should receive antimicrobials as they are likely to develop neutropenia. Oral fluoroquinolones are appropriate for clinically stable and afebrile patients, but if they are febrile, unstable, or already neutropenic, a broader antimicrobial selection should be considered.[4] Prophylaxis against herpes simplex virus disease using acyclovir and antifungals in severe cases and in patients who are persistently septic despite receiving antimicrobials should be considered. Patients may need blood products during the course of their illness. All blood products should be irradiated prior to administration to prevent transfusion-related graft versus host disease.[4]

Several organizations in the United States and internationally are involved in radiological/nuclear emergency preparedness and response. In the United States, those organizations include the REAC/TS, the Nuclear Regulatory Commission, the Centers for Disease Control and Prevention, the Department of Health and Human Services, the Environmental Protection Agency, the Occupational Safety and Health Administration, the National Institute of Occupational Safety and Health, the Food and Drug Administration, and the RITN. Internationally, the International Atomic Energy Agency (IAEA), the World Health Organization, and the International Commission on Radiation Protection play an important role and collaborate with organizations in the United States.[3]

TABLE 34.1 Acute radiation syndrome dose-symptom relationship

Syndrome	Dose	Prodromal stage	Latent stage	Manifest illness stage	Recovery
Hematopoietic	>0.7 Gy (>70 rads) (Mild symptoms may occur as low as 0.3 Gy or 30 rads)	Symptoms are anorexia, nausea, and vomiting. Onset occurs 1 hour to 2 days after exposure. Stage lasts for minutes to days	Stem cells in bone marrow are dying, although patient may appear and feel well. This stage lasts 1–6 weeks.	Symptoms are anorexia, fever, and malaise. Drop in all blood cell counts occurs for several weeks. Primary cause of death is infection and haemorrhage. Survival decreases with increasing dose. Most deaths occur within a few months after exposure.	In most cases, bone marrow cells will begin to repopulate the marrow. There should be full recovery for a large percentage of individuals from a few weeks up to 2 years after exposure. Death may occur in some individuals at 1.2 Gy (120 rads). The LD50/60† is about 2.5 to 5 Gy (250 to 500 rads)

(*Continued*)

TABLE 34.1 **Continued**

Syndrome	Dose	Prodromal stage	Latent stage	Manifest illness stage	Recovery
Gastrointestinal	>10 Gy (>1000 rads) (Some symptoms may occur as low as 6 Gy or 600 rads)	Symptoms are anorexia, severe nausea, vomiting, cramps, and diarrhea. Onset occurs within a few hours after exposure. Stage lasts about 2 days.	Stem cells in bone marrow and cells lining GI tract are dying, although patient may appear and feel well. Stage lasts less than 1 week.	Symptoms are malaise, anorexia, severe diarrhea, fever, dehydration, and electrolyte imbalance. Death is due to infection, dehydration, and electrolyte imbalance. Death occurs within 2 weeks of exposure.	The LD100† is about 10 Gy (1000 rads)
Cardiovascular/ CNS	>50 Gy (5,000 rads) (Some symptoms may occur as low as 20 Gy or 2,000 rads)	Symptoms are extreme nervousness and confusion; severe nausea, vomiting, and watery diarrhea; loss of consciousness; and burning sensations of the skin. Onset occurs within minutes of exposure. Stage lasts for minutes to hours.	Patient may return to partial functionality. Stage may last for hours but often is less.	Symptoms are return of watery diarrhea, convulsions, and coma. Onset occurs 5–6 hours after exposure. Death occurs within 3 days of exposure.	No recovery is expected.

Table acquired from CDC website.

†The dagger point was to define LD50/60 and LD100. The URL for the table is: https://www.cdc.gov/nceh/radiation/emergencies/arsphysicianfactsheet.htm

CASE CONCLUSION

The 42-year-old patient was already exhibiting components of three of the four sub-syndromes at the time of arrival. Specifically, headache which is an early finding in the neurovascular sub-syndrome, nausea can be seen as an early finding in the GI sub-syndrome, and a direct laceration concerning for possible cutaneous and subcutaneous contamination. As mentioned, symptoms typically begin to arise 12 to 48 hours after the initial contact (can arise within 2 hours) but the fact that this patient began to have symptomatology shortly after the inciting incident was a poor prognostic indicator. Ultimately this patient began to have neurovascular decline requiring mechanical ventilatory support for airway protection. His hospital course was ultimately complicated by severe septic shock secondary to bacteremia and fungemia as a product of a severe hematopoietic latent stage. The patient was unable to recover and expired three weeks after admission.

KEY POINTS TO REMEMBER

- Estimation of exposure dose can be done based on clinical and laboratory grounds and has important prognostic implications.
- Decontamination of patients who are contaminated with radioactive material should not take precedence over the performance of life-saving interventions.
- Supportive care is the mainstay of treatment in addition to preventing infections and promoting the recovery of bone marrow function.

Further Reading

CDC Radiation Emergencies. Acute radiation syndrome: a fact sheet for physicians. April 22, 2019. https://www.cdc.gov/nceh/radiation/emergencies/arsphysicianfactsheet.htm

Kazzi Z. Acute radiation injuries. In: Jeffrey Brent, Keith Burkhart, Paul Dargan, Benjamin Hatten, Bruno Megarbane, Robert Palmer, Julian White, eds. *Critical Care Toxicology.* Springer; 2016:605–618.

Nelson LS, Howland MA, Lewin NA, Smith SW, Goldfrank LR, Hoffman RS. (n.d.). *Goldfrank's Toxicologic Emergencies.* 11th ed. McGraw-Hill Education; 2019.

References

1. CDC Radiation Emergencies. Acute radiation syndrome: a fact sheet for physicians. April 22, 2019. https://www.cdc.gov/nceh/radiation/emergencies/arsphysicianfactsheet.htm

2. Ionization energy. Britannica. Updated May 29, 2020. Accessed April 6, 2022. https://www.britannica.com/science/ionization-energy.

3. Nelson LS, Howland MA, Lewin NA, Smith SW, Goldfrank LR, Hoffman RS. *Goldfrank's Toxicologic Emergencies*. 11th ed. McGraw-Hill Education; 2019.

4. Kazzi Z. Acute radiation injuries. In: Jeffrey Brent, Keith Burkhart, Paul Dargan, Benjamin Hatten, Bruno Megarbane, Robert Palmer, Julian White, eds. *Critical Care Toxicology*. Springer; 2016:605–618.

5. CDC. *Non-Ionizing Radiation*. Centers for Disease Control and Prevention. December 7, 2015. https://www.cdc.gov/nceh/radiation/nonionizing_radiation.html

6. López M, Martín M. Medical management of the acute radiation syndrome. *Reports of Practical Oncology and Radiotherapy*. 2011;16(4):138–146. https://doi.org/10.1016/j.rpor.2011.05.001

7. Dainiak N, Gent RN, Carr Z, et al. Literature review and global consensus on management of acute radiation syndrome affecting nonhematopoietic organ systems. *Disaster Med Public Health Prep*. 2011;5(3):183–201. https://doi.org/10.1001/dmp.2011.73

8. Goans RE, Holloway EC, Berger ME, Ricks RC. Early dose assessment in criticality accidents. *Health Physics*. 2001;81(4):446–449. https://doi.org/10.1097/00004032-200110000-00009

9. Armed Forces Radiobiology Research Institute. *Medical Consequences of Nuclear Warfare*. Armed Forces Radiobiology Research Institute; 1989.

Index

For the benefit of digital users, indexed terms that span two pages (e.g., 52–53) may, on occasion, appear on only one of those pages.

Tables, figures, and boxes are indicated by *t*, *f*, and *b* following the page number

2-PAM, 354–55, 357, 358, 359, 360
4-methylpyrazole, 14, 32–33, 35*b*, 36, 37
2,4-dichlorphenoxyacetic, 353, 364
25-hydroxycholecalciferol, 106
3,4-methylenedioxymethamphetamine,
    189, 250

abortifacient, 239–40
acetaldehyde, 260
acetaminophen, 1, 2–3, 3*f*, 12, 13–14,
    89–90
acetaminophen hepatotoxicity, 14, 239
Acetaminophen-induced nephrotoxicity, 13
Acetaminophen Overdose, 1–15, 7*b*, 9*t*
acetazolamide, 24, 108
acetoacetate, 260–61
acetone, 29, 31–32
acetylcholine (ACh), 312–13, 322–23,
    333, 351–61
acetylcholinesterase (AChE), 59–60, 197–
    98, 313, 352–55, 356–58, 361
acidosis
    elevated anion-gap, 4
    ketosis without, 31*f*
    metabolic, 230*t*
    renal tubular, 21
    respiratory, 364
activated charcoal (AC), 22–23, 120, 130,
    131, 142*t*, 143, 176–77, 228, 288,
    368, 369
acute cocaine toxicity, 306
acute coronary syndrome (ACS), 299, 304,
    308, 383
acute digitalis poisoning, 181
Acute digitoxin intoxication, 182

acute intrathecal baclofen overdose, 294
Acute intrathecal baclofen withdrawal, 295
acute methamphetamine-related disorders
    and toxicity, 257
Acute opiate overdose, 282
acute opioid withdrawal, 273–74, 278*t*
Acute radiation injuries, 397, 398
addiction, 157, 222, 281, 282, 299
adenosine, 225, 228, 230*t*, 231
agents
    antiarrhythmic, 141*t*
    antimuscarinic, 197–98
    cholinergic/organophosphate, 86
    depolarizing, 287
    dopaminergic, 59
    oxidizing, 381–82
    sedative-hypnotic, 270–71
    sympathomimetic, 54, 301
agonists
    α-adrenergic receptor, 54
    beta-adrenergic receptor, 54
    mu-receptor, 138, 186–87, 188, 190
alcohol, 28, 29–30, 204–5, 206, 211–22,
    259, 260–62, 265
    rubbing, 28
    volatile, 32
alcohol abuse disorder, 211, 212–13, 213*b*,
    216, 219, 260–62, 263–65
alcohol dehydrogenase (ADH), 28–29, 30,
    32–33, 34–36, 37, 260
alcoholic hallucinosis, 214
Alcoholic ketoacidosis, 263, 266
alcohol withdrawal, 212, 214, 216, 217,
    220, 221
    severe, 221

alcohol withdrawal seizures, 214, 215–16, 220

alcohol withdrawal syndrome. *See* AWS

aldehyde dehydrogenase (ALDH), 28–29, 36, 260

algal blooms, 341

allodynia, cold, 344–45

alpha-2 agonists, 86, 155, 304

alpha-antagonism, 86, 304

Alpha-neurotoxins act, 313

alpha particles, 389

alprazolam, 211, 219, 220, 221, 222

amitriptyline, 159–60, 165–66, 169, 191

Ammonia, 7*b*, 380*t*

amphetamines, 54, 69–70, 128, 185, 187, 189, 205, 250–53, 306

anaphylaxis, 194, 313, 324, 326–27, 334–35, 336, 337

ANAVIP, 315–16

Angel's trumpet, 51–55, 55*f*

anhidrosis, 51–55, 57–58

anion gap, 1, 30, 31–32, 31*f*, 35*b*, 37, 56–57, 81–82, 263

   high, 12, 13, 21, 30, 37, 79, 197, 263

antagonism

   beta-adrenergic, 228

   kappa-opioid receptor, 152

antagonists

   adenosine, 228, 231

   beta-adrenergic, 229, 232

anticholinergic, 50, 51–55, 57–58, 59–60, 63, 167, 168, 197–98

antidotes, 33, 35*b*, 37, 38, 46, 47, 238, 239, 240, 369

antiepileptic, 166, 229, 286*t*, 291, 357

antihistamines, 54–55, 194, 195*t*, 196, 199, 252, 336, 348*t*

antimuscarinic, 168, 195*t*, 195–96, 199

antipsychotics, 51–54, 59, 60, 67–68, 74, 205–6, 253, 255, 303–4

antivenom, 314, 315–16, 317, 318, 326–27, 328, 329, 330, 334–36

aortic dissection, 251–52, 302

APAP, 1–3, 4–5, 6*t*, 7, 8, 9–11, 12

aphrodisiac, 173

ARDS (acute respiratory distress syndrome), 50, 56–57, 82, 250, 271, 365, 366, 379, 381, 383, 385

aromatherapy, 236–37, 238–40

arrhythmias, 86, 91–92, 161, 162–64, 165–66, 169, 231, 250, 287–88, 358

ARS (acute radiation syndrome), 389, 390, 392, 394, 397, 398

Arthropods, 337

Atropa belladonna, 51–55

atropine, 51–55, 94, 97, 197–98, 199, 354, 356–58, 359, 360

AWS (alcohol withdrawal syndrome), 212–18, 219, 220, 221, 261–62, 265

baclofen, 283–95

barbiturates, 71, 72–73, 166, 217–18, 220, 229, 230*t*, 253, 270–71, 370

bark scorpion, 322–24, 325, 327, 328, 329

bath salts, 189, 202

benzodiazepines, 51–54, 58–60, 72–73, 198, 205–6, 215–16, 217, 218, 219–21, 229, 253, 254, 291, 303, 357

benzodiazepine withdrawal syndrome. *See* BWS

benzoylecgonine, 188–89, 301–2

benztropine, 144–45

beta-2 agonism, 88, 224–25, 226, 227, 229, 231, 383

beta-blocker (BBs), 86, 88–89, 90–92, 93, 94, 98, 99, 303–4

beta-carotene, 103, 104

beta-hydroxybutyrate, 260–61

beta-neurotoxins, 313

bicarbonate, 22, 24, 81–82, 122, 163–64, 167, 263, 383

bioaccumulation, 341–44

bites, pit viper, 314, 316

bivalve mollusks, 341–44

Black Widow Envenomations, 324, 331–38

blockade
  calcium channels, 87
  potassium channel, 98, 197
body packers, 128, 130, 131, 132, 133
body stuffers, 128, 129–32, 133, 251–
  52, 254
body temperature, 51, 59, 62, 72
bradycardia, 87, 88–90, 97–98, 286t, 287–
  88, 289, 355, 356–57
bradydysrhythmias, 90–91, 177b, 179, 351
bradypnea, 206, 269, 283–84, 355
brake fluid, 28, 36
Brodifacoum Poisoning, 114, 115–16f,
  118, 124
bromadiolone, 115–16f
bromocriptine, 51–54, 59, 69, 72–73
Brugada pattern, 89, 90, 99, 143, 195
buprenorphine, 151–52, 153–56, 157, 158,
  190, 277–78t, 279, 280
BWS (benzodiazepine withdrawal
  syndrome), 219, 222

caffeine, 223–33
calcium channel blocker. See CCBs
Calcium Channel Blocker Overdoses, 45,
  60, 85–99, 141t, 304, 336
cannabidiol, 188
cannabinoids, 188, 201–9
cannabis, 202, 208, 209
carbamates, 197–98, 351–61
carbamazepine, 162, 218
cardiac arrhythmias, 69–70, 87, 138, 140,
  144, 306
cardiac glycoside toxicity, 171–82, 174b
cardiac toxicity, 94, 98, 142t–43, 144–45,
  146, 147, 161, 199, 249–50
cardiomyopathy, 250, 255, 302
catecholamines, 57, 88, 165, 225, 226,
  227, 231, 250–51, 300, 322–23,
  324–25
cathinones, 189, 202, 252
CCBs (calcium channel blocker), 60, 86,
  87, 88–89, 90–93, 99, 304

Centruroides sculpturatus envenomation,
  322, 329, 330
charcoal, 8, 22–23, 32, 45, 86–87, 94, 97,
  120, 238, 241–42, 288
chlorine dioxide, 380t
chlorine gas, 381–82, 384, 385, 386
chlorophacinone, 115–17, 124
chlorpromazine, 67–68, 215–16
chlorpropamide, 43
chlorpyrifos, 352
Choking agents, 385
cholecalciferol, 101, 103, 106
cholinergic, 59–60, 98, 325, 326–27
cholinergic crisis, 352, 357
chronic effects of cocaine, 307
chronic ethanol use, 4
Chronic methamphetamine use, 250
Chronic methylxanthine use, 226
Chronic retinoid toxicity, 104–5
chronic THC use, 207
ciguatera poisoning, 341–44b, 348t,
  349, 350
cineole, 238, 240, 242
citalopram, 66–67, 71
CIWA-Ar, 213b, 215–16, 220
Clinical Opiate Withdrawal Scale (COWS),
  153, 154, 155, 156
clonazepam, 219, 222
clonidine, 86, 98, 155, 270–71, 277–78t
clonus, 49, 51–54, 57, 65, 70, 73
  ocular, 51–54, 57, 70
clove oil, 236–37, 238, 239, 241–42, 245
Clupeotoxism, 347, 349
coagulopathy, 119, 120, 122, 123, 204–
  5, 206–7, 250, 251–52, 262–63,
  313, 315–16
coca, 299
cocaine, 51–54, 128, 188–89, 205,
  297–308
cocaine-associated chest pain. See CACP
cocaine-associated chest pain (CACP), 299,
  302–4, 305, 306, 307, 308
codeine, 185, 187–88

coma, 18, 19, 32, 35*b*, 36, 286*t*, 293, 294, 341–44, 392, 394
combative, 49, 65, 247–48, 264, 366
conduction abnormalities, 90–91, 138, 161, 162–63, 287–88, 294
convulsions, 17, 288, 394
Cooper, 38
copperheads, 311, 313, 316
coquinas, 341–44
Coral snake envenomations, 313–14
cottonmouth, 315–16
COWS (Clinical Opiate Withdrawal Scale), 153, 154, 155, 156
crabs, horseshoe, 345, 345*b*
CroFab, 315–16
Crotalidae family, 311, 313–15, 317–18
Crotalus duressis, 316
CYP2C8, 140, 141*t*
CYP2E1 inducers, 7
CYP3A4, 140, 141*t*
CYP450 inducers, 109*t*
CYP450-mediated pathways, 152
cyproheptadine, 51–54, 59, 63, 71–72, 291, 294
cytotoxicity, 239, 245, 365, 373

d-amphetamine, 250
dantrolene, 51–54, 59, 60, 61, 63, 291, 336
death, 128, 138, 140, 239–40, 249–50, 313, 345–46, 355, 358, 364, 365, 367–68, 392, 394
  coma mimicking brain, 294
  mimic brain, 286*t*, 292, 293
decongestants, 189, 199
decontamination, 99, 108, 120, 143, 176–77, 254, 356–57, 360, 382, 392, 397
deferoxamine, 81, 82
dehydration, 6*t*, 19, 32, 51–54, 73, 174, 195, 197, 205–6, 251–52, 394
delirium, 57, 162, 201, 203–4, 206, 208, 213*b*, 214, 219, 353, 355
  agitated, 253–54

hyperactive, 253–54, 257
delirium tremens. *See* DTs
depression, 17, 27, 66, 113, 152, 157, 159–61, 247–48, 255, 270
  cardiac, 90–91
Dermatitis, 242, 245
desquamation, 390
dexamethasone, 108
dexmedetomidine, 291, 295, 304
dextroamphetamine, 250
dextromethorphan, 187–88, 189
dextrose, 4, 41–42, 44–46, 264
diacetyl-morphine, 187–88
dialysis, 10*t*, 22, 25, 33–35*b*, 36, 39, 176–77, 196, 228, 292
diarrhea, 238–39, 241, 278*t*, 341–45, 346, 347, 355, 358, 359, 366, 393, 394
diazepam, 211, 216–17, 219, 220, 253, 357
dicentric chromosomes, 393–94
dicyclomine, 51–55, 278*t*
diethylene glycol, 28, 36, 39
difethialone, 115–17
Digibind, 181
digitoxin, 173
digoxin, 86, 171–72, 173–74, 176, 178, 179–80, 181
digoxin clearance, 176
digoxin levels, 90, 174, 178, 180
digoxin toxicity, 173–75, 176, 177, 178, 179–80, 181, 182
Dihyrdopyridine, 87
diltiazem, 63, 85, 87, 97, 141*t*, 304
dimethyl-4,4, 365
dinitrophenol, 51–54, 56, 364
dinoflagellates, 341–44, 347*b*
Dinophysistoxins, 350
diphacinone, 115–17
diphenhydramine, 51–54, 189, 190, 193–99
diphenhydramine overdose, 194, 195–96, 198, 199
diquat, 364, 365, 366, 367–70, 371, 372

dizziness, 105, 239–40, 286*t*, 341–46, 349, 355
dobutamine, 51–54, 91–92
Domoic acid, 341–44
dopamine, 51–54, 57, 59, 62, 66, 67–68, 69, 72–73, 250–51, 289
dronabinol, 188
droperidol, 253, 264
Drug Addiction Treatment Act, 154
drug-induced hyperthermia, 63, 197
Drug-Induced Liver Injury, 112, 245
DSFab, 176–78, 179–80
DTs (delirium tremens), 214, 215–16, 217–18, 220, 221
dysfunction
   autonomic, 66, 68
   brainstem, 286*t*
   mitochondrial, 9–10, 10*t*
Dyskinesia, 301*b*
dysphagia, 57, 68, 71, 74
dyspnea, 19, 57, 120, 321, 377–78, 381
dysregulation, autonomic, 69
dysrhythmias, 173–74, 177*b*, 178, 179, 180, 226, 228, 229, 230*t*

ECMO, 86–87, 93, 144–45, 166–67, 168, 369, 370, 384, 386
edema, cerebral, 19, 24, 50, 56–57, 250, 365–66, 392
Elapidae snakes, 311, 313–14
elemental iron, 78, 79–80, 82
elimination, 2, 35–36, 104, 140, 176–77, 194, 196, 272, 285
   enhanced, 81, 166–67, 369
   extracorporeal, 229–30*t*
   first-order, 285
   prolonged, 118
emergency drug screens, 301–2, 307
encephalopathy, 6*t*, 36, 66, 130–31, 264–65, 286*t*, 328, 366
endoscopy, 120, 130, 368
envenomation, 313, 314–18, 332–35, 336
   arthropod, 334

black widow spider, 337
cottonmouth, 316
pit viper, 315–16
ephedrine, 51–54
epinephrine, 51–54, 60–61, 91–92, 97, 165, 326–27, 336, 348*t*
ergocalciferol, 103
escitalopram, 66–67, 71
esmolol, 228–29, 232, 233
Esophageal injury, 365–66, 375
esophagitis, 226, 230*t*
Essential oil poisoning, 236, 239–40, 241, 242, 245
essential oils, 235–45
ethanol, 4, 28–31, 32–33, 34, 37, 38, 260, 261
ethanol and 4-MP ADH blockade, 32–33
ethanol intoxication, 27, 263–64
ethanol levels, 37, 56–57, 90, 113, 186, 261
ethanol withdrawal, 27, 266
ethylene-2,2, 365
ethylene glycol, 28, 29, 30, 31–36, 37, 38
etonitazene, 186–87
Etretinate, 104–5
eucalyptol, 240
eucalyptus oil, 236–37, 238, 240, 242, 244, 245
eugenol oil, 239, 242
euglycemia, hyperinsulinemia, 92–93
extracorporeal membrane oxygenation therapy, 376
Extracorporeal removal of poisons and toxins, 12
Extracorporeal Treatments, 9–10, 12, 14, 230*t*, 295
Extracorporeal Treatments in Poisoning (EXTRIP), 9–10, 12, 14, 34–35*b*, 233, 295

fasciculations, 323–24, 325, 326, 327, 353, 354, 355, 356–57
fatty acids, 92–93

fatty acid synthesis, 260–61
FDA (Food and Drug Administration),
        138, 146–47, 153, 189, 224, 232,
        249, 277–78, 326–27
fentanyl, 51–54, 149–50, 151–52, 186–87,
        188, 189–90, 270, 271–72, 273, 280
Ferrous chloride, 78t
ferrous fumarate, 78t, 80
ferrous fumarate salts, 78–79
ferrous gluconate, 78
Ferrous lactate, 78t
ferrous sulfate, 78, 80
First-order elimination kinetics, 293
first-pass metabolism, 152, 161, 225
fish, puffer, 345, 345b, 349
Fluconazole, 141t
Flumazenil, 206, 289, 295
fluoxetine, 65, 66–67, 71
Foeniculum, 242
fomepizole, 10, 12, 13, 32–33, 36,
        37, 38–39
Food and Drug Administration. See FDA
Formaldehyde, 380t
formic acid, 35–36
furanylfentanyl, 190

GABA agonists, 166
GABA-A receptors, 29–30, 212–13, 216,
        217, 218, 219, 261–62
GABA-B receptors, 294
GABA inhibition, 162, 166
gambiertoxins, 341–44
gamma-aminobutyric acid (GABA), 29–30,
        72–73, 74, 161, 212–13, 220, 229,
        253, 261–62, 333
gamma-hydroxybutyric acid (GHB),
        205, 270–71
gamma rays, 389, 393–94
Gap
        osmolal, 33
        osmole, 264
gastric lavage, 108, 120, 237, 348t
gastritis, hemorrhagic, 29

glimepiride, 43
glucagon, 86–87, 91
glucose, decreased, 19
glucose metabolism, 92–93
glucuronidation, 2–3, 237
glucuronides, 18–19, 239
GLUT-2 transporters, 43–44
glutamate, 333
glutamate N-methyl-D-aspartate, 220
glutathione, 2–3, 4, 239–40, 365
glyburide, 43, 46
glycogenolysis, 88–89
glycolic acid oxidase, 29
glycolysis, 19
Glycopyrrolate, 357
glyphosate, 364, 366, 368, 370, 371,
        374, 376
GMAWS (Glasgow Modified Alcohol
        Withdrawal Scale), 213b, 215–16
Grapefruit juice, 141t
Grouper, 344b
guanylate cyclase, 93
Guarana, 224
guaranine, 224
GWI (Gulf War Illness), 358, 359, 361

hair loss, 390
hallucinations, 54–55, 67–68, 162, 193,
        206, 213b–14, 227, 242, 251–52, 289
hallucinogens, 69–70
haloperidol, 51–54, 67–68, 139f, 144–45,
        247–48, 253, 264, 303–4
HCO₃, 263, 363
heart blocks, 90, 174, 286t, 344b
heart failure, 171–72, 173–74, 178, 250,
        255, 304, 370, 381, 383
hematemesis, 79
hematuria, 114, 119
hemodialysis, 9, 11, 22, 24, 34–36, 37,
        166–67, 369, 370
        emergent, 4–5, 12, 36
Hemp plants, 188
hepatic phase II, 2–3

hepatitis, 279
hepatotoxicity, 2, 10, 13, 14, 82, 111, 241, 242
herbicide glyphosate, 364, 372, 374
Herbicide Ingestions, 364, 365–68, 369, 371, 373–74, 375–76
herbicides, 363–76
hERG, 140, 142–43, 147
heroin, 128, 151–52, 185, 187–88, 271–72
High Dose Insulin, 98
Hiroshima, 392
histamine, 67–68, 141t, 161, 312–13, 346
human leukocyte antigen (HLA), 393–94
Hunter Serotonin Toxicity Criteria, 57, 63, 70, 75
hydralazine, 326
hydrocarbons, 236–37, 240, 245
hydrocephalus, 105
hydrochloroquine, 109t
hydrocodone, 188
Hydrogen chloride, 380t
Hydrogen fluoride, 380t
Hydrogen sulfide, 380t
Hydroquinone, 117
hydroxyzine, 215–16, 278t
hyperactivity, 249, 323
hyper-adrenergic state, 250–51
hyperagitated state, 253–54
hyperbaric oxygen exposure, 372
hypercalcemia, 101, 103, 105, 106, 108–9t, 111, 112, 174
hypercarotenemia, 107
Hypercium perforatum, 51–54
hyperglycemia, 80, 88–89, 97, 227
hyperkalemia, 56, 60, 86, 176–77, 179, 180, 182, 227, 229, 251–52
Hyperkalemia in acute digitalis poisoning, 181, 182
hyperlipidemia, 377–78, 383, 387
    retinoid-induced, 108
hypermetabolic state, 56, 58
hypernatremia, 168
hyperphosphatemia, 106

hyperpolarization, 285, 344
hyperreflexia, 51–54, 57, 66–67, 70
hypersalivation, 68, 197–98, 199, 286t, 288, 323–25, 326, 353
hypertension, 66–67, 68, 87, 275, 278t, 286t, 287–88, 301b, 302, 304, 323–24, 325, 333
hyperthermia, 19, 50, 51, 54–58, 68, 69–70, 72–73, 251–52, 289, 303–4
Hyperthermia-inducing agents, 50–54
hyperthermia of sympathomimetic toxicity, 54
hyperthermic, 24, 60–61, 72, 195, 249
hypertonia, 51–54, 57, 70
hypertonic saline, 136f, 145, 163–64, 169
hyperventilation, 19, 108, 164, 169, 301b
hypervitaminosis, 110, 111, 112
hypocalcemia, 35–36, 103
Hypochlorous acid, 381–82
hypoglycemia, 21–22, 23–24, 36, 43, 44–45, 46, 92–93, 94
    persistent, 43
hypoglycemic therapies, 47
hypokalemia, 21–22, 23, 92–93, 144, 174, 179, 180, 227, 228, 230t, 231
hypomagnesemia, 92–93, 174, 179, 227, 228, 230t
hyponatremia, 69–70, 251–52
hypoparathyroidism, 102–3, 110
hypophosphatemia, 92–93, 227
hypotension, 6t, 23–24, 87, 88–91, 98, 164–66, 196–97, 229
Hypotension in TCA overdose, 164–65
hypothalamus, 51–55, 68, 289
hypothermia, 86, 203–4, 272–73, 286t, 289
hypothyroidism, 86, 105, 270–71
hypoventilation, 22, 25
hypovitaminosis, 109t
hypoxia, 56–57, 60–61, 130–31, 270, 271, 348t, 360, 369, 382, 383

ibuprofen, 191, 224–25
ice water immersion, 58–59, 63, 197, 254

ILE (intravenous lipid emulsion), 99, 142*t*, 144–45, 295
immunosuppression, 11, 141*t*
Imodium, 146–47
Indinavir, 141*t*
Indirect-acting sympathomimetics, 54
inhalation poisoning, 348*t*
inotropy, 88–89, 91, 92–93, 173–74, 301
INR, 8*b*, 9, 21–22, 56–57, 107, 113, 118, 121, 122, 393–94
insecticide/pesticide, 352, 356–57
insect repellent, 239–40
insensible losses, 72–73
insulin, 43–44, 92–93
    high-dose, 92–93
insulin overdose, 47
intracardiac pacemaker, 182
intracellular calcium, 90, 179
intrathecal baclofen withdrawal, 289, 294, 295
intrathecal overdoses, 288–89, 292
Intravenous N-acetylcysteine dosing, 10*t*
Iodine, 389
iodine-131, 389
ionizing radiation, 389–90, 393–94, 398
ipecac syrup, 120
ipratropium bromine, 383
iron, 57, 77–83
Iron ingestions, 78–79, 80–81, 82, 83
irreversible bond, 354–55
irrigation, whole-bowel, 22–23, 80–81, 90–91, 94, 99, 120, 130, 131
irritant gases, 379–81, 380*t*–81, 382, 383, 384, 385
irritant gas exposure, 379, 381, 382, 383, 384, 385
ischemia, 18, 56–57, 97, 250, 251–52, 254, 301, 303, 304, 305–6
isoniazid, 7, 236
isopropanol, 28–36
isoproterenol, 142*t*, 144
isotonitazene, 186–87, 192
isotretinoin, 101, 104–5, 111

Ito cells, 104
Itraconazole, 141*t*

Jaundice, 6*t*

K+-ATPase channel, 347
KCH criteria, 7*b*, 8*b*, 9
K-dependent clotting factors, 117, 119–20
ketamine, 189, 218, 253–54
ketoacidosis, 30–31
ketoconazole, 109*t*
ketones, 29, 236–37, 240–41
kidney dysfunction, 285, 289
kidney failure, 12, 35*b*, 47, 56–57, 174, 176–77, 182, 301–2, 367–68, 370
kinetics
    first-order, 18–19
    slow dissociation, 152
    unpredictable, 129
    zero-order elimination, 18–19, 118, 225, 285
King's College Criteria, 7*b*, 8*b*, 9, 14

labetalol, 89, 189, 254
lactate dehydrogenase, 29
lactated ringers, 360
lactic acid, 7*b*, 8*b*, 21, 36, 56–57, 80–82
    elevated, 1, 4–5, 9–10, 12, 14, 30–31, 36, 56, 79, 80
lamotrigine, 189
latrodectism, 334, 338
Latrodectus antivenom, 334–36, 337
Latrodectus envenomation, 332–36
Latrodectus species, 332, 337
lavandin extract, 245
lavender, 238–39, 242, 245
lavender oil, 238–39, 245
lethargy, 6*t*, 79, 80, 81, 82, 171–72, 175, 217–18, 239–40
leukocytosis, 56–57, 71, 80, 81–82, 227, 230*t*, 333–34
Levodopa withdrawal syndrome, 62
lidocaine, 145, 165–66, 168, 179, 229, 303

lidocaine infusion, 145
linezolid, 51–54, 62, 66, 289
lipid emulsion, 99, 144–45, 166–67, 196, 199, 295
lipophilic nature, 56, 89, 98, 118, 144–45, 161, 194, 251, 285
liquid chromatography-mass spectrometry, 186
lisinopril, 171–72, 297–98, 377–78, 387
liver failure, 4–5, 10–11, 12, 13, 14, 50, 79, 250
liver transplant, 2, 9, 11, 12, 13, 15
location, high-altitude, 311
long-acting anticoagulant rodenticide (LAARs), 123, 124, 203–4, 208, 209
long-acting VKAs, 115–16f, 120, 122
loop diuretics, 108–10
loperamide, 138–43, 144–45, 146, 147, 148
    antidiarrheal medicine, 138–40, 142t, 143, 144–45, 146–47
lorazepam, 73, 183, 216, 217, 219, 222, 235, 242, 247–48, 283–84
Low doses of radiation, 392
low-level nerve agent exposure, 361
L-type calcium channels, 43–44, 45, 87, 88–89
lung injury, toxic inhalation-induced, 384
Lyme disease, 86
lymphocytopenia, 391f

malignant hyperthermia, 50, 51, 56, 58, 60, 61, 63, 289
malnourishment, 4, 7, 105, 216
management of toxic hyperthermia, 51–54, 55f, 57–60, 61, 63
marijuana, 185, 187, 189, 202, 300
Marine-based toxins, 350
marine dinoflagellates, 341–44
MAT (multifocal atrial tachycardia), 226, 230t
MDA, 250
MDAC, 228

MDMA, 49, 189, 190, 250, 252, 289
Measured Osmolality, 30–31
Mellanby effect, 261
mental status, altered/depressed, 88–89, 201, 203–4, 206, 240, 241–42, 272–73, 356
menthofuran, 239–40
Menthol, 242
meperidine, 51–54, 66, 138–39f
mesocorticolimbic dopaminergic system, 300
metallic taste, 346
metalloproteinases, 312–13
metformin, 47, 189, 297–98, 387
methadone, 153, 155, 158, 188, 189–90, 192, 201, 272, 277–78, 280
methamphetamine, 127–28, 189, 190, 247–57
methamphetamine toxicity, 131, 249–50, 253, 255
methamphetamine use, 249–50, 251–52, 253–54, 255, 256, 257
methanol, 28, 29–30, 31–33, 36, 37, 38
methanol toxicity, 28, 29–30, 32–33, 34–36, 37, 38, 39
methylene blue, 93, 99
methylenedioxymethamphetamine, 250
methyl ester, ecgonine, 301–2
methylphenidate, 51–54, 250
Methylpyrazole, 38
Methyl salicylate, 18, 240–41
methylxanthine poisoning, 223–33
methylxanthines, 224, 225, 226, 227–28, 229–30t, 231, 232
methysergide, 72
metonitazeme, 186–87
metoprolol, 63, 85, 136f, 232
microcephaly, 105
midazolam, 193, 291–92, 326, 327
miosis, 270, 272–73, 286t, 353, 354
Mojave rattlesnake, 315–16
monoamines, 54, 300

morphine milligram equivalents
(MME), 271–72
morphine sulfate, 185, 187–88, 271–
72, 281
mortality, 20–21, 43, 59, 60, 156, 277–79,
303–4, 305, 369
MOUD (Medication for Opioid Use
Disorder), 151, 153
muscle fasciculations, 321, 357
muscle rigidity, 51–54, 56, 59, 62, 68,
69–70, 72
muscle spasticity, 285
muscular fasciculations, 325, 355
muscular flaccidity, 289
muscular hypertonicity, 289
myasthenia gravis, 352, 358
mydriasis, 54–55, 66–67, 195t, 272–73,
286t, 353
myocardial sensitization, 173–74
myocarditis, 323, 333
myoclonus, 51, 57, 66–67, 227, 286t,
289, 325
myoglobin, elevated, 57, 78
myotonic jerks, 353
Myristica, 242
Myristicin, 242

Na+ channel blockade, 162–63, 164–66,
197–98, 199
Na+-K+-ATPase, 173–74, 176, 177, 227
N-acetylcysteine, 3–7, 7b, 8–10, 11, 12,
13–14, 239–40, 241–42
naloxone, 142t, 143, 152, 269, 270,
271, 273, 274, 275–77, 278–79, 280
NAPQI (N-acetyl-p-benzoquinone
imine), 2–4
narcolepsy, 189, 249
nateglinide, 43
National Institute on Drug Abuse (NIDA),
185, 256
National Poison Data System. *See* NPDS
N-desethylisotonitazene, 186–87
N-desmethyl-loperamide, 140, 142–43,
147

Nefazodone, 141t
Negative chronotropy, 87–88
Negative dromotropy, 87–88
Negative inotropy, 88
nerve agent poisonings, 361
nerve gas, 352
nervous system
adrenergic, 54
autonomic, 51, 323
parasympathetic, 352–53
sympathetic, 300, 352–53
nervous systems, central, 270, 353
neuroglycopenia, 19, 21–22, 23–24
neuroleptic, 50, 51, 62, 66, 68–69, 74, 75,
289, 292
neuroleptic malignant syndrome. *See* NMS
Neuroleptic Malignant Syndrome,
62, 65–75
neurological symptoms, 175, 203–4, 239–
40, 341–45, 349
neuromuscular, non-depolarizing, 72
neurotoxicity, 36, 37, 39, 98, 242, 313–15,
329, 341–44, 366
neurotoxicity Thujone, 242
neurotoxic shellfish poisoning, 350
neurotoxins, 313, 322–23, 328
neutropenic, 394
nicardipine, 326
nicotinamide adenine dinucleotide
phosphate, 365
nicotine, 232, 285
nicotinic symptoms, 352, 353, 354,
355, 356–57
NIDA (National Institute on Drug Abuse),
185, 256
NIDA-5 panel screens, 185
Nitazenes, 186–87
Nitrates, 303
nitric oxide synthesis, 93
nitrogen dioxide, 380t
nitroglycerin, 304
nitroprusside, 254
NMDA (N-methyl-D-aspartate), 19, 29–
30, 212–13, 216, 217, 218, 220, 261

NMS (neuroleptic malignant syndrome), 50, 51–54, 57, 59, 62, 66–70, 71–73, 74, 75, 289
Nonaccidental poisoning in children, 237–38
non-depolarizing paralytics, 287
Nondihydropyridine, 87
Non-Ionizing Radiation, 389, 398
noradrenaline, 307
norbuprenorphine, 152
norepinephrine, 23–24, 51–54, 66, 71, 91–92, 97, 161, 165, 167, 300, 333
NPDS (National Poison Data System), 28, 37, 50–51, 62, 86, 99, 115–17, 138, 249, 364, 372
NSAIDs, 278t, 334
nystagmus, 195t, 264–65, 323–24
    rotary, 323–24, 325
    vertical, 286t

octreotide, 45–46, 47, 262–63
oculocephalic, 283–84
oculomotor palsy, 264–65
oils
    peppermint, 238
    sage, 242
Okadaic acid, 341–44, 350
ondansetron, 228, 231, 278t
opiates, 185, 186–88, 196, 201
opioid agonists, 151–52
opioid epidemic, 151
opioid potency, 270
opioid properties, 138
opioids, 86, 128, 151–52, 153, 186–87, 188, 270, 271–72, 273, 274–76
    exogenous, 271
    full-agonist, 151–52
    high-affinity, 276
    long-acting, 155
    semisynthetic, 187–88
opioid tolerance, 275–76
opioid toxicity, 149–51, 270–71, 272–74, 274t–75, 277, 278–79, 280, 282

opioid use disorder (OUD), 153, 154, 156–57, 158, 270, 279, 280, 282
opioid withdrawal, 135–37, 138, 140, 143, 149–50, 151, 153, 154, 277–78, 280
Opium, 186
oral antidiabetic medications, 43
Organophosphate-induced delayed neuropathy (OPIDP), 358, 359
organophosphates, 236, 324–25, 352, 354–55, 356, 357, 359
osmol gap
    calculated, 30–31
    elevated, 30–31, 263
ototoxicity, 19
oxalate crystalluria, 29, 33
oxidative phosphorylation, 19, 51, 56, 58, 60, 63, 79, 240–41
oxidative stress, 3–4, 382
oximes, 357
oxybutynin, 51–55
oxycodone, 151–52, 188
oysters, 341–44, 349
Ozdemir, 123

Pacific ciguatoxin-1, 341–44
palpitations, 171–72, 228, 346
Palythoa toxica, 347b
palytoxin poisoning, 347, 348t, 349, 350
Panax ginseng, 141t
pancreatitis, 93, 166–67, 325, 329, 365–66
pancytopenia, 390–91
papilledema, 105, 110
Paprika, 109t
paracetamol, 13, 14
paralytic, 341–44, 350
paramethoxyamphetamine, 250
Paraquat and diquat, 365–66, 367–70, 371, 373, 374, 375
paraquat poisoning, 365–66, 369, 370, 372, 373, 374, 375, 376
paresthesia, 242, 339–40, 341–45, 347, 359
Parkinson disease, 51–54, 69
Parkinsonism hyperpyrexia syndrome, 75

pathways
  kappa-mediated, 152
  mesocortical dopamine, 67–68
  mesocorticolimbic, 300
  sulfation, 3
PAWSS (Prediction of Alcohol Withdrawal
    Severity Scale), 214
PCC, four-factor, 123
pennyroyal oil, 239–40, 241–42
Peppermint, 242
Pesticide Poisonings, 352, 361, 364, 366,
    371, 373
P-glycoprotein inhibition, 140, 141t,
    146, 147
pharmacobezoars, 80–81
pharmacodynamics, 140, 162, 209, 219
pharmacokinetics, 140, 219, 293, 329
phenobarbital, 109t, 215–16, 217–18,
    220, 221
phentolamine, 304
phenylephrine, 23–24, 54, 91–92, 189, 276
phenylethylamines, 249, 250
phenylpiperidine, 138
phenylpropanolamine, 51–54
phenytoin, 166, 179
Phosgene, 380t
phosphodiesterase, 225, 231
phospholipase A2, 312–13, 372
phytoplankton, 341
pink oleander, 173
pneumomediastinum, 365–66, 373–74
pneumonitis, 32, 130, 164, 176–77, 237–
    38, 241–42, 392
pneumopericardium, 373–74
pneumoperitoneum, 81–82
pneumothorax, 365–66
polonium-210, 389
poppy seeds, 186, 187–88
potassium channels, 66–67, 89, 94, 140,
    142–43, 195
potassium efflux, inhibiting, 44
potassium shifting, 227
priapism, 289, 333, 334–35, 337

prochlorperazine, 228
prolonged PR intervals, 107, 287–88
Prolonged QTc, 90, 94
promethazine, 189, 228
propofol, 72–73, 166, 218, 229, 230t,
    253, 291
propranolol, 88–89, 90, 94, 98, 99
propylene glycol, 28, 30–31, 36, 166
pseudodiphtheria, 365–66, 373
pseudoephedrine, 189, 252
Pseudomonas aeruginosa, 346
pseudotumor cerebri, 110
psychosis, 54, 203–4, 205, 214, 253,
    255, 286t
psychostimulants, 249–50
pulmonary edema, 19, 24, 81, 242, 251–
    52, 271, 275, 282, 323–24, 365
pulmonary fibrosis, 365, 368, 370,
    390, 392
Pulmonary Irritants, 377–86
pupils, 27, 49, 65, 114, 149–50, 159–60,
    193, 195t, 201, 283–84, 286t
purpura, 6t, 119
pyramidal involvement, 359
pyridostigmine bromide, 358
pyridoxine, 35–36

QRS, prolonged, 136f, 140, 159–60, 162–
    63, 197–98
QRS duration, 136f, 165–66, 169
QRS interval, narrow, 73, 163–64
QTc prolongation, 71, 74, 140, 143, 144,
    165–66, 195, 228, 229, 231, 251–52
QT intervals, shortened, 107, 174
Quinidine, 141t
Quinine, 141t
Quinone, 117
quinone reductase, 117

radiation, 377–78, 389–94
radiation exposure, 390–91, 393
Radiation Injury Treatment Network
    (RITN), 394

radicals, free, 365, 371, 379, 389
radioactive iodine I-131, 387, 389
rattlesnakes, 309, 311, 313, 315–
16, 317–18
    pigmy, 311
    timber, 311, 313
receptors, 67–68, 88, 93, 165, 186–87,
194, 216, 219, 220, 261–62, 285
    5-HT2A, 66–67
    adrenergic, 88, 300
    alpha-adrenergic, 67–68, 161
    altered muscle fiber, 287
    beta-2, 88–89
    beta-adrenergic, 225
    cholinergic, 326–27
    dopamine, 67–68
    glutamate, 29–30, 212–13
    kappa-opioid, 152, 271
    neuronal presynaptic, 333
    serotonin, 51, 66, 250–51
redox cycling, 363–76
the red tide, 341
reflexes, 66, 90, 240
    absent, 283–84, 286t
    diminished, 366
    negative oculocephalic, 286t
release
    antidiuretic hormone, 251–52
    calcium-dependent calcium, 43–44
repaglinide, 43
respiratory alkalosis, 19, 21, 22, 136f,
227, 240–41
respiratory arrest, 270, 323
respiratory depression, 140, 142t, 143, 151,
217–18, 220, 270–71, 272–73, 280,
286t, 287
respiratory depression reversal, 275,
277, 280
respiratory failure, 130–31, 241–42, 287,
313, 323–24, 341–44, 345b, 348,
358, 366, 367
retinoids, 103, 105
retinol, 103, 104

retinol activity equivalents (RAE), 102–3
reversal, cold temperature, 344b
rhabdomyolysis, 50, 54, 56–57, 69–70, 72,
73, 195, 204–5, 206, 227
rigidity, 51–54, 57, 70, 289, 333
    lead pipe, 51–54, 68, 74
Rumack-Matthew Nomogram, 5–6, 12
ryanodine receptor type, 59, 289

salicylates, 18–24, 25, 51–54, 56–57, 89–
90, 240–41
salicylate toxicity, 18–19, 21, 22, 23,
24, 25, 58
Salicylic acid, 18
    ionized, 23
salivation, 321, 323–24, 351, 353, 355
Salivation/Sialorrhea, 354
sarcoplasm reticulum, 56, 59, 60, 88, 173–
74, 289
Saxitoxin, 341–44
schizophrenia, 67–68, 190, 205
Scombroid, 346, 348t, 350
scorpion antivenom, 329
scorpion envenomations, 321–30
scorpionism, 324–25, 326–27
scorpions, 322, 324, 325, 327–28, 329
Sea bass, 344b
seafood-related toxins, 339–50, 345b,
347b
secretions, 74, 173, 356–57, 358
sedative-hypnotics, 50, 211–22
Sedative-Hypnotic Withdrawal, 212, 213b,
215–16, 217–18, 219–20, 221
seizures, 69–70, 162–64, 166, 195t, 197–
98, 205–6, 231, 235–36, 240–41,
242, 253, 289–91, 341–44, 355–57,
363–64, 366
    prolonged, 166
    refractory, 230t, 240
seizures and serotonin syndrome, 69–70
serotonergic agents, 51, 66–67, 69–70,
74, 254
serotonin, 66–67, 161, 289, 300, 312–13

serotonin norepinephrine reuptake inhibitors (SNRIs), 50–51, 71, 161
serotonin reuptake inhibitors, 50–51, 66, 74, 161
serotonin syndrome, 63, 65–75, 289, 292
serotonin toxicity, 50, 51–54, 57, 59, 61, 62, 63, 66–67, 70, 71
serotonin toxidrome, 325
serum alkalinization, 144, 164–65, 168, 169
Serum digoxin concentration (SDC), 175–76, 177b, 178, 180
serum sickness, 326–27, 334–35, 336
severe hyperthermia, 58–59, 254
severe lipophilic intoxications, 295
shellfish, 339–40, 341–44
shellfish and seafood-related toxins, 339–50, 345b, 347b
shellfish poisoning, toxic, 341, 349, 350
SIADH (Syndrome of Inappropriate Antidiuretic Homone release), 69–70, 251–52
sialorrhea, 57, 74
snakebite, 311–12, 314–15, 316–17, 318–19, 334–35, 338
snake neurotoxin, 313
snakes, coral, 311, 313
sodium bicarbonate, 23, 24, 142t, 144, 163–66, 168, 303, 383
sodium channel blockade, 88–89, 94, 98, 161, 162, 168, 197, 300, 303
sodium channel blockers, 357
sodium channels, cardiac, 89, 169
sodium dithionite, 367, 374
sodium hydroxide, 367
spiders, brown recluse, 334
splenomegaly, 101
status epilepticus, 214, 286t, 292, 293, 294, 358
steroids, cardioactive, 180, 181
stimulant use disorder, 254
stroke
    exertional heat, 50

methamphetamine-related, 250
strontium-90, 389
subcutaneous emphysema, 373–74
succinylcholine, 56, 72, 287
sulfation, 2–3, 237
sulfhydryl groups, 2–4
sulfonylurea-induced hypoglycemia, 44, 46, 47
sulfonylurea overdose, 43, 44–45, 46, 47
sulfur dioxide, 380t
superoxide dismutase, 365
superwarfarins, 115–17, 118, 119–22, 123
supplementation, 120–21, 264
    folic acid, 35–36
supplements
    dietary, 103, 110, 112, 232
    ergocalciferol, 103
    unregulated, 102
supportive care, aggressive, 24, 34, 208, 241–42, 292–93, 371
surfactant, 237, 371
sympathetic nerve activity, 216, 217, 251–52, 271, 304
sympatholysis, 253–54
sympathomimetics, 50, 51–54, 57–58, 59–60, 66, 236, 255, 289, 300, 324
synthetic cannabinoid (SC), 124, 188, 202, 202t, 203–6, 207, 208, 209

tactile illusions, 213b
tea tree oil, 238, 245
temperature, 17, 27, 49, 50, 56, 57, 58–59, 65, 70, 72–73, 159–60
    elevated body, 58–59
teratogenicity, 102–3, 105–6
terbutaline, 51–54
terpinen-4-ol, 238
tetanus, 295, 324, 328
tetrahydrocannabinol, 188
tetrahydrocannabinol-9-carboxylic, 188

tetrahydrofolate, 29
tetrodotoxin, 345, 345*b*, 348*t*, 349, 350
THC (Tetrahydrocannabinol), 188, 202,
    202*t*, 203, 204–5, 208
THC-9-COOH, 188
theobromine, 224, 226, 231
theophylline, 224–26, 227, 228, 230*t*,
    231, 233
thermoregulation, 51, 68, 254
    impaired, 51–54
thermoregulatory centers, 58–59
thiamine, 27, 35–36, 211, 215–16,
    260–61, 263, 264–65
thioridazine, 67–68
Thujone, 242
Thyme, 242
thyrotoxicosis, 50
tinnitus, 19, 240–41
Tokyo subway sarin attack, 361
tolbutamide, 43
tolerance, 105, 207, 225, 274–75
tonic-clonic jerking movements, 191, 213*b*
tonic-clonic seizure, 159–60, 211, 235
Toxic Alcohol Management, 27–39, 31*f*
toxic alcohol metabolism, 28–29, 34
toxic alcohols, 28–31, 32–33, 35–36, 38,
    205, 263
toxic hyperthermia, 50, 51–54, 55*f*, 56–60,
    61, 63
toxidromes, 5, 19, 25, 50, 88–89, 162,
    177*b*, 195–96, 236, 354, 355
    cholinergic, 356
    opioid, 130, 186–87
    sympathomimetic, 130, 168, 249,
        251–52, 325, 355
toxins
    heat-stable, 344, 347
    marine, 341, 348
    scorpion, 329
tramadol, 51–54, 188, 189
transferrin, 78
transplant, 8*b*, 11, 14, 394

tricyclic antidepressant overdose, 50–51,
    159–69, 189–90, 191
tricyclic antidepressants, 50–51, 66, 71,
    140, 161, 169, 189–90, 195–96
triggerfish, 345
tyrosine hydroxylase, 250–51

UDS (urine drug screen), 184, 186, 187,
    188–89, 190, 191, 192, 204–5, 301–2
UGT (UDP-glucuronosyl transferases), 2–3
uncouplers of oxidative phosphorylation,
    50, 51–54, 56, 58, 60, 63, 240–41
uranium-238, 389
urine alkalinization, 23

vasoconstriction, 165, 301, 303, 304, 308
vasodilation, 23–24, 32, 79, 87, 90–92,
    162, 194, 226, 229, 304
vasopressors, 23–24, 60–61, 90, 91–93, 94,
    97, 98, 229, 232, 276, 287–88
vasospasm, 250, 302, 303–4, 306
venlafaxine, 66–67, 71, 75, 189
venom, 311–14, 315–16, 322–23, 326–
    27, 333
verapamil, 87, 90, 304
vitamin, 101–12, 109*t*, 117, 119–21, 123
Vitamin A, 103, 105–6, 107, 109*t*, 111
vitamin D2, 103, 109*t*
vitamin D3, 101, 103, 109*t*
vitamin K1, 124
Vitamin K antagonists (VKA), 115–18,
    119–20, 121–22, 123, 125
vitamin toxicity, 111
VKA. *See* Vitamin K antagonists

Wernicke's syndrome, 264–65
wintergreen, oil of, 18, 236–37, 240–
    41, 242
withdrawal
    alprazolam, 219, 222
    barbiturate, 212
    benzodiazepine, 219–20, 221, 222

withdrawal (*cont.*)
    buprenorphine-precipitated, 155, 158
    drug/alcohol, 292
withdrawal of alcohol in chronic
    users, 214

Xanthid crabs, 347*b*
xanthoderma, 107, 112

zolpidem, 211, 219–20, 222
Zombie outbreak, 208, 209